GeoJournal Library

Volume 132

Series Editor
Barney Warf, University of Kansas, Lawrence, KS, USA

CW01466455

Now accepted for Scopus! Content available on the Scopus site in summer 2021.

This book series serves as a broad platform for scientific contributions in the field of human geography and its sub-disciplines. The series, which published its first volume in 1984, explores theoretical approaches and new perspectives and developments in the field of human geography.

Some topics covered by the series are:

- Economic Geography
- Political Geography
- Cultural Geography
- Historical Geography
- Health and Medical Geography
- Environmental Geography and Sustainable Development
- Legal Geography and Policy
- Urban Geography
- Geospatial Techniques
- Urban Planning and Development
- Land Use Modelling
- and much more

Publishing a broad portfolio of peer-reviewed scientific books, GeoJournal Library invites book proposals for research monographs and edited volumes. The books can range from theoretical approaches to empirical studies and contain interdisciplinary approaches, case studies and best-practice assessments. The books in the series provide a great resource to academics, researchers and practitioners in the field.

Beata Sirowy • Deni Ruggeri
Editors

Urban Agriculture in Public Space

Planning and Designing for Human
Flourishing in Northern European Cities
and Beyond

Springer

Editors
Beata Sirowy
Department of Urban
and Regional Planning
Norwegian University of Life Sciences
Ås, Norway

Deni Ruggeri
Department of Plant Science
and Landscape Architecture
University of Maryland
College Park, MD, USA

ISSN 0924-5499   ISSN 2215-0072   (electronic)
GeoJournal Library
ISBN 978-3-031-41552-4   ISBN 978-3-031-41550-0   (eBook)
https://doi.org/10.1007/978-3-031-41550-0

This work was developed within the project "Cultivating Public Space: urban agriculture as a basis for human flourishing and sustainability transition in Norwegian cities", funded by the Research Council of Norway, BYFORSK programme, grant number 270725. Project duration: 2017-2022.

Illustrations:
Beata Sirowy: Title page + p. xix + Partitions: Part 1, Part 3, Part 4
Deni Ruggeri: p. v + Partitions: Part 2, Part 5

This Springer imprint is published by the registered company Springer Nature Switzerland AG
The registered company address is: Gewerbestrasse 11, 6330 Cham, Switzerland

Paper in this product is recyclable.

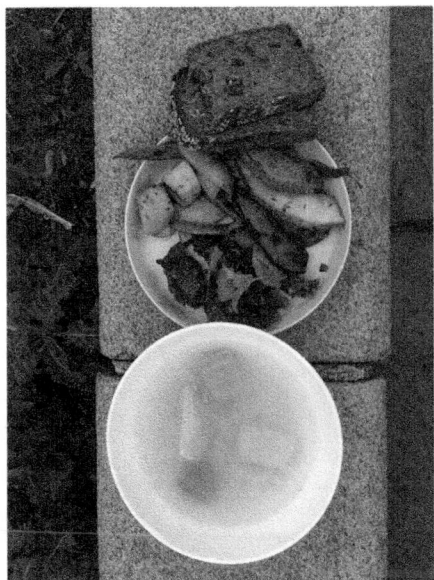
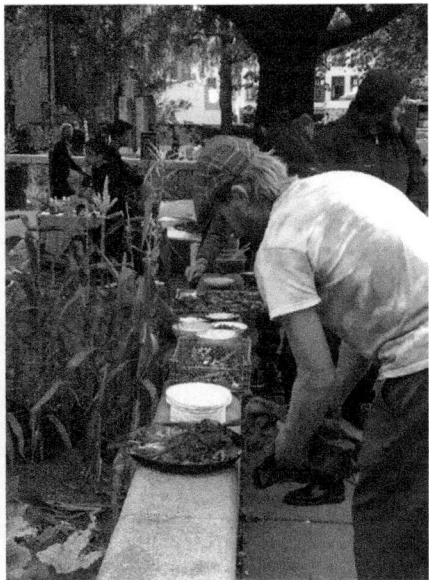

Foreword: Why Public Urban Agriculture?

In public perception, urban agriculture has evolved over the past two decades from an exotic phenomenon to an established urban component. It has found its way into many municipal agendas. New actors and networks support the cultivation of food in and around the city. Many research projects in the European context (Lohrberg et al. 2016) have addressed urban agriculture. Nevertheless, there are still many gaps in knowledge, and many specific features of urban agriculture have not yet been sufficiently captured and understood, particularly with regard to regional differences and explanatory models. It is therefore even more gratifying that the present book has filled such a gap, namely the importance of public space for urban agriculture in Northern and Central Europe.

Indeed, two aspects are surprising: first, why are so many projects of urban agriculture – especially forms of urban gardening – located in the public space, which is not suitable for the pure production of food, think of soil conditions, spatial restrictions, vandalism and so on? Second, why has this contradiction not yet been investigated in depth, why have the public virtues of urban space not been looked at more closely?

Having addressing these questions, is a great merit of this book. Going beyond single case studies, the authors have put conceptual approaches to agriculture in the public sphere: human flourishing, civic friendship, communities of virtue. In addition, they successfully differentiated the concept of publicness, so that it can be applied to urban agriculture.

The authors thus demonstrate that public space is not always conducive to food production; however, it is essential to achieving many of the benefits that potentially characterize urban agriculture. The authors do not focus on such forms of urban agriculture that are not oriented toward publicness, be it a suburban farm, indoor, roof top or backyard farming, or allotments. This leads me to the question of how to classify the phenomenon "urban agriculture goes public" in terms of its general evolution. My thesis regarding European cities is that agriculture has been present in *urban* space for centuries, acting as a constant companion of urban development

(Fig. 1). However, production in *public* space has been exceptional. This changed through the urban gardening movement, which since the turn of the millennium has deliberately sought out public space to test new forms of collective and sustainable food production and demonstrate them as an alternative to the conventional production of food, but also to the economy-driven production of urban space.

Agriculture in the city, as recent publications show (Daviron et al. 2019, Landsteiner and Soens 2020), is not an invention of the twenty-first century, but a centuries-old phenomenon. Based on several case studies, Lohrberg et al. (2022) demonstrate that agricultural production in different forms shaped urban development since the Middle Ages and developed rich forms until the age of industrialization.

These forms can be assigned to spatial patterns: small-scale, intensely practiced horticulture has often blended into the fortifications of cities – an outstanding example being the *bostans* in Istanbul (Başer and Tunçay 2010). These vegetable plots, run as family-based businesses, benefited from the fact that the firing field in front

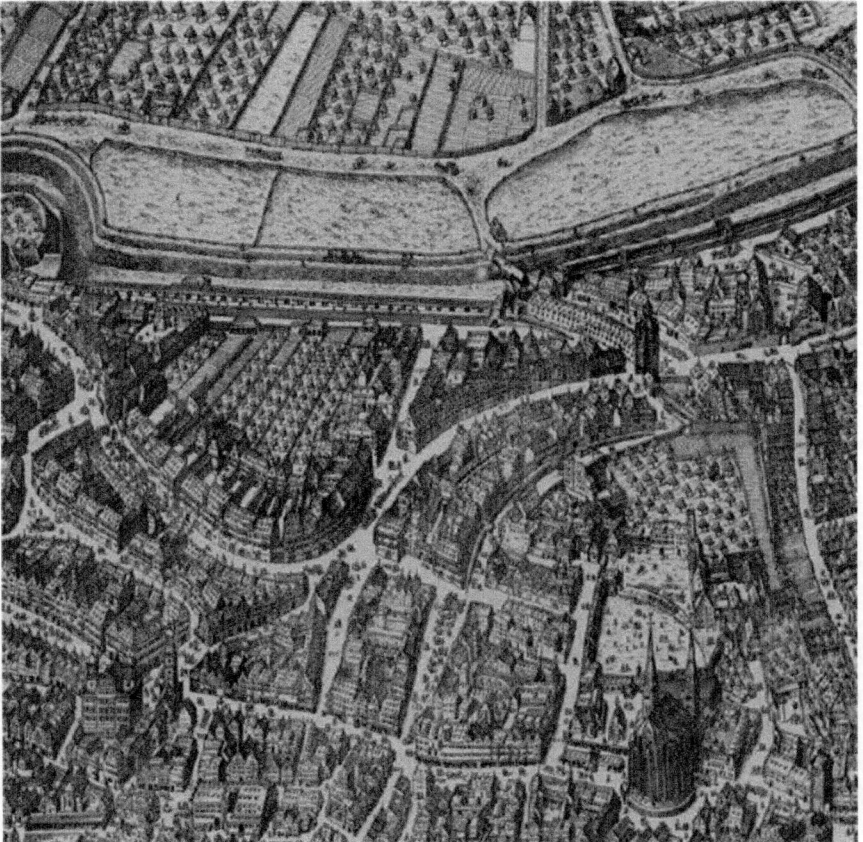

Fig. 1 Wolfgang Kilian, "Augusta Vindelicorum/Augspurg," 1626 (detail)

of the walls was not allowed to be built on, but a large urban market was located just behind the walls. Another spatial pattern is the conversion of marsh and river landscapes close to cities into vegetable and fruit growing areas, as we know from French cities such as Amiens and Bourges (Brunet et al. 2022). Again, it was the large purchasing power of the city that allowed high investments to meliorate these hardly accessible areas. Following the same pattern, urban river valleys in Spain have also been transformed by horticultural practices, not based on drainage but on sophisticated irrigation systems, as shown by the "Vega de Granada" (Kerfers et al. 2022).

Another typical aspect of pre-industrial urban agriculture is its strong links to the specific natural conditions of the city, its soils, geology, and weather. In the nineteenth century, for example, a 300 hectare peach-growing orchard ("Mur à Pêches") was established in the Parisian suburb of Montreuil to take advantage of the local gypsum deposits (Hamid Kargari et al. 2022). The gypsum was extracted as a building material for the growing metropolis, and many landowning villagers used the quarries' overburden to build heat-retaining trellis walls to cultivate the highly priced peaches for the Parisian market (Fig. 2).

The walls, three to four meters high, are in a way symbolic of urban agriculture of earlier eras. Although cultivation in the city was widespread, it mostly took place in protected spaces, behind walls, fences, ditches, hidden in the city's block interior. Cultivation was also exclusive in social terms. Horticulture was organized in many places – for example, in the German town of Bamberg – by guilds that internally

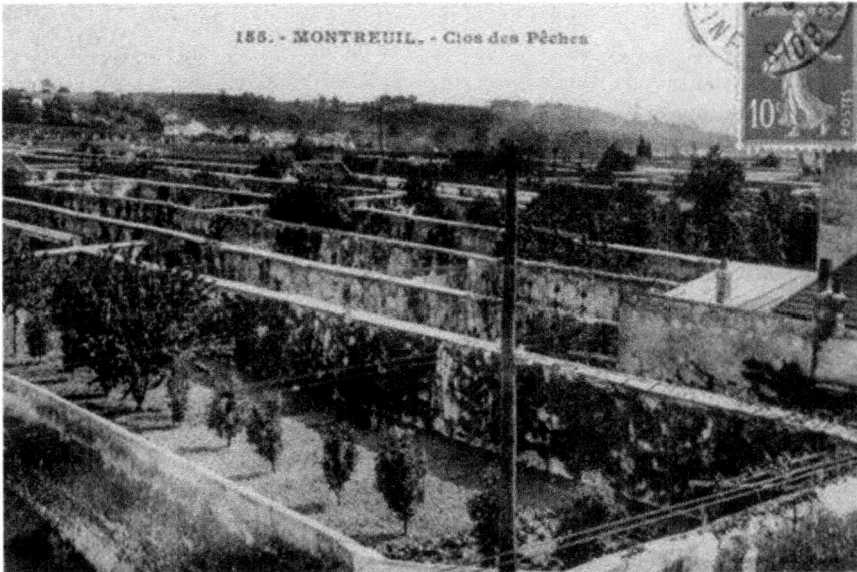

Fig. 2 Peach wall compartments (stamp in use from 1907 to 1922), taken from Lohrberg et al. (2022:176)

passed on knowledge about cultivation, crop species, and genetic information (seeds), but protected this from outside access (Keech and Redepenning 2022). The public space – as a place that is open and accessible to the public – played no role in these forms of production. Streets and markets were used intensively for the sale of goods, but cultivation took place primarily in private or communally-occupied spaces.

Beginning with the industrial revolution, new, globally oriented transportation systems – railroads, steam shipping – emerged, causing the diverse local forms of urban agriculture to decline or disappear as produce could be shipped easily into the city from other areas. However, new forms of urban agriculture also entered the scene, like greenhouses and allotment gardens. The latter were strongly oriented toward the self-sufficiency of growers. Initially condemned as illegal land grabs, allotment gardens established themselves as an integral part of welfare-oriented urban planning, especially after the first World War (Lohrberg 2001). Designed on the drawing board, the sites were managed cooperatively, but again, not as a public space in the strict sense. High hedges, bordered entrances, and narrow paths were designed to make the space feel as it was reserved for a specific community, a perception that still characterizes many contemporary allotment sites.

Industrialization not only changed the forms of urban agriculture, but it also led to a changed perception of agriculture in the city. While, as shown, it was previously a natural part of the urban fabric, it is then described as its opposite (Siebel 2015). As Isendahl (2012) has elucidated, the mindset-leading discipline of urban sociology, which emerged at the beginning of the twentieth century, has systematically ignored urban agriculture. In particular, he refers to the Chicago School of Sociology, as the first to take an in-depth look at metropolitan living conditions. The scholars were fascinated by Chicago's dynamic growth, fuelled by industrialization and migration from Europe. When observing and describing the people's working and housing conditions, researchers operated in an environment where urban agriculture must have played a de facto minor role. While research on this phenomenon is limited, Steel (2013) demonstrates that Chicago's food supply at that time was highly globalized. In particular, railroads made it possible to benefit from the outstanding production potential of the Midwest, bringing in grain and livestock in large masses and quantities. With its meat packing district, Chicago set new standards in industrial animal slaughtering and made meat a mass commodity: "For the first time, cities had a cheap, reliable source of food." (Steel 2013).

Obviously, modern urban sociology emerged in a city that had pioneered the industrialization of food production like no other. The analytical description of the almost hyperreal urban conditions in Chicago therefore inevitably led to an image of the city in which urban food cultivation no longer played a role. Here, according to Isendahl (2012), lies the root of a "dogmatic separation in modernist thought between city folk/townspeople and agriculturalists, between the urban and the agrarian" (Fig. 3). With respect to the rich histories of urban agriculture – which was just sketched in this chapter – Isendahl (ibid.) uncovers this mindset as a "limited … understanding of the diversity of the constitution of cities."

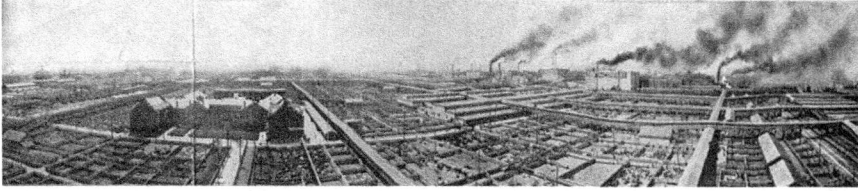

Fig. 3 Panoramic view of Chicago Union Stock Yards – From the Water Tower. Charles J. Bushnell, "Some Social Aspects of the Chicago Stock Yards: Industry at the Chicago Stock Yards", American Journal of Society VII (September, 1901):146

However, this limited understanding was quite influential during the twentieth century, affecting the dominant urban policies of many countries, with fatal consequences especially for cities in the global South. Here, urban agriculture played a crucial role for food safety and food sovereignty but was negated or obstructed by official urban development policies. In the 1990s, the mindset changed, when the United Nations officially recognized urban agriculture as key for some of its development programs (UNDP 1996). However, today, the idea of equating urban agriculture with poverty and backwardness still lingers. For example, Chinese city governments still aim at containing urban food cultivation as something unmodern and incongruous as Zhao (2021) has illustrated for the city of Nanjing.

Such processes are also occurring in Europe. Pickard (2022) found evidence that in Sofia's socialist policies, urban agriculture played a prominent role, e.g., people were allowed by a specific law to grow their own food on unused urban land. In the 1990s, with the introduction of free-market principles also for urban development, these rights were cancelled. Today, urban agriculture actors face obstacles and constraints in many places. They miss the former acknowledgment of urban agriculture.

To conclude, in the Western-influenced development model of the city, a contra-agrarian attitude is still inscribed. This explains why in the last two decades urban agriculture has been so strongly oriented toward the public sphere or the public space. The actors of urban agriculture "go public" to not only practice but also demonstrate their agenda in a mindset-oriented way. As a contested space, public space serves this aim. Activities that are permanently accepted here can claim to be settled in urban society as well. Spatial presence leads to social acceptance. Unlike media space, public space as a physical space cannot be reproduced at will. This uniqueness makes it so attractive for demonstrative purposes.

In this respect, the step of urban agriculture going public can also be understood as part of its overall evolution: the industrialization of the city and, with it, the Western development model of the city have taken urban agriculture its self-evidence of earlier centuries. This terrain still needs to be reclaimed, in a double sense: as a space for integrated production as well as for interpretive

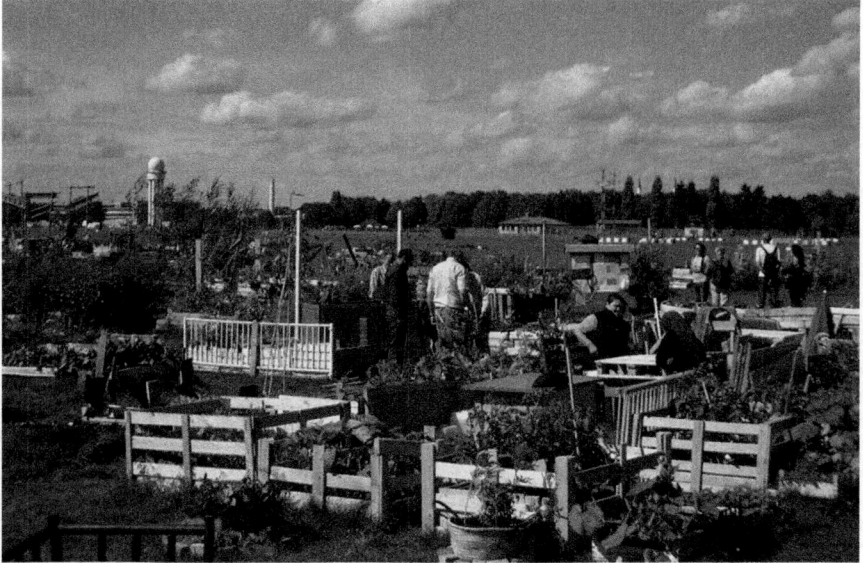

Fig. 4 Community garden "Allmende-Kontor," Berlin-Tempelhof, photo taken by Frank Lohrberg, 2017

purposes (Fig. 4). I thank the authors of this book for having illuminated this evolutionary step of urban agriculture in such a vivid and multifaceted publication.

RWTH Aachen University   Frank Lohrberg
Aachen, Germany

Literature

Başer, B., & Tunçay, H. E. (2010). Understanding the spatial and historical characteristics of agricultural landscapes in Istanbul. *ITU AZ, 7*(2), 106–120.

Brunet, L., Laufhütte, N., Timpe, A., & Christenn, K. (2022). From Marshes to Market Gardens: Hortillonnages d'Amiens and Marais de Bourges. In F. Lohrberg, K. Christenn, A. Timpe, & A. Sancar (Hrsg.), *Urban agricultural heritage* (pp. 72–79). Birkhäuser. https://doi.org/10.1515/9783035622522

Daviron, B., Perrin, C., & Soulard, C.-T. (2019). History of urban food policy in Europe, from the ancient city to the industrial city. In *Designing urban food policies* (Vol. 2019, pp. 26–51). Springer.

Hamid Kargari, A., Wehnert, K. C., Christenn, K., & Timpe, A. (2022). Murs à Pêches de Montreuil: Rediscovering Urban Agricultural Heritage. In F. Lohrberg,

K. Christenn, A. Timpe, & A. Sancar (Hrsg.), *Urban agricultural heritage* (pp. 176–181). Birkhäuser. https://doi.org/10.1515/9783035622522

Isendahl, C. (2012). Investigating urban experiences, deconstructing urban essentialism. *Connecting Past and Present, 25.*

Keech, D., & Redepenning, M. (2020). Culturalization and urban horticulture in two World Heritage cities. *Food, Culture & Society, 23*(3), 315–333. https://doi.org/10.1080/15528014.2020.1740142

Kerfers, A., Rahimi, A., Timpe, A., & Christenn, K. (2022). La Vega de Granada: A cultural landscape built around irrigation. In F. Lohrberg, K. Christenn, A. Timpe, & A. Sancar (Hrsg.), *Urban agricultural heritage* (pp. 106–111). Birkhäuser. https://doi.org/10.1515/9783035622522

Landsteiner, E., & Soens, T. (Hrsg.). (2020). *Farming the city: The resilience and decline of urban agriculture in European History* (Resilienz und Niedergang der städtischen Landwirtschaft in der europäischen Geschichte 16). StudienVerlag.

Lohrberg, F. (2001). *Stadtnahe Landwirtschaft in der Stadt- und Freiraumplanung.* Stuttgart.

Lohrberg, F., Lička, L., Scazzosi, L., & Timpe, A. (Hrsg.). (2016). *Urban agriculture Europe* (p. 231). Jovis.

Lohrberg, F., Christenn, K., Timpe, A., & Sancar, A. (Hrsg.). (2022). *Urban agricultural heritage.* Birkhäuser. https://doi.org/10.1515/9783035622522

Pickard, D. (2022). The role of centralized policy planning for Bulgarian urban agricultural heritage from the socialist period. In F. Lohrberg, K. Christenn, A. Timpe, & A. Sancar (Hrsg.), *Urban agricultural.* Birkhäuser.

Siebel, W. (2015). *Die Kultur der Stadt.* Suhrkamp Verlag.

Steel, C. (2013). *Hungry city: How food shapes our lives.* Random house.

UNDP – United Nations Development Programme. (1996). *Urban agriculture. Food, jobs and sustainable cities* (Publication Series for Habitat II, Vol. 1). New York

Zhao, L. (2021). Exploring the spatial planning dimensions of urban informal food systems in Nanjing, China. *Urban Agriculture & Regional Food Systems, 6*(1), e20012.

Preface

In Europe, as in the rest of the world, urban agriculture takes on a variety of forms – from rooftop and balcony cultivation to allotment gardens, and from suburban farms to inner-city installations. Urban agriculture projects range in their social, economic, and environmental scope and value-driven motivations, as in their adaptation to local climatic, cultural, and political conditions. Our book does not aim to address European urban agriculture in all this complexity. Instead, it focuses on *urban agriculture initiatives occupying public spaces in dense, inner-city neighborhoods,* a specific setting, and one that received little attention from researchers to date. We are interested in uncovering urban agriculture's potential impacts on individual and community well-being, and seek to understand the best planning, design, policy, and management practices that can help to successfully integrate urban agriculture in public space.

Since the turn of the twenty-first century, urban agriculture has been a prominent theme in urban research, but we continue to know little about its impacts on well-being of individuals and communities. Furthermore, researchers have focused their attention to semi-private community gardens, where benefits and access are limited to active urban farmers. Despite its inherent potentials to engage the wider public and enhance the quality of urban life at the neighbourhood and district levels, there is not yet a significant body of research investigating the establishment of urban agriculture projects in urban public space. Although the empirical focus of this publication is on Norway, specifically the Oslo region, our work branches out to include experiences and projects from Northern European countries like Denmark, the Netherlands, and the United Kingdom, including a short detour in the USA. We seek to identify what might be both idiosyncratic and common across different contexts and places. The result is a rich documentation of the diversity of urban agriculture expressions in contemporary compact city development, and the identification of a series of useful critical questions, strategies, and practices that can help expand and strengthen its presence in neighborhoods and communities across the metropolitan landscape.

The book is based on the outputs of a research project entitled "Cultivating Public Space: urban agriculture as a basis for human flourishing and sustainability transition in Norwegian cities". Funded by the Research Council of Norway, based at the Norwegian University of Life Sciences, the project ran between 2017 and 2022. It involved an interdisciplinary and international collaboration between academics, activists, and public and private sector actors interested in uncovering research evidence of the transformative potential of urban agriculture to enhance well-being and activate public life. The project's inter-disciplinary perspectives reflected in this book range from urban planning to design, from public health to agroecology, and from human geography to philosophy.

By including a diversity of voices and cultural perspectives, we wanted to make this book engaging and relevant to an international audience of researchers, policy makers, urban designers, planners, educators, community activists, residents, and public space users of the sustainable, compact city of today and the future. In Norway and Northern Europe, the urban agriculture we have explored in this book shows a very strong social motivation, with food production as a secondary concern. Our insights can be also useful for audiences from other world regions motivated to implement urban cultivation for food production, social and environmental justice, and health, offering examples of the positive integration of well-being concerns into the planning, design, and management of productive public landscapes.

Norwegian University of Life Sciences   Beata Sirowy
Ås, Norway

University of Maryland   Deni Ruggeri
College Park, MD, USA

Contents

Editors and Contributors

About the Editors

Beata Sirowy is an independent urban scholar. She worked as a senior research fellow at the Department of Urban and Regional Planning, the Norwegian University of Life Sciences (2012–2023) and was the leader of the research project Cultivating Public Space (2017–2022) whose findings are presented in this book. Her educational background consists of philosophy (MA) combined with architecture and urban planning (MSc), and her research interests lie at the intersection of these domains. Her Ph.D. thesis (2010) addresses the theme of user-oriented architectural practice from a phenomenological perspective. She has published on the hermeneutics of art and the built environment; ethical aspects of architecture and planning; and the role of public space in sustaining human well-being and resilience in cities. She was a Visiting Scholar at UC Berkeley twice – at the Institute of Urban and

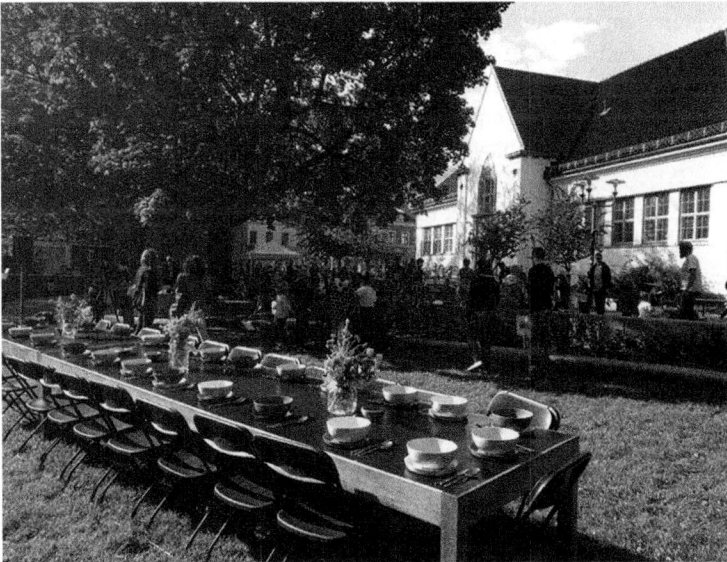

Urban agriculture at Schouss Plaza, Oslo. (Photo: B. Sirowy)

Regional Development (2019/20) and at the Department of Philosophy (2022). She currently works on a book addressing the relevance of Confucian concepts for contemporary urban development.

Deni Ruggeri (Ph.D., 2009) is Associate Professor of Landscape Architecture at the University of Maryland, College Park, USA. His research focuses on social and psychological dimensions of landscape architecture, livability in urban design, participatory design and co-creation, and biophilic, health- supporting design. Prof. Ruggeri is the author of 25 journal articles and book chapters, and co-edited the book *Defining Landscape Democracy. A Path to Spatial Justice* (2018). He serves as the Executive Director of the Environmental Design Research Association (EDRA), for which he has been Chair of the Board of Directors. From 2015 to 2018, Prof. Ruggeri has coordinated the Landscape Education for Democracy (LED) Erasmus Plus project, an educational program on the ethics, theories, and practices of democratic design and planning funded by the European Union. Prof. Ruggeri has held associate professorships at the Norwegian University of Life Sciences and the University of Oregon. He has been Assistant Professor at Cornell University, and has lectured at the University of California, Davis, and University of California, Berkeley.

Contributors

Adam Curtis works with sustainability and social design, exploring the ways in which shifts towards a greener world can also spur social justice. He has over a decade of experience in both the USA and Norway in grassroots organising, project management, and research. With MA in Development, Environment and Cultural Change from the University of Oslo, Adam has focused his work on the connections between sustainable transitions and social change. He currently acts as CEO for Nabolagshager, managing a portfolio of international research projects and social programming spanning topics from sustainable food systems to inclusive design.

Arild Eriksen is an architect educated at Bergen School of Architecture (2004). After several years as an employee at architectural offices in Norway, he co-founded the architectural office Eriksen Skajaa Arkitekter in 2010. The office took the initiative for participation processes with different groups of users, including former squatters. The office also worked with urban agriculture, and Arild was one of the founders of the urban beekeeping organization ByBi in Oslo. In 2018, he started Fragment architectural office that continues working with the political and community-oriented focus. He has taught at the Oslo School of Architecture, Bergen School of Architecture, Norwegian University of Life Sciences, and IBA Thüringen in Germany. He is currently writing a book on "the edible neighborhood" with Helene Gallis, with funding from the Horizon 2020 project Edicitynet.

Katinka Horgen Evensen is associate professor at the Department of Landscape Architecture, Norwegian University of Life Sciences. She received her doctoral degree in Environmental Psychology and Public Health from the Norwegian University of Life Sciences. She is part of the research group Green Space Management and Aesthetics (FUGE) at the Department of Landscape Architecture, Norwegian University of Life Sciences. Her research focuses on health-promoting environments like restorative and recreational urban green spaces. She has taken part in research projects on perceived safety in public parks and green space management, and on recreational value of urban cemeteries.

Helene Gallis founded the urban agriculture and social entrepreneurship company *Nabolagshager* in 2013, and has previously worked with sustainability issues in Spain, USA, Germany, and Norway with organizations such as Worldwatch Institute and The United Nations Development Programme. She has experience from a wide field, including sustainable production and consumption, policy development, entrepreneurship, and strategic communication. Helene is educated in sustainability and communication from Australia, Ecuador, Mexico, and Spain, with expertise in urban ecology, corporate social responsibility, and green entrepreneurship. She published the book *DYRK BYEN! – håndbok for urbane bønder* in 2015, which was Norway's first book on urban farming projects.

Pavel Grabalov is an urban researcher with a recently awarded Ph.D. degree from the Faculty of Landscape and Society, Norwegian University of Life Sciences. His Ph.D. thesis (2022) was devoted to the role of cemeteries across different urban contexts: "Urban cemeteries as public spaces: A comparison of cases from Scandinavia and Russia." His research interests revolve around interrelations between people and their environments and how these interrelations are captured or ignored by urban planning and development policies.

Kelvin Knight is reader in Ethics and Politics at London Metropolitan University, where he directed CASEP, the Centre for Contemporary Aristotelian Studies in Ethics and Politics, from 2009 until its departure in 2021. He is currently also chief researcher in the Institute of Management and Political Science at Mykolas Romeris University. Having authored *Aristotelian Philosophy: Ethics and Politics from Aristotle to MacIntyre* and many related essays, whilst editing or co-editing five books on contemporary Aristotelianism, he is now completing a book on the history and philosophy of human rights.

Bettina Lamm is associate professor of Landscape Architecture and Urban Design at the University of Copenhagen. Her research addresses the interaction between the lived life and our surrounding landscapes. She studies how temporary interventions and art strategies can contribute to a reprogramming of the interim landscape through presenting new site readings and experiences. Through a practice based research approach, she tests collaborative design-build methods, exploring how community based design processes can contribute to the cultivation of both people and places. Her approach has thus a social, aesthetic, and political agenda.

Geir Lieblein is agroecologist and professor of Agroecology at the Norwegian University of Life Sciences (NMBU). From his early work on field crops, he has progressively expanded into farming and food systems research, and more recently the effect of food on human bodies and further on education and learning. He has worked with a wide range of researchers and extra-university stakeholders on several continents. He is co-author of more than 60 publications in peer-reviewed journals and books. He co-founded the Agroecology Group and the MSc program in Agroecology at NMBU. In 2000 he introduced visionary thinking and in 2015 student project work in urban agriculture cases in different cities in Southern Norway as part of the MSc Agroecology program.

Frank Lohrberg is landscape architect and professor for Landscape Architecture at RWTH Aachen. His doctorate (2001) dealt with Urban Agriculture and City Planning. Since 2002, he is principal of lohrberg stadtlandschaftsarchitektur, the office focuses on landscape architecture. Since 2010, he has been the chair of the Institute of Landscape Architecture at RWTH Aachen University. Prof. Lohrberg has run several national and EU-funded research projects focusing on urban agriculture and green infrastructure. Currently his institute coordinates the H2020 project "EFUA-European Forum on Urban Agriculture."

Melissa Anna Murphy is an architect and urban space scholar currently serving as deputy head of the Department of Culture, Religion and Social Studies at the University of South-Eastern Norway. She received her doctoral degree in urban and regional planning from the Norwegian University of Life Sciences, where she contributes lectures in urban development and place-making. Her research focuses on socio-material urban experiences in the city tied to democracy, diversity, inclusion, and agency. Much of her work aims to trace phenomena from policy and urban planning to urban design, spatial management, and everyday life in urban spaces.

Anna Marie Nicolaysen is a researcher and teacher in the Agroecology group, Department of Plant Sciences, at the Norwegian University of Life Sciences. Her research interests lie in the food system and its connections to culture and health. Her work with action research in a community-based research organization in Hartford, CT, had a focus on inner-city populations' HIV risk and farmworker health (six journal publications). Her Ph.D. in medical anthropology from the University of Connecticut (2012) was on conversion to organic agriculture among smallholders in India (one book and two journal articles). As part of the Agroecology group at NMBU, her attention is on teaching and research in action learning in farming and food systems including urban agriculture, where she has been engaged in the research projects Cultivating Public Space and Adapt. Currently she is involved in the Sustainability Arena GreenSmart at NMBU with a module on Urban Agriculture and Society.

Inger-Lise Saglie is professor in Urban and Regional Planning at the Department of Urban and Regional Planning, Faculty of Landscape and Society, Norwegian University of Life Sciences. She is trained as an architect and has worked in practice with building design at Akershus County Council and city planning in Oslo and Tromsø. In her research, she has worked with environmental issues in urban and rural settings, planning theory and planning processes, as well as planning legislation.

Vebjørn Egner Stafseng is educated at the University of Oslo (B.A. Culture and Communication 2015) and NMBU (M.Sc. Agroecology 2019). He is now a PhD student with the Agroecology group, Department of Plant Science, NMBU, with a focus on transition processes for inclusive and robust urban gardening in public spaces. Previously he has worked on research projects on urban agriculture in connection with heritage studies, public health, and environmental learning. In his current position, he is also a teacher in the MSc Agroecology program with a special focus on the collaboration with external actors in the food system for educational cases for the students. He has also been active in the establishment of a National Centre for Urban Agriculture at NMBU with the aim to facilitate research-informed development of urban agriculture in Norway.

Anne Tietjen is associate professor of Landscape Architecture at the University of Copenhagen. She works with urban and rural transformation through spatial design, focusing on the politics and agency of design. Her work is situated within relational spatial design and planning theory, specifically based on new materialism and actor-network theory. She has carried out extensive research on strategic urban and rural planning, urban/rural public space, and heritage in planning. Anne's work bridges theory and practice at the intersection of landscape architecture, urban design, and planning. Her design-based research in this field has been informed by 12 years of international experience in architecture and urban design practice.

Esben Slaatrem Titland is a Norwegian cartoonist and illustrator living in Oslo, and an occasional urban farmer. He has an education from the School of Arts and Crafts in Oslo and the Einar Granum Art School. After a period of work with several self-produced fanzines, he made his debut in 2008 with the booklet *Båter mot bølgene* (*The boats against the waves*). The publication won the Sproing prize for the best debut that year (a national prize awarded to honor good cartoonists and promote the general interest in cartoons published in Norway). Since then, he has published several comic books and contributed with illustrations to a number of research based publications.

Chiara Tornaghi is associate professor of Urban Food Sovereignty and Resilience at the Centre for Agroecology, Water and Resilience, Coventry University, UK. She works at the intersection between urbanism/urbanisation and agroecology/food sovereignty, with particular interest in fostering practices that challenge and transform neoliberal, resource-extractive, colonial, and patriarchal food and knowledge system, inspired by principles of agroecology, feminism, biocultural diversity, and more-than-human health.

Kimberly Weger works with participation and social inclusion, exploring how the theories of deliberative democracy can be applied within urban agriculture and placemaking projects. Kim comes from Canada and has her M.A. degree in Political Science from the University of Calgary, with research on community participation in development in Ghana. After finishing her career as an international athlete in speed skating, Kim worked in Germany in an international sport development project, and currently works with Nabolagshager on national and international projects connecting people, ideas, and research, and translating sustainability theories into practice.

Chapter 1
Setting the Stage: Urban Agriculture, Public Space, and Human Well-Being

Beata Sirowy and Deni Ruggeri

> *The ultimate goal of farming is not the growing of crops, but the cultivation and perfection of human beings.*
>
> — Masanobu Fukuoka, *The One-Straw Revolution (1975)*

1.1 The Multidimensional Benefits of Urban Agriculture to Public Life and Well-being in Cities

Over the past few decades, urban dwellers have shown greater interest in growing food. This has been accompanied by a resurgence of strategies and policies addressing urban agriculture at different governance levels and geographical scales from the transnational to the municipal and the local. While the benefits of urban agriculture to the resilience of food supply have been documented (FAO, 2019), the popularity of urban agriculture and its increased acceptance have allowed the emergence of new forms of cultivation that integrate opportunities for community building (Carolan & Hale, 2016), place-keeping and stewardship (Piso et al., 2019), and access to greener and more inclusive public spaces (Wadumestrige et al., 2021). Contemporary urban agriculture functions as an arena for hands-on learning new sustainable food production cycles and more informed consumption choices (Puigdueta et al., 2021).

Urban agriculture is also an important arena for health promotion, through increased physical activity, stress reduction, and restorative experiences (Koay & Dillon, 2020).

B. Sirowy (✉)
Department of Urban and Regional Planning, Norwegian University of Life Sciences, Ås, Norway
e-mail: beata.sirowy@gmail.com

D. Ruggeri
Department of Plant Science and Landscape Architecture, University of Maryland, College Park, MD, USA
e-mail: druggeri@umd.edu

© The Author(s) 2024   1
B. Sirowy, D. Ruggeri (eds.), *Urban Agriculture in Public Space*, GeoJournal Library 132, https://doi.org/10.1007/978-3-031-41550-0_1

It benefits the environment by enhancing biodiversity in highly urbanised areas (Clucas et al., 2018) and enriching the experiential qualities of urban landscapes through innovative landscape architecture and urban design solutions (Viljoen & Bohn, 2014). Local food production might not be able to satisfy the entirety of our needs, but it can specialise in producing nutritious food and social economy by making resources available to inspire new forms of cooperative food production (Wadumestrige et al., 2021). When taken as a gestalt of all the previously listed benefits, today's urban agriculture emerges as a multifaceted practice with systemic benefits across many domains of human well-being from the individual household and the immediate community to the public health sustainability, and resilience of an entire city's population (Langemeyer et al., 2021).

To leverage its greatest impact, opportunities to join in urban agriculture practices should be widely accessible to all segments of urban population, close to everyone's home. Worldwide, due to the scarcity of and high value of land in dense inner-city areas, integrating urban agriculture in existing and planned public spaces may be the most feasible and impactful strategy. Our book wants to support this process by providing theoretical and practical insights on the integration of urban agriculture in public space development – addressing its well-being, design, organisation, educational, and urban planning implications. The relationship between public space and urban cultivation yields benefits to both. Public space offers conveniently accessible land for urban agriculture projects. In turn, urban cultivation can enhance the inclusiveness and multifunctionality of public space, which is crucial in addressing liveability and adaptation of urban neighbourhoods (Gehl, 2010; Madden, 2018).

Urban agriculture integrated in public space differs from private and semi-private projects (allotment gardens, backyard projects, rooftop gardens, or commercial farms) in management models and design, but perhaps most prominently in *the accessibility to a broad range of users*, not only those individuals primarily engaged in urban agriculture projects, but also secondary and tertiary users, like locals who may occasionally visit and participate, the passers-by and those who may be affected in more indirect, subtle or symbolic ways. The broader accessibility means more extensive impacts on urban population in terms of:

(a) Symbolic representation
  As Frank Lohrberg point out in his Foreword to this volume, urban agriculture actors occupy public space to not only practice cultivation, but also to demonstrate their mindsets, values, and agendas in a contested public domain. This in turn may lead towards a societal transition, as the activities that are permanently accepted in public space can claim to be settled in urban society at large, making urban agriculture both a space for food production and a space for interpretive purposes (ibid.).

(b) Individual well-being
  Urban agriculture situated in public space has a potential to benefit a greater diversity of individuals and their needs, and empower those who have often been neglected by city planning and policy. It offers opportunities for cultivating of virtues and sustaining capabilities as discussed in Chap. 2 and illustrated through our empirical studies (Chaps. 4 and 6).

(c) Community well-being

This type of impacts includes opportunities for cultivation of civic friendship and communities of virtue (Chap. 3), placemaking (Chap. 7), participatory action learning (Chaps. 8 and 9), co-creation and bottom-up participation (Chaps. 5 and 11), biocultural diversity and social justice (Chap. 13).

Embedding urban agriculture in public space, is not immune to disputes and compromises. In Chap. 4, the authors propose a framework for an analysis of different dimensions of publicness of urban agriculture projects and possible conflicts among these.

In the neoliberal city restrictions to the use of public space by certain users and the displacement of noncommercial, community-oriented uses, and those catering to low-income families and fragile individuals make the presence of non-commercial uses of public space like urban agriculture essential to ensure a heathy, inclusive and democratic public life (Nemeth & Schmidt, 2011). Further, additional threats to the inclusiveness of public space come from the compact city development model, which since the 1990s has been dominant in Norway and other European countries (Hanssen et al., 2015). This model of urban development typically offers high-quality, accessible outdoor areas that fail to perform as *democratic* public spaces, i.e. as sites that encourage social exchange (not just casual encounters) between social groups (Hajer & Reijndorp, 2001:11), identity and symbolic significance construction, and the claiming and eventual renegotiating of shared values and beliefs. The densities required by the compact city also greatly limit space availability for agricultural production, biodiversity, and ecology, making public space a natural ground for cultivation of highly productive urban ecosystems.

Urban agriculture initiatives have a great potential to sustain a collective stewardship of accessible and inclusive public landscapes (Murphy et al., 2022). As authors McIvor and Hale (2015:727) argue, urban agriculture is 'well positioned to help citizens cultivate lasting relationships across lines of difference and amidst significant power differentials—relationships that could form the basis of a community's collective capacity to shape its future'. By engaging residents in the cultivation of community bonds, urban agriculture has great potential as a systemic, collaborative, emergent, and constantly evolving civic practice necessary to tackle the 'wickedness' of community development in the face of uncertainty (Rittel & Webber, 1973).

Urban agriculture can be an instrument for the exercise of the right to the city (Lefebvre, 1996), a principle reaffirmed in 2016 by The New Urban Agenda adopted at the United Nations Conference on Housing and Sustainable Urban Development (Habitat III). The United Nations define the right to the city as 'the right of all inhabitants … to occupy, use and produce just, inclusive and sustainable cities' (UN, 2017:26). Further, they describe it 'as a common good essential to the quality of life' (ibid.), emphasising in this context the importance of public space as an arena for social interactions and political participation, sociocultural expression, diversity, and social cohesion. By offering citizens opportunities for participation in urban decision-making and appropriation of urban spaces based on their needs, urban agriculture projects can contribute positively to these objectives and to advance livability in cities.

The right to the city has recently evolved into an emerging dialogue around the right to landscape and landscape democracy (Egoz et al., 2018). Landscape democracy views access to the landscape as a foundation for equity in advancing human health, delight, respite, and healing. Far from being just a theory, landscape democracy speaks of an ethos, a way of being. It refers to the community-based practices and interactions that cultivate democratic dialogue and action. Central to landscape democracy is the idea that it can be achieved through mutuality and cooperation, entailing rights and responsibilities for everyone (Council of Europe, 2000:2). To build a more equitable and inclusive society, citizens must actively practice their role as community members, learning how to dialogue, learn, and interact to form a shared understandings of what it means to be a community. As a socially oriented practice of landscape stewardship, urban agriculture is the ideal ground for learning and practicing landscape democracy. By connecting people around the shared task of growing food in public and semiprivate spaces, urban agriculture offers a critical space for collective action and the exercise of a right but also a responsibility essential to prepare ourselves to increasingly unpredictable socio-economic and ecological challenges.

Viewing urban public space as a locus of individual and social well-being, we situate ourselves in the neo-Aristotelian tradition, including the capability approach (Nussbaum, 2011) and virtue theory (MacIntyre, 2007, 2016). These approaches call for a non-reductionist, multidimensional, and cross-sectorial framework to evaluate the quality of urban landscape in terms of its ability to sustain human flourishing, both on the individual and communal level (Chaps. 2 and 3). The neo-Aristotelian tradition offers a more convenient vantage point to approach human well-being in cities on the micro-level of a neighbourhood, than the perspective of social justice based on the Rawlsian approach, which concentrates on 'macro' questions of equitable distribution of burdens and benefits in urban development (Fainstein, 2010). Simultaneously, this book acknowledges the importance of socially just arrangements for human well-being in cities – including securing an equitable access to high-quality, safe, inclusive public spaces, with a diversity of functions, addressing the needs of different segments of urban population. A systematic integration of publicly accessible urban agriculture interventions in urban development is illustrated in Chaps. 11 and 12, focusing on strategic planning and public policy in Norway.

The motivation behind this book is a deep concern for human well-being in cities. It is, however, essential to remember that we cannot discuss well-being in separation from the question of human-nature interaction. Cities are essentially socio-ecological systems, and any decision-making aimed at sustainable and resilient urban development should always consider an urban system's different components and scales (Walker & Salt, 2012). Many important questions emerging in this context, that could be addressed through the lenses of urban agriculture, belong to the quickly developing domain of food geography. It is a domain concerned with a variety of topics—from our relation with food, changing consumption patterns and the nature of our supply chains, to the spatial patterns of our food production, the ever-pressing need for sustainable agriculture, and the complex relationships between food, place, and space (Kneafsey et al., 2021). While the subject lays beyond the necessary boundaries we set for our work, Chap. 13 addresses some of these issues advocating urban agriculture practices that challenge commodification of food, promoting biocultural diversity, and cultivation of knowledge practices that heal the nature/society rift.

Given the richness and diversity of urban agriculture forms in public space, we decided to narrow our scope to projects integrated in densely populated neighbourhoods, in Norwegian and selected Northern European cities, with only brief excursions in the North American continent. This focus prevents us from drawing broad generalizations across the variety of urban agriculture forms worldwide, yet from our unique point of view, we are able to speculate about main differences in the motivations for urban agriculture in our European context and the rest of the world. Globally, we observed an urban agriculture deeply involved in strengthening local food supply and food justice (improving access to fresh and healthy food), reducing climate impacts of food production by establishing short supply chains, and sustaining livelihoods through opportunities for income generation and employment (FAO, 2022). In Northern Europe the main motivation is primarily social – pertaining to different aspects of individual and social well-being in cities, discussed throughout this book. Despite our choice to begin with the contexts closest to us, we hope our findings will be relevant as a source of inspiration, or comparison for researchers, decision makers, and civil society actors seeking to advance the well-being and empowerment of urban communities globally, suggesting strategies and actions that could be exploited in a variety of geographical, cultural, and socio-economic contexts.

1.2   The Structure and Content of This Book

The structure of this book reflects the unfolding of our research project Cultivating Public Space (CPS), starting with its conceptual foundations (Chaps. 2 and 3), followed with discussions of urban agriculture cases (Chaps. 4, 5, 6, and 7), educational contexts (Chaps. 8, 9, and 10), planning/policy dimensions (Chaps. 11 and 12), and concluding with critical reflections on future urban agriculture trajectories (Chaps. 13 and 14). Still, all chapters were written independently by different project partners and could be read individually. This book emerges from a Norwegian context where our project originated (Chaps. 6, 7, 8, 10, 11, and 12) but has expanded to include international urban agriculture cases from the Netherlands, Denmark, the United Kingdom, and the United States (Chaps. 4, 5, 9, and 13). Its novelty lies in the interdisciplinary and cross-sectorial perspectives included, ranging from urban planning to design, from public health to agroecology, from human geography to philosophy. We have also included a variety of voices – academics, scholars-activists (Chap. 13), and practitioners (Chaps. 7 and 10).

With our multifaceted, yet locally situated discussions we respond to the knowledge gap about a holistic understanding of urban agriculture, the social groups benefiting most from it, and the government support mechanisms created in support of it (Wadumestrige et al., 2021). Given that urban agriculture is highly influenced by idiosyncratic local factors, 'studying more about opportunities and challenges for urban agriculture under different socio-economic contexts and different agriculture models could be more beneficial to connect farming practices in cities with urban planning' (ibid., p.1).

Part I: *Conceptual Foundations: Urban Agriculture for Human Flourishing* offers the theoretical foundations for our investigation rooted in the Aristotelian/ neo-Aristotelian perspectives on individual and communal well-being in cities.

In Chap. 2, Beata Sirowy proposes an operationalisation of human well-being in cities based on the Aristotelian notion of *eudaimonia* and elements of Martha Nussbaum's capability approach, referring also to the theory of affordances. This operationalisation may be used to evaluate the potential of public spaces (both actual and planned) to sustain human flourishing – an alternative to valuation models driven by an instrumental rationality, such as cost-benefit analysis. In the framework she proposes, the relationship between affordances, capabilities, and virtues in urban placemaking can be understood as a continuous process of negotiating a space's optimum set of affordances – environmental and social – so it sustains a variety of central capabilities and offers opportunities for cultivation of related virtues, moral and intellectual. This model calls for citizen participation in the process of altering the affordances of their environments for the benefit of all.

By problematising eudaimonic well-being in cities, this chapter contributes to a growing discussion on the relationship between the qualities of the built environment and human well-being in cities. This research typically focuses on the range of pathways through which the built environment may affect human well-being, not so much on the operationalisation of well-being, and typically adopts a hedonic view of human well-being. The author postulates that the distinction between eudaimonic and hedonic well-being needs to be pronounced more clearly in urban research, and more attention needs to be paid to the eudaimonic well-being construct which is much more concerned with the achievement of full human potential than the hedonic models.

In Chap. 3, authors Beata Sirowy and Kelvin Knight expand on the discussion of human flourishing (eudaimonic well-being) started in Chap. 2 with considerations of virtues (excellences of character and understanding) and civic friendship. In determining *how* to better integrate these concepts in urban development, they employ the neo-Aristotelian concept of practices, as distinct from organisational institutions and introduce a concept of communities of virtue (MacIntyre, 2016, 2007). They posit that the development of urban public space should be viewed in terms of citizens' participative practices, not just (as is typically the case) administratively conceived functions. This approach to the development of urban public space addresses individual and communal well-being to a much higher extent than the pragmatic multifunctionality demands prevalent in local policies.

Enhancing the conditions for participation in shared practices in urban settings facilitates the development of communities of virtue – localities consolidated by shared goals and standards of excellence, which are a setting for cultivating virtues (intellectual and moral) and development of civic friendship (ibid.) This discussion is illustrated with references to urban agriculture – understood as practice in the MacIntyrean sense, and therefore a potential setting for the development of communities of virtue that could be integrated in development of public space. Importantly, an urban agriculture project can potentially offer settings for cultivation of multiple, additional practices beyond food production – such as culinary arts, herbal medicine, mindfulness, carpentry, or even chess or raft building – as exemplified in some of our project cases (Chaps. 4, 5, 6, and 7).

Part II: *Public Urban Agriculture in Northern European Contexts* offers evidence from case studies of urban agriculture in Norway, Denmark, and the Netherlands. The focus is on the systematic integration of urban agriculture in public spaces to ensure access for large and diverse segments of the urban population to an increasingly privatised public realm. The major challenge here is reconciling the needs and expectations of different groups of users, i.e. how to facilitate urban agriculture projects that benefit the public (the secondary and tertiary users) while allowing individuals directly engaged in urban agriculture (the primary users) to fulfil their objectives.

In Chap. 4, Melissa Anna Murphy and Pavel Grabalov explore how urban agriculture can contribute to the capabilities of gardeners and the larger urban community. They tell the story of urban agriculture case studies in Aarhus (Denmark) and Rotterdam (the Netherlands) to understand how different municipalities facilitate urban agriculture and how various urban agriculture initiatives perform in public spaces. In their analysis, they draw on a conceptualisation of publicness focused on the interactions in and products from physical space that link people. With an emphasis on an understanding of the public that is greater than the gardeners involved, the authors identify four trajectories in publicness supported by urban agriculture, serving the public through (a) increasing access and animation in public space, (b) contributing to social services, (c) producing and distributing food, and (d) building communities to spread cultivation knowledge. While not mutually exclusive, the four trajectories place different strains upon the public space ideal of physical access. The authors conclude that food production and social services may be ill-suited to urban spaces that demand high levels of public access. However, these benefits can reach a broader public if appropriately situated and facilitated.

In Chap. 5, Bettina Lamm and Anne Tietjen introduce four urban agriculture projects started between 2011 and 2013 in and around the city of Copenhagen and their efforts to cultivate food and community. The sites share a common emphasis on urban agriculture as a tool for cultivating citizenry. All four urban gardens were community-based efforts, open to the wider public, yet they varied widely in their organisation, management, funding, and context. While two of the gardens were started by cultural activists, the others were the initiative of municipal agency and a private land developer. All of them shared a vision to not only grow produce, but also create spaces for social inclusion and community gatherings. Looking into their underlying value system and organisational structure allows us to compare how the different typologies of urban agriculture would impact people's ability to thrive. The authors are particularly interested in the agendas pursued by the communities who managed the gardens, how these agendas related to the specific site and context, and how the communities negotiated public access requirements with creating an enduring gardening community. The fact that some of the gardens did not become permanent is a reflection on city's prioritisation of urban agriculture goals, and clearly reflects a weakness in the policy and implementation about the needs to build resilient and lasting community bonds. These sites have nonetheless been testing grounds for new forms of relationships between individuals and community groups.

In Chap. 6 Katinka Horgen Evensen and Vebjørn Egner Stafseng present eight case studies from the Oslo metro area, in which they explore ways of integrating urban agriculture in public spaces. The authors collected experiences of project initiators and managers from urban agriculture initiatives of various typologies, scales, and organisational models; from the city farm to small experimental cultivation projects. They learned that the main motivation behind those urban agriculture projects was the creation of social meeting places and learning arenas for cultivation and ecological knowledge. Urban agriculture in Oslo has also been a tool in local urban space development to improve city dwellers' well-being, activate and make unused space safer, and integrate cultivation in green space management in innovative ways. The authors conclude with a discussion of factors that can support or hinder the practice of urban agriculture in public space. They contend that the most pressing design challenge may be to enhance and ensure for urban agriculture projects an image and perception of being truly public and welcoming to all.

In Chap. 7 Helene Gallis, Kimberly Weger, and Adam Curtis share Norwegian experiences of a pioneering urban agriculture social non-profit enterprise *Nabolagshager* (Neighbourhood Gardens). The chapter is a rich memoir of the stories associated with the development of urban agriculture projects in Oslo seen through the lens of its founder, activist Helene Gallis. The chapter makes the case for a more systematic application of placemaking principles to enhance the social well-being impact of urban agriculture projects. Gallis argues that combining placemaking with urban agriculture can enable community members, residents, and marginalized groups to participate in the co-creation of urban agriculture and exercise their human capabilities. The stories highlight the transformative impact of placemaking principles – key among them that of triangulation. They are told here as inspiration for innovative new forms of reappropriation and co-production of democratically conceived, accessible, and inclusive public spaces.

Part III: *When Education Gets in the Urban Agriculture Mix* addresses various educational experiences related to action research, practice, and engaged-learning efforts inspired by the Cultivating Public Space project. In these processes project partners and students entered into a rich and transformative dialogue with and across communities of urban farmers, residents, and design and planning professionals. The theories, knowledge, and explanations emerging from the research were tested, redefined, and reinterpreted against the real-life experiences of urban agriculture practitioners. The students' work fed back into the CPS research, supporting the generation of an urban agriculture toolbox that was developed as a part of the project.

In Chap. 8, Vebjørn Egner Stafseng, Anna Marie Nicolaysen, and Geir Lieblein describe the participatory action learning process involving NMBU Agroecology students and faculty to envision a change in seven urban agriculture sites and communities in the Oslo region. The chapter critically reflects on the visions that emerged through co-creation and the forces that could hinder or support the ideas that emerged. The process reveals a rich educational experience that greatly benefited students, project partners, and locals but also a resistance by urban agriculture coordinators against solidifying their organic, adaptable efforts into generalisable steps and actions for the future. They fear that a fixed vision might prevent adaptation and, in the long run, restrict urban agriculture's ability to be resilient and long-lasting. The authors find that policy and plans from municipalities may also play a critical role in limiting the development of new and diverse forms of urban agriculture in favour of uniformity and standardisation.

In Chap. 9, Deni Ruggeri reflects on the educational experiences connected to the Cultivating Public Space project. From the onset, the project has sought to engage students in creating a toolbox for urban agriculture in public space. By embedding the research findings, activities, and knowledge co-produced by the project partners within the global classroom, students played an instrumental role in translating the research findings into concrete sustainable development and urban regeneration strategies based on urban agriculture. This required thinking of it as more than just a collection of objects – boxes, tool sheds, fences, and paths – but as holistic multifunctional landscapes to cultivate food, health, and community. Another crucial finding relates to the uniqueness of each urban agriculture site and the need to build upon each context's distinctiveness, placeness, and identity to shape stories of future transformation that communities can coalesce around and activate.

Chapter 10 by Arild Eriksen, with Deni Ruggeri and Esben Slaatrem Titland, approaches urban agriculture from the perspective of an architect and urban farmer/beekeeper practicing bottom-up, participatory design in Oslo. It touches on a few critical dimensions of urban agriculture in public space, which relate to the private and corporate claim on these landscapes, and their potentiality as multifunctional and abundant contributors to sociocultural and ecological diversity, food security, health, and democratic discourse. The authors conclude with a reflection on their efforts to develop an urban agriculture toolbox, drawing from knowledge collected by the Cultivating Public Space researchers, supplemented with the analyses and solutions produced by a multidisciplinary group of students enrolled in a project-funded continuing education course taught by the authors at the Norwegian University of Life Sciences in 2018/19. Rather than a collection of prescriptive design solutions, the toolbox has an innovative form of a graphic novel produced in cooperation with cartoonist and urban farmer Esben Slaatrem Titland and presents a rich account of the motivations, personal sacrifices, successful actions, and setbacks emerging from our urban agriculture case studies that other urban agriculture actors might empathise with and be inspired by. It is an Open Access publication, available here (in Norwegian): Byens Bønder.

Part IV: *Planning for Urban Agriculture in Norway* addresses motivations of urban agriculture municipal actors in Norway to support urban agriculture initiatives and policy developments in major Norwegian cities. Although urban planners are generally keen on integrating urban agriculture in a city development, it has been limitedly integrated into policy and planning. More extensive research is needed on how cities can legally and effectively integrate urban agriculture into spatial planning holistically, filling a critical knowledge gap in our understanding of how food production and delivery may become more strategically planned, financed, and governed.

In Chap. 11, Inger-Lise Saglie dives into planning documents and strategic urban agriculture planning efforts from three of Norway's largest cities: Oslo, Bergen, and Trondheim. The paper seeks evidence in the documents and in the discourses used by municipal leaders and government officials interviewed on motivations for their urban agriculture policies and strategic efforts. The author groups policy key motivations into five categories. First, urban agriculture is set into an urban greening development discourse, particularly in Oslo and Bergen; second, food production and alternative food systems are important policy motivations, particularly in Trondheim and Bergen, where urban agriculture is engaged in a dialogue with peri-urban, professionalised agriculture; third, urban agriculture as social meeting spaces and community building; fourth, urban agriculture as a tool for municipal welfare and employment training services; and fifth, as a practice of active citizenship and co-creation in city development.

In Chap. 12, Inger-Lise Saglie seeks to answer the question: "How have Norwegian public policies for urban agriculture emerged and got institutionalized?" In Norway, urban agriculture has been initially associated with citizen activism and local, volunteerism-driven bottom-up initiatives. However, municipalities have been interested in the development of strategic urban agriculture public policies. The three Norwegian cities introduced in the previous chapter – Oslo, Bergen, and Trondheim – show many common traits in the institutionalisation of urban agriculture policy. There are also marked differences regarding the role of voluntary groups and bottom-up and top-down processes, degree of networking, relationship to professionalised peri-urban agriculture, and the implementation. Oslo shows a politically driven participatory approach with plans and visions for developing urban agriculture as a social activity in green/urban spaces. In Bergen, the non-profit/volunteerism sector has an active role in strategy development and in directing practice through their competence centre. In Trondheim, the policy is co-produced and refined yearly in partnership with professional farmers, a unique example of a synergy between tradition and innovation. Having been at the forefront of developing public policies for urban agriculture in Norway, the cases of Oslo, Bergen, and Trondheim offer insights into the state of the art in the policy development around urban agriculture in Scandinavia.

Part V: *A Way Forward for Urban Agriculture in Cities and Communities* serves as a moment of reflection on the current state of urban agriculture and ponders on its future trajectories. It also seeks to suggest a series of threads for an emergent dialogue around principles and practices that may facilitate or hinder urban agriculture's progress towards making the greatest impact on individual and communal well-being, and becoming an integral and permanent part of the resilient city of tomorrow.

In Chap. 13 Chiara Tornaghi reminds us to be vigilant about the way urban agriculture is applied in our cities and of the potential deleterious consequences of advancing urban agriculture without being aware of the systems it affects, from ecology to community, justice and human rights. The author sets out to describe an agroecological approach to urban farming, which combines resource conservation, regeneration, and biodiversity, while also advancing reparation by tackling past injustices and the hegemony of profit over human flourishing. The chapter offers useful recommendations for an agroecology-inspired urban agriculture in public space: biocultural diversity, knowledge practices that heal the nature/society rift, and the creation of urban agriculture practices that challenge commodification. It also reflects on the epistemology of urban agriculture and the need for it to be defined in terms of the stories and experiences of the people it affects, especially the underserved.

Chapter 14 by Beata Sirowy and Deni Ruggeri concludes with a short reflection on the future trajectories for urban agriculture in the compact city, building upon the findings of CPS research project. Cities are changing rapidly under new and old pressures, and they are reorganising and planning in response to the local consequences of global challenges, like the recent COVID-19 pandemic. What does a resilient urban agriculture look like in the future Norwegian/Northern European and global city? The goal is to co-design, plan, and implement forms of urban agriculture that can increase productivity and reduce land consumption, while also serving as a social arena for the cultivation of citizens' virtues and community identity and collective action to celebrate human capabilities. No strategic plan, policy, design, and implementation can succeed unless it is adapted and enriched by the uniqueness of the context in which it embeds itself. Aside from the diversity urban agriculture approaches and practices shared, this book's most important contribution may be simple sharing of stories and experiences of urban agriculture practices in public space that illustrate motivations, successes, failed attempts, and the adaptations necessary to make it a part of our daily life.

References

Carolan, M., & Hale, J. (2016). "Growing" communities with urban agriculture: Generating value above and below ground. *Community Development, 47*(4), 530–545.

Clucas, B., Parker, I. D., & Feldpausch-Parker, A. M. (2018). A systematic review of the relationship between urban agriculture and biodiversity. *Urban Ecosystem, 21*, 635–643.

Council of Europe. (2000). *Council of Europe Landscape Convention*. European Treaty Series – No. 176. Florence.

Egoz, S., Jørgensen, K., & Ruggeri, D. (Eds.). (2018). *Defining landscape democracy: A path to spatial justice*. Edward Elgar Publishing.

Fainstein, S. (2010). *The just city*. Cornell University Press.

FAO. (2019). *FAO framework for the urban food agenda*. Rome. https://www.fao.org/3/ca3151en/ca3151en.pdf

FAO. (2022). *Peri-urban agriculture sourcebook—From production to food systems*. Rome. https://www.fao.org/3/cb9722en/cb9722en.pdf

Fukuoka, M. (1978 [1975]). *The one-straw revolution: An introduction to natural farming*. Rodale Press.

Gehl, J. (2010). *Cities for people*. Pan American Copyright Conventions.

Hajer, M., & Reijndorp, A. (2001). *In search of new public domain*. NAi Publishers.

Hanssen, G. S., Hofstad, H., & Saglie, I. L. (Eds.). (2015). *Kompakt byutvikling. Muligheter og utfordringer*. Universitetsforlaget.

Kneafsey, M., Maye, D., Holloway, L., & Goodman, M. (2021). *Geographies of food*. Bloomsbury Publishing.

Koay, W. I., & Dillon, D. (2020). Community gardening: Stress, Well-being, and resilience potentials. *International Journal of Environmental Research and Public Health, 17*(18), 6740.

Langemeyer, J., Madrid-Lopez, C., Beltran, A. M., & Mendez, G. V. (2021). Urban agriculture—A necessary pathway towards urban resilience and global sustainability? *Landscape and Urban Planning, 210*, 104055.

Lefebvre, H. (1996). *Writings on cities*. Basil Blackwell.

MacIntyre, A. (2007). *After virtue: A study in moral theory*. University of Notre Dame Press.

MacIntyre, A. (2016). *Ethics in the conflicts of modernity: An essay on desire, practical reasoning and narrative*. Cambridge University Press.

Madden, K. (2018). *How to turn a place around: A Placemaking handbook*. Project for Public Spaces.

McIvor, D. W., & Hale, J. (2015). Urban agriculture and the prospects for deep democracy. *Agriculture and Human Values, 32*, 727–741.

Murphy, M., Parker, P., & Hermus, M. (2022). Cultivating inclusive public space with urban gardens. *Local Environment, 28*, 1–18.

Nemeth, J., & Schmidt, S. (2011). The privatization of public space: Modeling and measuring publicness. *Environment and Planning B: Planning and Design, 38*, 23–25.

Nussbaum, M. (2011). *Creating capabilities. The human development approach*. Belknap Press of Harvard.

Piso, Z., Goralnik, L., Libarkin, J., & Lopez, M. (2019). Types of urban agricultural stakeholders and their understandings of governance. *Ecology and Society, 24*(2), 18.

Puigdueta, I., Aguilera, E., Cruz, J. L., Iglesias, A., & Sanz-Cobena, A. (2021). Urban agriculture may change food consumption towards low carbon diets. *Global Food Security, 28*, 100507.

Rittel, H. W., & Webber, M. M. (1973). Dilemmas in a general theory of planning. *Policy Sciences, 4*(2), 155–169.

United Nations. (2017). *The New Urban Agenda*.

Viljoen, A., & Bohn, K. (2014). *Second nature urban agriculture: Designing productive cities*. Routledge.

Wadumestrige, D., Chethika, G., Geetha, M., & Kensuke, F. (2021). Promoting urban agriculture and its opportunities and challenges—A global review. *Sustainability, 13*(17), 9609.

Walker, B., & Salt, D. (2012). *Resilience thinking: Sustaining ecosystems and people in a changing world*. Island press.

Part I
Conceptual Foundations: Urban Agriculture for Human Flourishing

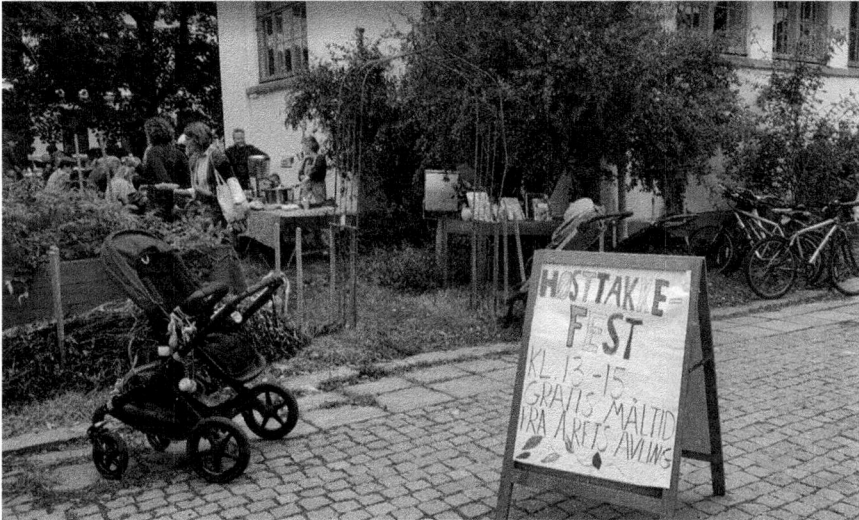

Chapter 2
Capabilities and Beyond: Towards an Operationalization of Eudaimonic Well-Being in a Public Space Context

Beata Sirowy

2.1 Introduction: Addressing Well-Being in Cities

Since 1990 the United Nations Development Programme has undertaken to produce an annual report on the human dimension of development, consistently asserting that "the process of development should … create a conducive environment for people, individually and collectively, to develop their full potential and to have a reasonable chance of leading productive and creative lives in accord with their needs and interests" (UNDP, 1990: 1). This is an important goal for urban development worldwide, especially considering that by 2050, the global urban population is expected to nearly double. Human activities and their impacts are increasingly concentrated in cities, and this poses immense sustainability challenges of environmental, social, and economic nature, all of these impacting human well-being. Addressing these challenges, The New Urban Agenda (UN, 2017) articulates a vision for a better and more sustainable urban future – "one in which all people have equal rights and access to the benefits and opportunities that cities can offer" (ibid., p. iv). It postulates that "cities can be the source of solutions to, rather than the cause of, the challenges that our world is facing today" (ibid.). In this context, the improvement of well-being in cities – both in developed and developing countries – emerges as an important objective, which is also central to the UN Sustainable Development Goals (SDGs) (UN, 2015).

To address human well-being in cities in an adequate way, we need a better understanding of this construct. Growing scholarship on the relationship between the quality of the built environment and quality of urban life (Marans & Stimson, 2011; Pfeiffer & Cloutier, 2016; Wang & Wang, 2016; Shekhar et al., 2019; Mouratidis, 2021) typically focuses on the range of *pathways* through which the

B. Sirowy (✉)
Department of Urban and Regional Planning, Norwegian University of Life Sciences, Ås, Norway
e-mail: beata.sirowy@gmail.com

B. Sirowy, D. Ruggeri (eds.), *Urban Agriculture in Public Space*, GeoJournal Library 132, https://doi.org/10.1007/978-3-031-41550-0_2

built environment may affect subjective well-being of urban dwellers, not so much on the *operationalization* of well-being. The concept of subjective well-being (SWB) commonly used in this field is usually taken as unproblematic, defined in terms of the "personal evaluation of quality of life" (Diener et al., 2018; Mouratidis, 2021), as opposed to objective (economic) well-being measured by quantitative indicators such as income. This distinction is not satisfactory, as both these constructs fall into the category of hedonic well-being.

I argue that the concept of human well-being in cities is not sufficiently understood. In particular, the essential distinction between eudaimonic and hedonic well-being needs to be expressed more explicitly in urban research. In this chapter I address this distinction and propose a preliminary operationalization of eudaimonic well-being in the context of urban agriculture, informed by the virtue tradition (Aristotle, 2009), elements of the capability approach (Nussbaum, 2011), and the theory of affordances (Gibson, 1979; Rietveld, 2012). Chapters 4 and 6 further contribute to refining and contextualizing of these operationalizations through case studies of urban agriculture in Norway and other Northern European countries.

2.2 The Distinction Between Eudaimonic and Hedonic Well-Being

Eudaimonia is often translated as happiness but it differs substantially from today's understanding of this word in terms of pleasurable, often transitory experiences (hedonic happiness). For ancient Greeks, *eudaimonia* denoted human flourishing – the actualization of our full potentials, a rewarding and fulfilled human life, which was necessarily one lived in accordance with virtues – excellences of character and understanding (Aristotle, 2009). Importantly, virtue is not so much about what a person *does* in specific situations but what a person *is* in the totality of their life (Taylor, 2002: 44).

Eudaimonic well-being (human flourishing) needs to be clearly distinguished from hedonic well-being (or subjective well-being) related to "the frequency and intensity of emotional experiences such as happiness, joy, stress, and worry that make a person's life pleasant or unpleasant" (Christodoulou et al., 2013:2; Kahneman & Deaton, 2010). Human flourishing is not about positive emotional experiences (which usually have a transitory nature) but about the actualization of one's potentials, perception of meaningfulness of one's life, growth. Positive emotions are usually present here, but the contentment is based upon a person's effort of self-cultivation and sense of purpose. It is "the lasting realisation of what has been wrought" (Taylor, 2002:119).

The theme of eudaimonic well-being has been addressed within psychology for a long time – already in 1930s psychologists investigated issues such as self-actualization, creativity, becoming, meaning, and human potential. The interest in these issues has led to the emergence of humanistic psychology in mid-1950s

(Schneider et al., 2015), objecting to the reductionist investigation of the human mind and behavior embraced by behaviorism and psychoanalysis. Humanistic psychology perspectives had major influence on psychotherapy practice since 1950s (Perls et al., 1951; Frankl 1946/1959; Rogers, 1961) but their impact on empirical research within psychology was limited due to an absence of credible assessment tools to measure the diverse aspects of human flourishing they described (Ryff, 2017). This situation has changed in 1980s with the first attempts to operationalize eudaimonic well-being construct and develop tools for its assessment (Deci & Ryan, 1985; Ryff, 1989). Research on eudaimonic well-being gained momentum in early 2000s. Ryan and Deci (2001:141) in their review of well-being studies within psychology note that these have been informed by two general perspectives:

> the hedonic approach, which focuses on happiness and defines well-being in terms of pleasure attainment and pain avoidance; and the eudaimonic approach, which focuses on meaning and self-realization and defines well-being in terms of the degree to which a person is fully functioning. These two views have given rise to different research foci and a body of knowledge that is in some areas divergent and in others complementary.

The interest in the topic of eudaimonic well-being in psychology has been steadily growing (Ryan et al., 2008; Huta & Ryan, 2010; Huta & Waterman, 2014; Huta, 2016; Vittersø, 2016; Cromhout et al., 2022), but these discussions have had limited impact outside this disciplinary domain. Eudaimonic well-being is little understood within the policy context, and its operationalization is considered challenging. Accordingly, researchers and decision-makers most often use the construct of hedonic well-being for policy monitoring, informing, and analysis purposes within different policy domains (Stone & Mackie, 2013), perhaps with an exception of lobal-level strategies, as reflected in Human Development Reports published annually by the United Nations Development Programme since 1990. Yet, several studies in psychology suggest that eudemonic well-being is relatively more important for the overall psychological functioning and life satisfaction (McMahan & Estes, 2011; Ryff, 2017; Ruini & Cesetti, 2019). This point at the necessity of extending the urban well-being discussion beyond hedonic models.

2.3   Well-Being as an Ethical Construct

Most basically, the question of urban well-being is an ethical question of "what makes a good urban life?" and can be only answered against the background of a broader normative outlook. In this I follow Upton (2002) who argues that spatial planning needs to be understood fundamentally as a form of applied ethics: it is concerned with values, and therefore it is necessary to develop an understanding of how the ethical frameworks and their concepts inform the making of places.

The normative orientation of contemporary urban discourse comes primarily from Western modern ethics and its principle-based (deontological) and outcome-based (consequentialist) systems.

In both these perspectives, the question of human well-being is predominantly viewed in terms of hedonic well-being (Taylor, 2002:119). The example of a deontological perspective is the Rawlsian theory of distributive justice (Rawls, 1971), in the urban context primarily concerned with the just distribution of burdens and benefits of urban development and securing individual liberties (Fainstein, 2010; Soja, 2010). Consequentialist thinking, on the other hand, is chiefly concerned with achieving the greatest utility for the greatest number (however ambiguous this notion may be) and has informed the development of cost-benefit analysis – a valuation tool widely used in urban decision-making.

The third major orientation in modern ethical discourse is the virtue tradition in its diverse formulations. The Aristotelian virtue ethics was the dominant approach in Western moral philosophy until the Enlightenment, when deontologist and consequentialist perspectives gained the central position in the ethical discourse. It re-emerged in the late 1950s in Anglo-American philosophy as a response to increasing dissatisfaction with the prevailing forms of deontology and consequentialism. As Anscombe (1958:1) points out: "Anyone who has read Aristotle's *Ethics* and has also read modern moral philosophy must have been struck by the great contrast between them." Subsequently, she argues that the dominant ethical positions neglect several topics that had always figured in virtue ethics' perspective, such as motives and moral character of an individual, moral education, moral wisdom, or a concept of a good human life. In her view, ethics – if it is to be meaningful – should revive these concepts.

Virtue ethics differs from deontological and consequentialist perspectives in that it is not concerned with abstract rules of conduct. In Greek Antiquity, where this tradition has its roots, the key question of ethics was the question of a fulfilling life (*eudaimonia*) and a closely associated idea of virtue (the excellence of character and understanding). It investigates what is "good" (i.e., leads to human flourishing) rather than what is "right" from the perspective of a moral law. The central questions are here: "How should I live?", "What kind of person should I aspire to be?" "How to cultivate the excellence of character?" Taylor (2002:6) describes this perspective as "the ethics of aspiration" and the two other modern ethics' perspectives concerned with the moral law as "ethics of duty." This is of course a simplified model: the ethics of duty and the ethics of aspiration to some extent overlap, and as Nussbaum (1999:163) observes, both deontology and consequentialism contain treatments of virtue. Taylor's distinction however gives a good idea of the difference in the fundamental orientation. For early Greek and Roman moral thinkers, ethics was essentially "the art of living" rather than a search for universal moral laws.

There is nonetheless a great diversity among formulations of virtue theories and a great deal of disagreement between some of them (Nussbaum, 1999). Certainly, rather than refer to a diffuse category of "virtue ethics," it is better to talk about "a class of ethical theories that share a common emphasis on virtues as central features of their account of morality" (Ivanhoe 2013: 50). Other unifying factors include "a concern for the role of motives and passions in good choice, a concern for character, and a concern for the whole course of an agent's life" (Nussbaum, 1999:163). In Russell's (2012: 2) view, the major trait of virtue theories is their focus "not so much on what to do in morally difficult cases, as on how to approach all of one's choices with such personal qualities as kindness, courage, wisdom, and integrity."

One of the most common objections to virtue ethics includes the charge of cultural relativity: the critics often point out that different cultures embody different virtues; hence in the virtue ethics perspective actions can be evaluated as right or wrong only relative to a particular cultural context. This charge, however, is related to a more general, metaethical problem of justification and can be also directed to consequentialism and deontology. In fact, it seems that virtue ethics, with its practice-oriented and context-sensitive approach, has less difficulty with cultural relativity than the other two perspectives. As Sen and Nussbaum (1993) argue, cultural disagreement arises mostly from local understandings of virtues, but virtues themselves are not relative to culture.

2.4 Eudaimonic Well-Being and Capabilities

Operationalizing eudaimonic well-being (human flourishing) in Cultivating Public Space research project we borrowed from Nussbaum (2011). We used the list of ten central human capabilities (i.e., ways of being and doing that people have reasons to value) to categorize the key dimensions of eudaimonic well-being in the urban context. The link to capabilities is strictly speaking not necessary in an operationalization of eudaimonic well-being, yet it offers a robust starting point and an advantage of connecting to an established discourse that has been very influential in social sciences research.

The capability approach has its origins in the works of the Nobel Prize winner Amartya Sen (1974, 1979) who criticized the limitedness of the traditional economic models and evaluative accounts largely based on utilitarianism and Rawlsian theory. He argued that these models fail to grasp the activities we are able to undertake ("doings") and the kinds of persons we are able to be ("beings"). He called these ways of being and doing *capabilities*, describing them also as the *real freedoms* to achieve our desired doings and beings. In line with the Aristotelian vision, the capability approach has its focus on the ends (ways of being and doing we have reasons to value) rather than on the means (resources/public goods we can access), arguing that resources and goods are important, but alone do not guarantee that people are able to convert them into the desired doings and beings.

The key questions to be asked when inquiring about capabilities are: "What am I able to do and to be? What are my real options?" (Nussbaum, 2011:106). Accordingly, this framework brings to the analysis the idea of assets relevant for people and groups to fulfill their aspirations – such as being well-nourished, educated, and healthy. What is important, this approach emphasizes the freedom people have to shape their lives in meaningful ways and the importance of the enabling or disabling environment for the pursuit of well-being (Frediani & Hansen, 2015:3–4). This freedom can be understood in terms of opportunities, abilities, and choices of individuals and groups to pursue different well-being dimensions (ibid.).

Nussbaum (2011) emphasizes the distinction between *functionings* and *capabilities*. It is basically a distinction between the realized (choices) and the effectively possible (opportunities), or between the achievement of actual "beings" and "doings" people have reason value and freedom to realize these "beings" and "doings." Having an opportunity to play, one may not realize it for personal reasons. Similarly, a person with a plenty of food available may choose to fast. According to Nussbaum (ibid.), capability, not functioning, should be the appropriate political goal of public policy, since it respects citizens' freedom of choice. This view has been criticized by authors pointing out that it is challenging to maintain a clear distinction between capabilities and functionings (Wolff & De-Shalit, 2013). Firstly, it is difficult to determine at what point an opportunity is too remote to constitute a capability – for example, do I have a capability for play if relevant recreational facilities are located at a substantial distance from my home, but I could travel to the area where these are more available? Second, some capabilities necessarily build upon certain functionings. For example, the capability to play to a large extent presupposes bodily health as a functioning. The third problem is epistemological – functionings unlike capabilities can be easily observed and therefore are easier to account for in research and policy. This, according to Wolff and de-Shalit (2013) provides a pragmatic reason to focus on functionings rather on capabilities. I can add to this discussion another argument supporting the focus on functionings over capabilities in the discussions of human well-being. Eudaimonia (human flourishing) is essentially about functionings (the realization of one's potentials), rather than about capabilities (freedom to realize these).

Nussbaum (2003:42) considers the list of central capabilities as "open-ended and subject to ongoing revision and rethinking, in the way that any society's account of its most fundamental entitlements is always subject to supplementation (or deletion)." In a similar tone, Alkire (2005:127) argues:

> The first observation to make about the capability approach is that operationalizing it is not a one-time thing. Some critics seem to be nostalgic for an approach that would cleanse the capability approach from all of the value choices and provide an intellectual breakthrough … But many of the residual value judgments in the capability approach will need to be made on the ground over and over again. … That was what Sen means by fundamental or assertive incompleteness.

The capability approach has been criticized for too strong focus on individual well-being. Yet, capabilities are not only enhancing individual lives but the collective life – influencing the ability of individuals to participate in democratic life of a society and to shape meaningful social relationships, as is further elaborated in our discussion of civic friendship and communities of virtue in Chap. 3 and supported by findings from our empirical studies presented in this book.

While extensively applied in domains such as political economy, social welfare, or education, there have been few attempts to utilize the capability approach in the context of spatial planning and urban design (Frediani & Hansen, 2015:3). I see a substantial potential of this approach in regard to programming and evaluation of the quality of public spaces. Nussbaum (2011:163) acknowledges that the quality of environment plays an important role in capability approach, being crucial for human well-being.

2.5 Addressing Public Space: Environmental and Social Affordances

The theory of affordances offers a convenient point of departure for operationalization of eudaimonic well-being in the public space context. Similarly to capability approach, it is concerned with the activities we are able to undertake ("doings") and the kinds of persons we are able to be ("beings") but addresses these in the spatial and social contexts of our immediate surroundings.

The term "affordance" was coined by James Gibson (1966). In his book *The Ecological Approach to Visual Perception (1979:127)*, Gibson explains:

> The *affordances* of the environment are what it *offers* the animal, what it *provides* or *furnishes*, either for good or ill. The verb *to afford* is found in the dictionary, the noun *affordance* is not. I have made it up. I mean by it something that refers to both the environment and the animal in a way that no existing term does. It implies the complementarity of the animal and the environment.

In this perspective, elements and features of our surroundings aren't just objects, but microenvironments that afford us (and other living beings) possibilities. For instance, a rigid flat surface affords support and locomotion to terrestrial animals. The water surface of a lake does not afford support to a terrestrial animal, but it does afford it to some insects. Thus, the same part of an environment may afford different things to different species or organisms. This is because affordances are relational in nature, they are both a fact of the environment and a fact of the organism. In this, they cut across the dichotomy of subjective-objective. Urban agriculture projects – depending upon their design, organization, and functional program – offer affordances such as food growing, physical exercise, learning, restorative activities, play, etc. They also offer a rich variety of affordances for non-human organisms (see Chap. 13).

Gibson's focus was environmental affordances. He didn't systematize theoretically the notion of social affordances, but he gave several examples of these, using this notion in two different senses (de Carvalho, 2020). The first group are affordances depending on social conventions – for example, the postbox is an object that "affords letter-mailing to a letter-writing human in a community with a postal system" (Gibson, 2015:130). An agent from a culture without a postal system cannot perceive the postbox as an object affording letter-mailing. The second group of social affordances are possibilities for interaction that other persons or animals afford. Through these affordances a person or an animal shows up to an observer not as a physical object but as an agent with the capacity to reciprocate. According to Gibson (2015:126), these are "the richest and most elaborate affordances of the environment." Rietveld (2012: 207) defines this category of affordances as "possibilities for social interaction offered by an environment: a friend's sad face invites comforting behavior, a person waiting for a coffee machine can afford a conversation, and an extended hand affords a handshake." Social affordances are of crucial importance in addressing the communal dimension of urban agriculture.

Importantly, affordances depend on our perceptions and abilities – different people may identify different affordances in the same space, based on their bodily abilities, skills, cultural background, and age. For example, for a person with good cooking skills, the crops from an urban garden present more affordances for nutritious and tasty meals than for someone who has no knowledge on this matter. This is very much related to the discussion of conversion factors in the capability approach: the extent to which a person is able to convert available options (capabilities) into functionings is based on personal, social, and environmental factors (Sen, 1992).

2.6 Toward an Operationalization of Eudaimonic Well-Being in the Urban Agriculture Context

In the following I present a preliminary operationalization of eudaimonic well-being in the context of public space that was developed within Cultivating Public Space research project. I aimed to create a conceptual tool to evaluate well-being impacts of urban agriculture projects, but this operationalization may be used more generally to evaluate the potential of any kind of public space (both actual and planned) to sustain human flourishing – an alternative to valuation models driven by an instrumental rationality, such as cost-benefit analysis.

The operationalization was informed by elements of three perspectives: the virtue tradition, the capability approach, and the theory of affordances. The operationalization process paralleled the construct-oriented approach to personality assessment (Ryff, 2017), but in this case it was concerned with public space assessment. The process began with conceptually based definitions of well-being dimensions to be operationalized – Nussbaum's (2003, 2011) list of ten central capabilities. I continued with the question: *What kind of environmental and social affordances need to be granted by a given urban agriculture project to sustain the well-being dimensions indicated by each of the capabilities?* These preliminary insights (Table 2.1) were further contextualized/validated in the course of empirical research in our project (see Chaps. 4 and 6). This was the first stage of the operationalization.

Table 2.1 Sustaining capabilities through affordances of urban agriculture: a preliminary operationalization of eudaimonic well-being dimensions in the context of urban agriculture projects

	Capability	Nussbaum's definition (2003:41–42)	Preliminary operationalizations: environmental and social affordances of urban agriculture
1.	Life	"Being able to live to the end of a human life of normal length; not dying prematurely, or before one's life is so reduced as to be not worth living."	-Experienced safety of urban agriculture projects and their surroundings -Effective crime prevention measures
2.	Bodily health	"Being able to have good health, including reproductive health; to be adequately nourished; to have adequate shelter."	-Opportunities for physical/restorative activities -Access to green areas -Access to local organic food -Opportunities for gaining nutrition knowledge
3.	Bodily integrity	"Being able to move freely from place to place; to be secure against violent assault, including sexual assault and domestic violence"	-Experienced safety of urban agriculture projects and their surroundings -Effective crime prevention measures
4.	Senses, imagination, thought	"Being able to use the senses, to imagine, think, and reason … Being able to use imagination and thought in connection with experiencing and producing works and events of one's own choice, religious, literary, musical, etc. Being able to use one's mind in ways protected by guarantees of freedom of expression…. Being able to have pleasurable experiences and to avoid nonbeneficial pain."	-Opportunities to experience/influence tactile and symbolic qualities of design and aesthetics -Freedom of expression/self-expression -Opportunities for local political engagement -Opportunities for engaging into artistic/creative practices -Opportunities for contemplative/mindful activities
5.	Emotions	"Being able to have attachments to things and people outside ourselves; to love those who love and care for us, to grieve at their absence; in general, to love, to grieve, to experience longing, gratitude, and justified anger. Not having one's emotional development blighted by fear and anxiety."	-Opportunities for meaningful relations and interactions with others -Opportunities for self-expression -Measures limiting anxiety and fear in social interactions
6.	Practical reason	"Being able to form a conception of the good and to engage in critical reflection about the planning of one's life."	-Opportunities for learning -Opportunities for deliberation on values/goals/visions -Opportunities for engagement in development, managing and programming of urban agriculture projects -Flexible and adaptable planning and design of urban agriculture projects

(continued)

Table 2.1 (continued)

	Capability	Nussbaum's definition (2003:41–42)	Preliminary operationalizations: environmental and social affordances of urban agriculture
7.	**Affiliation**	"A. Being able to live with and toward others, to recognize and show concern for other human beings, to engage in various forms of social interaction; to be able to imagine the situation of another. … B. Having the social bases of self-respect and nonhumiliation; being able to be treated as a dignified being whose worth is equal to that of others. …"	-Opportunities for development of a sense of belonging and meaningful relations with others -Inclusive/nondiscriminatory way of organizing projects -Inclusive meeting places for all segments of society
8.	**Other species**	"Being able to live with concern for and in relation to animals, plants, and the world of nature."	-Opportunities for forming relation to nature – cultivation of plants, beekeeping, etc. -Opportunities for encountering wild nature in cities
9.	**Play**	"Being able to laugh, to play, to enjoy recreational activities."	-Opportunities to engage into leisure, recreation, and play activities -Opportunities for celebrations -Opportunities to engage into cultural activities
10	**Control over one's environment**	"A. Political. Being able to participate effectively in political choices that govern one's life; having the right of political participation, protections of free speech and association. B. Material. Being able to hold property (both land and movable goods), and having property rights on an equal basis with others; … In work, being able to work as a human being, exercising practical reason, and entering into meaningful relationships of mutual recognition with other workers."	(a) Political: -Opportunities for participation in decision-making -Opportunities for expression of political views -Opportunities for deliberation on values/goals/visions (b) Material -opportunities for engagement in managing, planning, development and programming of urban agriculture projects; -opportunities for employment/job training

The second stage of operationalization has been delineated conceptually but would benefit from a follow-up empirical research for further contextualization. It extends the operationalization of well-being in terms of capabilities with the consideration of virtues which is largely absent in capability scholarship. The key question here is: *What kind of virtues can be linked to each of the central capabilities, and what kind of environmental and social affordances would support the cultivation of these virtues?*

Virtues are moral or intellectual excellences (see Chap. 3 for more in-depth discussion of this theme). Different sets of virtues that can be encountered in virtue literature since Antiquity. Here, I use a contemporary categorization of Peterson and Seligman presented in their book *Character Strengths and Virtues* (2004) identifying six key virtues and related character strengths:

- Wisdom and Knowledge: Creativity, Curiosity, Open-mindedness, Love of Learning, Perspective.
- Courage: Bravery, Persistence, Integrity, Vitality.
- Humanity: Love, Kindness, Social Intelligence.
- Justice: Citizenship, Fairness, Leadership.
- Temperance: Forgiveness, Humility/Modesty, Prudence, Self-Regulation.
- Transcendence: Appreciation of Beauty and Excellence, Gratitude, Hope, Humor, Spirituality.

Table 2.2 provides an overview over the definitions of these (Peterson & Seligman, 2004:29–30).

Importantly, virtues benefit not only the individual but also the community, encouraging tangible outcomes like reverence for life, rich and supportive social networks, respect by and for others, satisfying and productive work, and material sufficiency – ultimately sustaining healthy communities and families (Peterson & Seligman, 2004:19).

Building upon the first stage of our operationalization (Table 2.1), where we focused on ten central capabilities (viewed as well-being dimensions to be addressed in urban gardens through their environmental and social affordances), I now deepen this discussion asking how these capabilities link to specific virtues and what kind of environmental and social affordances would be conductive/limiting to the cultivation of these virtues. For some capabilities these links are quite straightforward, for others, may be less evident but still can be identified with some interpretive effort. For example, the capability of practical reason can be directly linked to virtue of wisdom and related character strengths: curiosity, open-mindedness, love of learning, and perspective. It can be also linked to the virtue of justice and character strengths such as fairness and leadership. The capability of affiliation can be linked to virtue of humanity and character strengths such as love, kindness, and social intelligence. The capability of bodily health can be linked to virtue of temperance and character strengths such as such as prudence and self-regulation.

Table 2.2 Classification of virtues and character strengths based on Peterson and Seligman (2004:29–30)

Virtues	Character strengths
Wisdom and knowledge: "cognitive strengths that entail the acquisition and use of knowledge"	**Creativity** [originality, ingenuity]: "Thinking of novel and productive ways to conceptualize and do things; includes artistic achievement but is not limited to it"
	Curiosity [interest, novelty-seeking, openness to experience]: "Taking an interest in ongoing experience for its own sake; finding subjects and topics fascinating; exploring and discovering"
	Open-mindedness [judgment, critical thinking]: "Thinking things through and examining them from all sides; not jumping to conclusions; being able to change one's mind in light of evidence; weighing all evidence fairly"
	Love of learning: "Mastering new skills, topics, and bodies of knowledge, whether on one's own or formally; obviously related to the strength of curiosity but goes beyond it to describe the tendency to add systematically to what one knows"
	Perspective [wisdom]: "Being able to provide wise counsel to others; having ways of looking at the world that make sense to oneself and to other people"
Courage: "emotional strengths that involve the exercise of will to accomplish goals in the face of opposition, external or internal"	**Bravery** [valor]: "Not shrinking from threat, challenge, difficulty, or pain; speaking up for what is right even if there is opposition; acting on convictions even if unpopular; includes physical bravery but is not limited to it"
	Persistence [perseverance, industriousness]: "Finishing what one starts; persisting in a course of action in spite of obstacles; 'getting it out the door'; taking pleasure in completing tasks"
	Integrity [authenticity, honesty]: "Speaking the truth but more broadly presenting oneself in a genuine way and acting in a sincere way; being without pretense; taking responsibility for one's feelings and actions"
	Vitality [zest, enthusiasm, vigor, energy]: "Approaching life with excitement and energy; not doing things halfway or halfheartedly; living life as an adventure; feeling alive and activated"

Humanity: "interpersonal strengths that involve tending and befriending others"	**Love:** "Valuing close relations with others, in particular those in which sharing and caring are reciprocated; being close to people"
	Kindness [generosity, nurturance, care, compassion, altruistic love]: "Doing favors and good deeds for others; helping them; taking care of them"
	Social intelligence [emotional intelligence, personal intelligence]: "Being aware of the motives and feelings of other people and oneself; knowing what to do to fit into different social situations"
Justice: "civic strengths that underlie healthy community life"	**Citizenship** [social responsibility, loyalty, teamwork]: "Working well as a member of a group or team; being loyal to the group; doing one's share"
	Fairness: "Treating all people the same according to notions of fairness and justice; not letting personal feelings bias decisions about others; giving everyone a fair chance"
	Leadership: "Encouraging a group of which one is a member to get things done and at the same time maintain good relations within the group; organizing group activities and seeing that they happen"
Temperance: "strengths that protect against excess"	**Forgiveness and mercy:** "Forgiving those who have done wrong; accepting the shortcomings of others; giving people a second chance; not being vengeful"
	Humility/modesty: "Letting one's accomplishments speak for themselves; not seeking the spotlight; not regarding oneself as more special than one is"
	Prudence: "Being careful about one's choices; not taking undue risks; not saying or doing things that might later be regretted"
	Self-regulation [self-control]: "Regulating what one feels and does; being disciplined; controlling one's appetites and emotions"

(continued)

Table 2.2 (continued)

Virtues	Character strengths
Transcendence: "strengths that forge connections to the larger universe and provide meaning"	**Appreciation of beauty and excellence** [awe, wonder, elevation]: "Noticing and appreciating beauty, excellence, and/or skilled performance in various domains of life, from nature to art to mathematics to science to everyday experience"
	Gratitude: "Being aware of and thankful for the good things that happen; taking time to express thanks"
	Hope [optimism, future-mindedness, future orientation]: "Expecting the best in the future and working to achieve it; believing that a good future is something that can be brought about"
	Humor [playfulness]: "Liking to laugh and tease; bringing smiles to other people; seeing the light side; making (not necessarily telling) jokes"
	Spirituality [religiousness, faith, purpose]: "Having coherent beliefs about the higher purpose and meaning of the universe; knowing where one fits within the larger scheme; having beliefs about the meaning of life that shape conduct and provide comfort"

In the course of Cultivating Public Space project we have encountered different manifestations of virtues both in our empirical studies and classroom activities, and this discussion is further extended theoretically in Chap. 3 in the context of communities of virtue. Still, more research is needed to get a better understanding of how environmental and social affordances of public space can sustain the cultivation of virtues in specific contexts. This is a problem of identifying the enabling conditions for development of virtues and character strengths that Peterson and Seligman (2004: 11) delineate as an important concern for future research:

> We ... believe that positive traits need to be placed in context; it is obvious that they do not operate in isolation from the settings,... in which people are to be found. ... Some settings and situations lend themselves to the development and/or display of strengths, whereas other settings and situations preclude them. ... Enabling conditions as we envision them are often the province of disciplines other than psychology, but we hope for a productive partnership with these other fields in understanding the settings that allow the strengths to develop. Our common sense tells us that enabling conditions include educational and vocational opportunity, a supportive and consistent family, safe neighbourhoods and schools, political stability, and (perhaps) democracy. The existence of mentors, role models, and supportive peers—inside or outside the immediate family—are probably also enabling conditions. ... [A] future goal would be to characterize the properties of settings that enable strengths and virtues.

On the basis of our preliminary understanding of the relationship between affordances, capabilities, and virtues, urban placemaking for human flourishing can be understood as a continuous process of negotiating a space's optimum set of affordances – environmental and social – so it sustains a variety of central capabilities and offers opportunities for cultivation of related virtues, moral and intellectual. This model calls for citizen participation in the process of altering the affordances of their environments for the benefit of all.

The interconnected framework of capabilities, virtues, and affordances (Fig. 2.1) can be used to evaluate eudaimonic well-being impacts of public space. As our case studies illustrate, successful urban gardens are inclusive, inviting, and vibrant because they offer multiple affordances attracting diverse group of citizens, sustaining their capabilities, and inspiring cultivation of virtues in multiple ways.

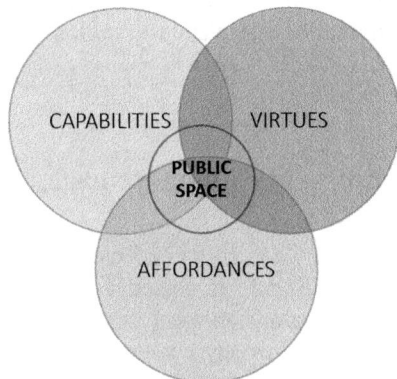

Fig. 2.1 The interconnected framework of capabilities, virtues, and affordances can be used to evaluate eudaimonic well-being impacts of any kind of public space

2.7 Beyond Capabilities

Despite our borrowing from the capability approach, the research of Cultivating Public Space project cannot be considered as capability research per se. In our attempts to operationalize human flourishing, we remain entirely within the Aristotelian tradition. The capability approach has been to some extent inspired by this tradition: in composing the list of central capabilities, Nussbaum (1999:40) asks an Aristotelian question, "What activities characteristically performed by human beings are so central that they seem definitive of a life that is truly human?" Yet, as she further admits, the guiding thought behind her approach is the liberal concept of freedom, "one that lies at the heart of [John] Rawls' project" (Ibid. p. 46).

Accordingly, the capability approach has been primarily concerned with a broader question of social justice and human rights, addressed typically on the national or even global level (Nussbaum, 2003, 2011). Its primary concern is with the material and institutional arrangements securing all individuals the liberty to realize their capabilities. The main emphasis here is on "well-being freedom" (opportunities/liberties to pursue ways of doing and being one has reasons to value) not so much the actual realization of these opportunities, i.e., "well-being achievement" (which is the core concern for virtue ethics and eudaimonic well-being discussion). The liberty concern in capability scholarship tends to overweight the well-being concerns (Sen & Nussbaum, 1993:38–39).

In our research we to some extent address the broader question of social justice in cities, looking into municipal policies enabling a systematic integration of urban agriculture projects in public space development (Chaps. 11 and 12). Our main interest however is "well-being achievement," i.e., human flourishing addressed on the level of an individual and a local community embedded in their immediate spatial settings.

Another point where we go beyond Nussbaum's capability approach is the emphasis on the importance of an individual effort of self-formation (the cultivation of virtue) and the quality of communal relationships (civic friendship) in the achievement of human flourishing (see also Chap. 3). As already indicated, capability scholarship typically focuses on *entitlements* of citizens, rarely addressing *responsibilities* related to self-formation and our relationships to others that are central to the virtue ethics tradition. Nussbaum (1994) to some extent addresses these issues in her earlier works on early Greek and Roman ethics.

2.8 Concluding Remarks

The virtue tradition is scarcely addressed in planning and urban discourse. In Cultivating Public Space research project we aimed to address this knowledge gap. By doing this, the project not only adds to the recently growing discussions within moral philosophy, addressing contemporary applications of virtue theories, but also responds to the demand for new conceptual frameworks that could help to tackle the problems and challenges confronting cities in an innovative way, as the intellectual apparatus, concepts, and mindset of traditional spatial planning prove to be deficient in today's complex realities (Ogilvy, 2002; Albrechts, 2010).

The virtue tradition offers a viable basis for an alternative, novel approach to operationalization of urban well-being, that can in turn inform evaluation and development of urban interventions. It demands incorporation of the ideal of human flourishing – a fulfilling individual and communal life – in planning practices and urban development strategies. In this perspective urban space is seen as an arena for the exercise of practical reason and the development of human capabilities and virtues, including "social virtues" such as solidarity and responsibility for the other. It also encourages a more respectful attitude toward natural environments (Cafaro & Sandler, 2005; Sandler, 2007; Zwolinski & Schmidtz, 2013). This view may substantially contribute to grounding an alternative model of economic development and inspire social change.

What is also important, virtue tradition implies a different approach to planning for sustainability than the dominant frameworks of consequentialism and deontology: the focus is on planning of the conditions for the desired actions, internalization of values, and their integration in lifestyles rather than on regulating/imposing the limits. Virtues act here as internal barriers. This is essentially a shift from a punitive structure of obligations and rules, toward character traits undermining a respectful attitude toward the environment. As Cafaro and Sandler (2005:3) put it, the "environmentally virtuous person is disposed to respond—both emotionally and through action—to the environment and the nonhuman individuals (whether inanimate, living, or conscious) that populate it in an excellent or fine way."

The virtue perspective offers an alternative to top-down perspectives, where an individual is typically viewed as *a recipient* of urban services. Here, she is also *an agent*, co-creating/cultivating public space and at the same time taking an active role in the cultivation of her character and contributing to the local community, which in turn leads to the achievement of a fulfilling life. Accordingly, we are concerned not just with individuals' *entitlements* and *liberties* (which is the focus of Nussbaum's capability approach) but also with their *responsibilities* related to the achievement of a fulfilling life and stewardship of shared urban spaces. The active role of citizens and the importance of the bottom-up approach in shaping urban spaces are emphasized in "the right to the city" discourse (Lefebvre, 1996; Mitchell, 2003); however, the theme of *responsibilities* in respect to self-formation/intellectual and moral excellence as the central aspect of human flourishing is also missing in this perspective. The theme of responsibilities of citizens is generally under-addressed in current urban research and sometimes considered problematic, which is indeed the case when it masks an effort of neoliberal urban authorities to transfer some of their responsibilities to local communities (Jonathan, 2013). Being aware of these ambiguities, it is crucial to underline that by neglecting the importance of individuals' responsibility in shaping meaningful lives, we may end up in a patronizing and disempowering approach to urban development.

My focus in this chapter is human well-being. It is however important to remember that this theme cannot be addressed in separation from the question of human-nature interaction, and we address it elsewhere in this book (see Chap. 13). Cities are essentially socio-ecological systems, and any decision-making aimed at a sustainable and resilient urban development should always consider different components and scales of an urban system (Walker & Salt, 2012).

References

Albrechts, L. (2010). More of the same is not enough! How could strategic spatial planning be instrumental in dealing with the challenges ahead? *Environment and Planning B: Planning and Design, 37*(6), 1115–1127.

Alkire, S. (2005). Why the capability approach? *Journal of Human Development, 6*(1), 115–135.

Anscombe, G. (1958). Modern moral philosophy. *Philosophy, 33*, 1–19.

Aristotle. (2009). *The Nicomachean ethics*. Oxford University Press.

Cafaro, P., & Sandler, R. (Eds.). (2005). *Environmental virtue ethics*. Rowman & Littlefield Publishers.

Christodoulou, C., Schneider, S., & Stone, A. A. (2013). Validation of a brief yesterday measure of hedonic well-being and daily activities: Comparison with the day reconstruction method. *Social Indicators Research, 115*(3), 907–917.

Cromhout, A., Schutte, L., Wissing, M. P., & Schutte, W. D. (2022). Further investigation of the dimensionality of the questionnaire for eudaimonic well-being. *Frontiers in Psychology, 13*, 795770.

de Carvalho, E. M. (2020). Social affordance. In J. Vonk & T. Shackelford (Eds.), *Encyclopedia of animal cognition and behavior*. Springer.

Deci, E. L., & Ryan, R. M. (1985). The general causality orientations scale: Self-determination in personality. *Journal of Research in Personality, 19*(2), 109–134.

Diener, E., Oishi, S., & Tay, L. (2018). Advances in subjective well-being research. *Nature Human Behaviour, 2*(4), 253–260.

Fainstein, S. (2010). *The just city*. Cornell University Press.

Frediani, A., & Hansen, J. (Eds.). (2015). *The capability approach in development planning and urban design*. The Bartlett Development Planning Unit.

Gibson, J. (1966). *The senses considered as perceptual systems*. Allen and Unwin.

Gibson, J. (1979). *The ecological approach to visual perception*. Houghton Mifflin Harcourt (HMH).

Gibson, J. (2015). *The ecological approach to visual perception, classical edition*. Psychology Press.

Huta, V. (2016). Eudaimonic and hedonic orientations: Theoretical considerations and research findings. In J. Vittersø (Ed.), *Handbook of eudaimonic well-being* (pp. 215–231). Springer.

Huta, V., & Ryan, R. M. (2010). Pursuing pleasure or virtue: The differential and overlapping well-being benefits of hedonic and eudaimonic motives. *Journal of Happiness Studies, 11*(6), 735–762.

Huta, V., & Waterman, A. S. (2014). Eudaimonia and its distinction from hedonia: developing a classification and terminology for understanding conceptual and operational definitions. *Journal of Happiness Studies, 15*, 1425–1456.

Ivanhoe, P. (2013). Virtue ethics and the Chinese Confucian tradition. In D. Russell (Ed.), The Cambridge Companion to Virtue Ethics (pp. 49–69). Cambridge University Press. https://doi.org/10.1017/CCO9780511734786.004.

Jonathan, J. (2013). Resilience as embedded neoliberalism: A governmentality approach. *Resilience, 1*(1), 38–52.

Kahneman, D., & Deaton, A. (2010). High income improves evaluation of life but not emotional well-being. *Proceedings of the National Academy of Sciences of the United States of America., 107*(38), 16489–16493.

Lefebvre, H. (1996). *Writings on cities*. Blackwell.

Marans, R. W., & Stimson, R. (2011). An overview of quality of urban life. In *Investigating quality of urban life* (pp. 1–29). Springer.

McMahan, E. A., & Estes, D. (2011). Hedonic versus eudaimonic conceptions of well-being: Evidence of differential associations with experienced well-being. *Social Indicators Research, 103*, 93–108.

Mitchell, D. (2003). *The right to the city. Social justice and the fight for public space*. Guilford Press.

Mouratidis, K. (2021). Urban planning and quality of life: A review of pathways linking the built environment to subjective well-being. *Cities, 115*, 103229.

Nussbaum, M. (1994). *The therapy of desire: Theory and practice in hellenistic ethics*. Princeton University Press.

Nussbaum, M. (1999). *Sex and social justice*. Oxford University Press.

Nussbaum, M. (2003). Capabilities as fundamental entitlements: Sen and social justice. *Feminist Economics, 9*(2/3), 33–59.

Nussbaum, M. (2011). *Creating capabilities: The human development approach*. Belknap of Harvard UP.

Ogilvy, J. (2002). *Creating better futures: Scenario planning as a tool for a better tomorrow*. Oxford University Press.

Perls, F., Hefferline, R., & Goodman, P. (1951). *Gestalt therapy: Excitement and growth in the human personality*. The Gestalt Journal Press: New Edition.

Peterson, C., & Seligman, M. (2004). *Character strengths and virtues: A handbook and classification*. American Psychological Association; Oxford University Press.

Pfeiffer, D., & Cloutier, S. (2016). Planning for happy neighborhoods. *Journal of the American Planning Association, 82*(3), 267–279.

Rawls, J. (1971). *A theory of justice*. Harvard University Press.

Rietveld, E. (2012). Bodily intentionality and social affordances in context. In F. Paglieri (Ed.), *Consciousness in Interaction. The role of the natural and social context in shaping consciousness*. John Benjamins.

Rogers, C. (1961). *On becoming a person: A therapist's view of psychotherapy*. Constable.

Ruini, C., & Cesetti, G. (2019). Spotlight on eudaimonia and depression. A systematic review of the literature over the past 5 years. *Psychology Research and Behavior Management, 12*, 767.

Russell, D. (Ed.). (2012). *The Cambridge companion to virtue ethics*. Cambridge University Press.

Ryan, R. M., & Deci, E. L. (2001). On happiness and human potentials: A review of research on hedonic and eudaimonic well-being. *Annual Review of Psychology, 52*, 141.

Ryan, R. M., Huta, V., & Deci, E. L. (2008). Living well: A self-determination theory perspective on eudaimonia. *Journal of Happiness Studies, 9*(1), 139–170.

Ryff, C. D. (1989). Happiness is everything, or is it? Explorations on the meaning of psychological well-being. *Journal of Personality and Social Psychology, 57*(6), 1069.

Ryff, C. D. (2017). Eudaimonic well-being, inequality, and health: Recent findings and future directions. *International Review of Economics, 64*(2), 159–178.

Sandler, R. (2007). *Character and environment: A virtue-oriented approach to environmental ethics*. Columbia University Press.

Schneider, K. J., Pierson, J. F., & Bugental, J. F. T. (Eds.). (2015). *The handbook of humanistic psychology: Theory, research, and practice*. Sage Publications.

Sen, A. (1974). Informational bases of alternative welfare approaches: Aggregation and income distribution. *Journal of Public Economics, 3*(4), 387–403.

Sen, A. (1979). Equality of what? In S. M. McMurrin (Ed.), *Tanner lectures on human values* (pp. 197–220). Cambridge University Press.

Sen, A. (1992). *Inequality re-examined*. Clarendon Press.

Sen, A., & Nussbaum, M. (1993). *The quality of life*. Clarendon Press.

Shekhar, H., Schmidt, A. J., & Wehling, H. W. (2019). Exploring wellbeing in human settlements-A spatial planning perspective. *Habitat International, 87*, 66–74.

Soja, E. (2010). *Seeking spatial justice*. University of Minnesota Press.

Stone, A., & Mackie, C. (Eds.). (2013). *Subjective well-being: Measuring happiness, suffering, and other dimensions of experience*. National Academies Press (US). Available: https://www.ncbi.nlm.nih.gov/books/NBK179225/

Taylor, R. (2002). *Virtue ethics: An introduction*. Prometheus books.

UN. (2015). *The 2030 agenda for sustainable development*.

UN. (2017). *The new urban agenda*.

UNDP. (1990). *Human development report*. Oxford University Press.

Upton, R. (2002). Planning praxis: Ethics, values and theory. *The Town Planning Review, 73*(3), 253–269.

Vittersø, J. (Ed.). (2016). *Handbook of eudaimonic well-being*. Springer International Publishing.

Walker, B., & Salt, D. (2012). *Resilience thinking: sustaining ecosystems and people in a changing world*. Island press.

Wang, F., & Wang, D. (2016). Place, geographical context and subjective well-being: State of art and future directions. In *Mobility, sociability and well-being of urban living* (pp. 189–230). Springer.

Wolff, J., & De-Shalit, A. (2013). On fertile functionings: A response to Martha Nussbaum. *Journal of Human Development and Capabilities, 14*(1), 161–165.

Zwolinski, M., & Schmidtz, D. (2013). Environmental virtue ethics: what it is and what it needs to be. In D. Russell (Ed.), *The Cambridge companion to virtue ethics* (pp. 221–239). Cambridge University Press.

Chapter 3
Cultivating Virtue: Neo-Aristotelian Concepts in Public Space Development

Beata Sirowy and Kelvin Knight

3.1 Introduction

We propose the Aristotelian concepts of *eudaimonia*—which we translate as human well-being or flourishing—and of the virtues (excellences of character and understanding) and civic friendship as guiding concepts for today's urban development, especially in the design and programming of urban public space. Taken together, they offer a coherent and, we believe, compelling framework for understanding how to enhance the lives of citizens and to build a "sense of We" across sociocultural and economic difference, which is crucial from the perspective of social cohesion.

By including the ideal of civic friendship in our conceptual framework, we add a new dimension to the discussion of eudaimonic well-being that has been gaining an increasing importance in social scientific research over the last decade (see also Chap. 2). On our Aristotelian account, civic friendship denotes an ethical and political virtue to be cultivated in any urban environment, as well as the kind of social relationship which such cultivation entails. We argue that civic friendship can be an important bonding and bridging factor in today's differentiated and fragmented societies.

B. Sirowy (✉)
Department of Urban and Regional Planning, Norwegian University of Life Sciences, Ås, Norway
e-mail: beata.sirowy@gmail.com

K. Knight
Mykolas Romeris Universit, Vilnius, Lithuania

London Metropolitan University, London, UK
e-mail: k.knight@londonmet.ac.uk

B. Sirowy, D. Ruggeri (eds.), *Urban Agriculture in Public Space*, GeoJournal Library 132, https://doi.org/10.1007/978-3-031-41550-0_3

In determining how best to integrate the above-mentioned notions in urban development, we employ the neo-Aristotelian concept of practices, as distinct from organizational institutions (MacIntyre, 2007: 186–203; Knight, 2008a, 2023), and introduce a concept of communities of virtue (cf. MacIntyre, 2016: 176–182). We propose that the development of urban public space should take account of citizens' participative practices, rather than only of functions that are administratively conceived. This way of approaching urban public space allows for addressing individual and communal well-being to a much higher extent than the framework of multifunctionality. Enhancing the conditions for participation in shared practices in urban settings facilitates the development of communities of virtue—localities consolidated by shared goals and standards of excellence, which are a setting for cultivating virtues (intellectual and moral), and development of civic friendship. Although state and corporate institutions are indispensable in supporting urban practices, the motivating goods they pursue differ from the goods internal to particular practices. This tension needs to be addressed and negotiated if we are to provide conditions for practices and communities of virtue to flourish.

In the final section of this chapter, we identify three concerns to be addressed in developing public space, based on neo-Aristotelian insights:

(a) Identifying practices that are to be supported within a given location
(b) Mapping threats to the internal goods of practices from institutions' pursuit of external goods and finding ways to mitigate these threats
(c) Facilitating the development of communities of virtue around selected practices

In line with Aristotle's emphasis on the importance of direct political engagement, all these domains should involve local citizens in participatory mapping of stakeholder needs and place values, codesign of necessary material infrastructure, and suchlike.

This discussion is illustrated with references to urban agriculture—understood as practice in the MacIntyrean sense and therefore a potential setting for the development of communities of virtue that could be integrated in development of public space. Importantly, an urban agriculture project can potentially offer settings for cultivation of multiple, additional practices—such as culinary arts, herbal medicine, mindfulness, carpentry, or even chess playing or raft building, as exemplified in some of our project cases (see Chaps. 4, 5, 6, 7, 9, and 13).

The chapter is divided into three parts. First, we introduce Aristotelian notions of *eudaimonia*, virtue, and civic friendship as guiding concepts for addressing individual and communal well-being in contemporary cities. We continue with the discussion of MacIntyre's concepts of practices, institutions, and communities of virtue, before concluding with a neo-Aristotelian approach to public space development and references to urban agriculture.

3.2   The Well-Being of Citizens in an Aristotelian Perspective

3.2.1   *Eudaimonia and the Virtues*

Eudaimonia is often translated as happiness, but it differs substantially from today's understanding of this word in terms of pleasurable, often transitory experiences (hedonic happiness). For ancient Greeks, *eudaimonia* denoted human flourishing—the actualization of our full potentials, a rewarding and fulfilled human life, which was necessarily one lived in accordance with virtues—excellences of character and understanding.

The idea of human flourishing is more than mere metaphor (MacIntyre, 2016, 24ff.). It is grounded in a teleological conception of living beings as having a natural potential, which is the specific good of each to actualize over their lifetime. This naturalistic ethic can be traced through Western intellectual history and can still be proposed as a solution to the aporia of rival moral philosophies (Irwin, 2007–2009 passim, 2020: 2). Since human beings are socially dependent, rational, language-using animals, the fulfilment of our individual potentials—that is, our flourishing as the kind of beings we naturally are—is conditional on our social conditions. More analytically, it is dependent upon the purposive social practices in which we engage with others. It is through such lifelong participation that we develop our dispositions and virtues, our own character and personality. With the progress of humankind, our social conditions are also increasingly determined by the historically given institutions in which personal virtues are necessarily subordinated to those institutions' constitutive rules, resources, and hierarchies.

Aristotle observes that everything has a *telos*: a natural purpose or final end and good. If we want to understand what something is, we should search for its *telos*. What is the *telos* for human beings? According to Aristotle, we are meant to fulfil our innermost potentials and thereby live happily, by cultivating both the moral and intellectual virtues. Someone who is not living a life that is virtuous is not living the life of a fulfilled human being. They are like a plant that does not flourish, an animal that is disabled, or an instrument that does not work, except that their dysfunctionality, their failure to actualize their own good or *telos*, is not due merely to their conditions but also to their own choice and intellectual error.

Someone who does live according to virtue is living a life that flourishes—they are being all that they can be, realizing their innermost potential. What does this involve? For Aristotle, humans are rational and social beings and therefore "political animals." Like other species, we come into being full of potential which, given favourable conditions, we are able to fulfil. The human good therefore includes much in common with the good life of other living beings, such as physical health, and still more that we share with other intelligent and sociable species. Even so, human abilities are of a higher order and wider range than those of any other species, and therefore so too are the excellences of which human beings are capable. These include the intellectual virtues actualized by those engaged in philosophical, practical, and scientific pursuits as well as the moral virtues that may be actualized by all of those engaged in the social activities and to some extent in one's solitary pursuits. Both types of virtues are essential for the political activity of organizing communal life and directing it to the common good. To cultivate the virtues is to cultivate oneself, and to achieve excellence is to flourish as a human being.

The importance of actualization of our potentials for our well-being is one of the central assumptions behind Martha Nussbaum's capability approach, viewing capabilities as an attempt to map central dimensions of human flourishing (Nussbaum, 2000, 2011; see also Chap. 2). Whilst capabilities discourse primarily focuses on societal or political arrangements supporting the actualization of human capabilities (material and institutional settings for realization of human flourishing), Nussbaum's earlier work emphasizes the importance of individual attitudes (emotions, values, judgements) and community in the achievement of *eudaimonia* (Nussbaum, 1994). In this she is very close to the Aristotelian vision.

Virtues are exercised and can only be cultivated and developed through different kinds of social interaction. Various kinds of community provide their members with opportunities to exercise and cultivate such moral virtues as courage, temperance, generosity, magnanimity, truthfulness, wit, justice, decency, and friendliness (Aristotle, 2014, 46–97, 104–107, 136–174: 1115a- 1138b, 1141b-1142b, 1154b-1172a,). In these communities people usually cultivate also intellectual virtues, including theoretical wisdom (*sophia*), scientific knowledge (*epistêmê*), the ability to make things (*techne*), and practical reason (*phronesis*): an experience-based ability to judge and act successfully with regard to "those things that are good or bad for man" (Aristotle, 2014, 103–104: 1141a22–28). These opportunities allow community members to grow and to flourish, through participation in common activities with common goals. To participate in such shared activity is to incur obligations to others that are voluntary. These include obligations of loyalty and solidarity to particular communities in which one participates. To share in actualizing a common good obliges one to act in the best way to achieve that good and to act in the best way toward others who are similarly obliged.

It is worthwhile paying more attention to the aforementioned division of virtues into intellectual virtues, or excellences of understanding, and moral virtues, or excellences of character. For us today, virtue has predominantly moral connotations. This makes it somehow less attractive as a conceptual tool in such domains as urban development. Emphasizing the knowledge dimension is very important in this context—virtue is as much about refining our character as it is about developing different kinds of understanding, practical reason, and hands-on skills.

Different types of intellectual virtues correspond to the ancient Greek division of knowledge into three main categories: theoretical, practical, and productive. Theoretical sciences are concerned with that which can be described by exact laws and include domains such as physics, mathematics, and metaphysics. The intellectual virtue to be achieved in their pursuit are theoretical wisdom (*epistêmê*)) or philosophic wisdom (*sophia*) which is a combination of *epistêmê* and intuitive understanding of first principles (*nous*). Poetical or productive sciences (*technai*) are concerned with producing an end result. Their aim is *poiesis*, production. The practical sciences are concerned with achieving the human good through right conduct. Here Aristotle situates politics and ethics. Their ideal is practical wisdom, *phronesis*, that unlike theoretical wisdom is always context-dependent and requires an extensive experience of particulars, typically gained throughout the years of life. Phronesis is a foundational virtue for the development of social virtues. Unlike his teacher Plato, Aristotle argued that best practice cannot result from the application of purely theoretical knowledge. Neo-Aristotelians often extend the objection further in arguing that such practices as agriculture are best understood by those who do the work.

3.2.2 Ethics and Politics

The concept of *eudaimonia* has, over the past couple decades, gained increasing attention within psychology and other social sciences dealing with human well-being (Ryan & Deci, 2001; Ryan et al., 2008; Huta & Waterman, 2014; Vitterso, 2016). This body of research is typically juxtaposing hedonic and eudaimonic form of human well-being in different contexts. The philosophical grounding of this discussion is usually limited to Aristotle's discussion of *eudaimonia* included in *Nicomachean Ethics*. *Politics*, however, gives additional insights into this concept.

Aristotle viewed ethics and politics as two interconnected fields of study, the former addressing the good of the individual, the latter the good of the *polis*, which he considered to be the best type of community. He was specifically interested in the role that politics and the political community can play in bringing about the virtuous life of citizens. In this he initiated a tradition of reasoning about politics as the activity of urban living: meeting the fellow citizens in public space and deliberating about what is good for their shared community. In this context he asserts, somehow shockingly for us moderns, that politics is the science of what is good for humans:

> For even if the good is the same for an individual and for a city, that of a city is evidently a greater and, at any rate, a more complete good to acquire and preserve. For while it should content us to acquire and preserve this for an individual alone, it is nobler and more divine to do so for a nation and city. And so our method of inquiry seeks the good of these things, since it is a sort of politics. (Aristotle, 2014, 13: 1095a6–11)

The good of *eudaimonia* participates in the good of political community through citizens' participative political practice, which Aristotle considers the most comprehensive form of the cultivation of moral virtue and exercise of practical reason. The conditions under which humans most truly flourish differ from those of beasts or gods in being social, institutional, and rationally, cooperatively purposive. Humans' moral virtues are those characteristics that are conducive to activity that is social, rational, cooperative, and, in a single word, *political*.

Politics is the shared reasoning and activity of citizens, *polites*, as such. As Strang (1998) puts it, "ancients called themselves 'political' not insofar as they were engaged in legislation or constitution-making, but insofar as they were engaged in direct deliberation, participation, decision-making, and follow-through." Their polis-life was participatory to a degree hitherto unheard of, and "its preeminent achievements were not laws as *products* but *actions* as embodiments of practical intelligence" (ibid.). The citizenry of a Greek polis might have been slave-owning patriarchs, but, in their social capacity as citizens, they were engaged in both making and executing collective decisions.

Following Aristotle, we propose the revival of such participative, political activity in our contemporary urban communities, even whilst differing from the original view in proposing that this be done in a way that is fully socially inclusive.

Another insight for today's thinking about cities is the importance of participation in the political domain for the good of citizens. As Aristotle says in the *Nicomachean Ethics* (1099b30), "the main concern of politics is to engender a certain character in the citizens and to make them good and disposed to perform noble actions." Unsurprisingly, most people living today's Western societies would disagree with that statement. We are used to regard politics (and politicians) as aiming at selfish ends, such as wealth, status, and power, rather than the "best end" of a virtuous life and the good of the community. Most of us would also see the idea that politics should be primarily concerned with creating a particular moral character in citizens as a dangerous intrusion on individual freedom, largely because we do not agree about what the "best end" is in our diversified and fragmented societies. Consequently, we expect of politics and the authorities that they keep us safe from other people (through the provision of police and military forces) so that each of us can pursue our own ends, whatever they may be. Development of individual character is left up to the individual, with possible support from family, religion, and other non-governmental institutions. In these ways the prevailing political and ethical beliefs differ from those of Aristotle.

If we are to apply Aristotle's insights under modern conditions, we must bear in mind that the ancient Greek *polis*—the kind of urban "political" community in which Greeks, Phoenicians, and some others organized their common life—was the community of citizens, not a separate institution constituted by a hierarchy of particular, professional roles. In translation of the term *polis*, we should also hyphenate our modern concepts of city and state. Whereas the Athens of which Aristotle wrote was politically independent and, on his account (since he took little interest in its maritime grain trade), economically self-sufficient, neither is the case with modern cities. For Aristotle, the *polis* was identical with the activity of its citizens, even though it also included both households and a variety of official positions. As the constitutive participants of a political community, Athenian citizens could determine their own laws, could decide collectively whether to go to war, and were responsible for their own defence. Only in the extraordinary circumstances in which citizens of Leningrad, Stalingrad, and Moscow once found themselves, as do, at the time of writing, the citizens of Mariupol, Kharkiv, and Kyiv, is it necessary to cultivate such martial virtues as those considered normal, and essential, by ancient Spartans, Athenians, and Romans. Similarly, our cities do not rule the surrounding agricultural land in the way that allowed Aristotle's many *poleis* to be economically autarchic.

What we now know as the sovereign state is a bureaucratic hierarchy of offices that is clearly separate from those who are subject to its impersonal rule and, indeed, is separate even from the private activities of those individuals who occupy those public roles professionally. In most cases, modern states may be defined, following Weber (1994: 310–311), by their monopolization of the means of legitimate physical violence. Whereas Aristotle defined the *polis* by its purpose or *telos* of actualizing the common good of its citizens, Weber stipulated that the state be defined only by reference to such particular means and not by any such specific purpose.

Despite these differences, we can still agree with the statement that an urban community "comes to be for the sake of living, but it exists for the sake of living well" (Aristotle, 2017, 12: 1252b29–30), and living the best kind of life for a human being requires participation in such a community. Such participation requires that citizens have sufficient political and legal freedom, sufficient material resources and free time, and sufficiently accountable and responsive civic authorities for them to be able to exercise effective agency over their own lives, individually, and over their own localities, collectively.

Even if excluded from practising martial virtues, we, as modern citizens, are normally free to reason with one another about how to exercise our moral agency and engage in collective action. Such an individual freedom, and the institutional conditions that secure it, can be considered today as a common good of citizenship. Conversely, we may very well reject Aristotle's proposition that workers, farmers, and others who lack time to devote to the activity of citizenship are therefore necessarily excluded from it. His supposition that citizens' living well also requires that they, as men, dominate their households, and therefore excluding women from the political domain should also be rejected. What remains is the idea that the good life is one lived in a civic community in accordance with virtue or excellence.

3.2.3   Civic Friendship

In our above conception of modern citizenship, we agree with Martha Nussbaum, Terence Irwin, and others that Aristotle's ideas of citizenship, virtue, and a political common good can, to some considerable extent, be applied to our contemporary conditions. We also agree with MacIntyre that such ideas are most easily applied to such localities as cities, towns, or even more particular neighbourhoods. It is at the local level that citizens can freely participate alongside one another in cooperative practices, together exercising their practical reasoning and judgement in deciding upon particular, revisable goals, and upon the performance of the tasks necessary for their actualization. This is the activity of civic friendship.

Aristotle argued that a *polis* is not just "a community of location" or an association "for the sake of preventing mutual injustice or for the sake of exchange." It is rather "the community in living well for both households and families." He acknowledged the household or *oikos* as a necessary constituent of the *polis* whilst regarding it as a fundamentally different, private (*idia*) sphere, being ordered to a lesser, economic good than the political community of the *polis*. In this context he talks about *politike philia*, civic (political) friendship, a form of friendship that can only arise amongst people inhabiting the same locality and connected to each other through different forms of social interaction. In Aristotle's time these included "brotherhoods, religious sacrifices, and the pastimes characteristic of living together," generating feelings of camaraderie amongst male heads of households. For him, such active friendships support the greater, civic friendship which is an essential aspect of "living well" (Aristotle, 2017, 65: 1280b29–39).

In his *Nicomachean Ethics*, Aristotle proposes that civic friendship "holds cities together and that legislators take it more seriously than justice" (Aristotle, 2014, 136: 1155a22). This type of friendship occurs when citizens "wish each other well for their own sake, do things for fellow citizens both individually and as a citizen body, and share in values, goals, and a sense of justice" (Schwarzenbach, 1996, 97). Such friendship is for Aristotle a criterion by which to distinguish just regimes from unjust ones; in tyranny there is least friendship (Aristotle, 2014, 150: 1161a31).

Whilst such a conception of citizenship can be traced through modernity as a declining tradition of republicanism and "civic virtue," it differs radically from that of what has become the dominant, Western political tradition of liberalism. Whereas the tradition that may be thought have begun by the time of Niccolò Machiavelli and culminated in that of Thomas Jefferson and Maximilien Robespierre (who still conceived of citizenship as a public, political activity), liberals understand it as a passive status involving legal rights over property and to privacy. For liberals, the most institutional forms that friendship takes are those of family, faith, and business.

Hannah Arendt (1958, 1968) is one who differed from this liberal conception, instead championing the republican tradition of civic virtue and of citizenship as political friendship. She assimilated this idea of community in contesting liberals' prioritization of private over public concerns. More recently, Sibyl Schwarzenbach has argued that civic friendship "must again be acknowledged as an essential factor unifying even the just modern state" because "in our time, the problem of social unity—of what it is that generally binds persons together in a just society—is emerging as of critical importance once again." Referring to "growing disparities in economic wealth, mounting violence, religious and racial tensions, the disintegration of traditional … familial relations, and staggering rates of systemic homelessness, drug dependency", she describes citizenship as a resource for "a fair and undogmatic social unity" (Schwarzenbach, 1996, 98–99). Citizens' common good should be therefore understood as more than that of freedom to reason about one's own ends and actions; it should also involve shared reasoning about ends and means, not against foreign "others" but in bettering shared conditions of life in a community of "civic friends."

Civic friendship can be seen as a factor grounding the sense of "We" across the difference. It emerges when we are interacting close with each other—it makes us more likely to acknowledge each other's values and claims as valid (Parkinson, 2012). This does not imply an imposed unity—we can be civic friends despite differences, mobilizing and working together for shared goods.

In practical terms, to facilitate the development of civic friendship, we need arenas for interaction beyond random encounters of urban life—spaces for doing things together, communicating, and deliberating on the common good. These include both formal, political arenas (such as townhall meetings) and informal, socially oriented public spaces, such as urban gardens or community kitchens. The latter has been the focus of our research project—Cultivating Public Space. We elaborate on this subject more later on in this chapter, extending the discussion with neo-Aristotelian concepts of practices and communities of virtue.

3.3 Alasdair MacIntyre on Productive Practices and Communities of Virtue

3.3.1 The Contemporary Reassertion of Aristotelian Concepts

The philosophical dominance that Aristotle's account of human conduct enjoyed from the late twelfth century onward ended during Europe's Enlightenment, after which Aristotelianism continued to be on the defensive for most of the nineteenth century. The reassertion of Aristotelian ethics and politics is identified by Nussbaum (2000) and Irwin (2009) with the work of the so-called British idealists, especially Thomas Hill Green, which led to a "New Liberalism" (see especially Nussbaum, 2000, 105–106, 112–116; Irwin, 2009, 536–624; Knight, 2011). These philosophical and political movements combined Aristotelianism's idea of the common good with Kant's philosophy of moral duty and Hegel's idea of the state as an ethical instrument. They thereby gave a philosophical grounding to the new idea of "the welfare state," an alternative to market-oriented liberalism.

Whilst this new kind of state was being democratically instituted, Elizabeth Anscombe and her husband Peter Geach led the way in using insights into linguistic practice from Ludwig Wittgenstein to update Thomistic Aristotelianism. Anscombe's "Modern Moral Philosophy" (1958) took a more uncompromisingly Aristotelian approach to ethics than that of political liberals. In her view, the dominant ethical positions neglect several topics that had been central in earlier ethics, such as those of character and the nature of a good human life. Ethics, if it is to be meaningful, should revive these concepts.

The principal question asked by Aristotle was "what is this for the sake of?" and, of humans, "what is the best life?", rather than to ask more abstractly, of particular situations and acts, "what is the right thing to do?" Hence, the specification of the rules of action is in this perspective of secondary interest. Ethics is seen as a domain "concerned with one's whole life – and not just the occasions when something with a distinctly 'moral' quality is at stake" (Russell, 2013: 2). Accordingly, "the focus is not so much on what to do in morally difficult cases, as on how to approach all of one's choices with such personal qualities as kindness, courage, wisdom, and integrity" (ibid.).

There is nonetheless a great diversity amongst understandings of Aristotelian ethics and politics (MacIntyre, 2020). Certainly, rather than refer to a diffuse "virtue ethics," it is better to talk about "a class of ethical theories that share a common emphasis on virtues as central features of their account of morality" (Ivanhoe, 2013: 50). Still more certainly, an Aristotelian ethics is one that regards virtues as real constituents of the human good.

Our Aristotelian approach to the development of public space is especially inspired by the way in which Alasdair MacIntyre has updated Aristotelian practical philosophy. He first did this in his 1981 *After Virtue: A Study in Moral Theory*, in which he identified Aristotle as the crucial figure in what he called "the tradition of the virtues." This was a work of intellectual history, exemplifying the idea that philosophy is inseparable from its past. This perspective enabled him to identify the basic, teleological structure of Aristotle's ethics as the beating heart of a continuing way of justifying morality, entirely separable from the historical specifics of Aristotle's own conception of the virtues. Further, MacIntyre shows why and how a contemporary Aristotelianism opposes patriarchal and other, institutionalized kinds of social injustice and domination (MacIntyre, 2007: 23–33, 74–78, 84–89, and 1998a; Knight, 2007: 102–225).

MacIntyre's argument remains that the best (and, to put it more strongly, the only philosophically sustainable) justification of moral precepts is that they command actions constitutive of one's good (understood in terms of human flourishing) and that habituation to courageous, truthful, prudent, just, and, in a word, virtuous acts is a necessary and constitutive "means" to the end that is the good life for a human being (MacIntyre, 2007: 184) as a rational, social, and, insofar as institutions permit, political animal.

3.3.2 Communities of Virtue and the Local Scale of Urban Politics

What most obviously distinguishes MacIntyre's ethics from that of almost all others who identify themselves as Aristotelians is his refusal to identify bureaucratic nation states as instruments of any genuinely common good. This is precisely why his understanding of a contemporary Aristotelianism is so apt for citizen-driven, locally based projects such as urban agriculture. He understands modern cities, towns, and villages as far more proximate than modern states to what Aristotle understood as a *polis*. On his account, individual freedom and rights secured by a nation state cannot be enough to secure democracy. A truly Aristotelian politics (*politike*) can only be practiced at a more local level, with opportunities for direct engagement, action, and deliberation. That said, he concedes that such a level can be extensive:

> A local political community with its own economy can be of considerable size, providing sophisticated forms of exchange, both between local producers and consumers and between both and more distant producers and consumers, and yet be made to serve the purposes of

the community. If we look at … those modern forms of association that have for some significant period of time sustained participatory achievement—forms of association as different as Donegal farming cooperatives, the state of Kerala in Southern India, the municipality of Bologna under Communist rule—we find excellent examples. (MacIntyre, 2008, 268)

In his *Ethics in the Conflicts of Modernity* (2016), MacIntyre elaborates two examples. One is the Danish fishing village of Thorupstrand, the other is the urban favela of Monte Azul in São Paulo, Brazil, where groups engage in

deliberative discussion on how to define and achieve the common goods with which they are concerned, on how to obtain the resources needed for their struggles, and how to mobilize political support, embarrassing national and municipal governments and elites that claim to be concerned for the poor, but who are strikingly unresponsive to the poor who do not organize politically. (MacIntyre, 2016, 181)

For the inhabitants of the Brazilian favela, the same virtues as for the villagers of Thorupstrand have been important: political prudence, justice, courage, and temperateness. Without these virtues the achievement of common goods of their communities (such as the maintenance and enhancement of commonly valued natural, educational, or other resources) would not have been possible.

The Nobel prize winner Elinor Ostrom argued for collective "self-organization and self-governance" against the neoliberal proposition that private ownership and management of scarce resources, such as fisheries or land, is the best way to avoid their depletion (Ostrom, 1990; Aligica, 2014) and "the tragedy of the commons" (Hardin, 1968), as the supposedly inevitable consequence of shared access and use. With Ostrom, we propose that resources are best governed and maintained through cooperation within the local communities who depend upon them.

That achievement of common goods enables individuals to identify and achieve their own good, as persons. Such a situation we call a community of virtue. It exists where and when people identify common goods and get their reasoning and actions together in pursuit of those goods, at the same time cultivating virtues and political friendship. Any such community needs to be on its guard against corruption by external interests and institutions.

3.3.3 Practices and Institutions

In *After Virtue* MacIntyre moved beyond the idea of shared practices with which Ludwig Wittgenstein had inspired much of post-war analytic philosophy. On Wittgenstein's account, to follow a rule is to engage in a shared practice (Wittgenstein, 2009, 87–88). For John Rawls, when developing his theory of justice, "practices" and "institutions" were therefore synonyms (Rawls, 1999a, b). MacIntyre went further than either in his social and ethical analysis, adding to Wittgenstein that to engage in a developed practice is to also actualize a shared good, whilst differing from Rawls in differentiating practices that prioritize the shared goods, from institutions, which prioritize the rules, along with the money, power, and status that accompany rules' application and enforcement. Therefore, on MacIntyre's account, institutional rationality differs from practical rationality. His stipulative definition of a practice is well-known:

> By a "practice" I am going to mean any coherent and complex form of socially established cooperative human activity through which goods internal to that form of activity are realized in the course of trying to achieve those standards of excellence which are appropriate to, and partially definitive of, that form of activity, with the result that human powers to achieve excellence, and human conceptions of the ends and goods involved, are systematically extended. ... Planting turnips is not a practice; farming is. So are the enquiries of physics, chemistry and biology, and so is the work of the historian, and so are painting and music. In the ancient and medieval worlds the creation and sustaining of human communities ... is generally taken to be a practice in the sense in which I have defined it. Thus the range of practices is wide: arts, sciences, games, politics in the Aristotelian sense, the making and sustaining of family life, all fall under the concept. (MacIntyre, 2007, 187–88.)

As MacIntyre argues, practices aim at their internal goods which are "good for the whole community who participate in the practice" rather than such goods external to the practice as money, status, or power which, when achieved, "are always some individuals' property and possession" (2007, 190–191). MacIntyrean practitioners, unlike modern bureaucratic managers, do not claim value neutrality; they are moral actors. Three virtues are central in their activities: truthfulness, justice, and courage. Courage is defined as "the capacity to risk harm or danger to oneself in connection with care and concern" (MacIntyre, 2007, 225). These virtues affect practitioner's relationship to their fellow practitioners and to others. Authority in this type of practice is derived not from power but from the mastery of the virtues internal to the practice. Those who have such an authority do not use it for purpose of domination and are not afraid to share their knowledge for the good of their community.

In the case of the practice of urban planning, internal goods can be linked to a good city, a city where major objective is the flourishing of its inhabitants and sustaining of their natural and cultural environments. The internal goods of planning practice can be also localized in the attempts to sustain disciplinary progress and to respond creatively to given problems, to move beyond the status quo.

Practices should not be confused with institutions, yet they usually require some institutional framework. For example, urban planning is conducted within planning institutions such as municipal planning offices (similarly—medicine is a practice; hospitals are institutions). "Institutions are characteristically and necessarily concerned with ... external goods," being structured in terms of money, power, status, and distributing them as rewards (MacIntyre, 2007, 194). Characteristically, the more that any person has of such external goods, "the less there is for other people" (MacIntyre, 2007, 190), unlike with internal goods.

Practices cannot survive without institutions but need to resist their acquisitiveness: "the cooperative care for common goods of the practice is always vulnerable to the competitiveness of the institutions" (ibid.). This is very much the case for planning, where planners in neoliberal institutions often experience value conflicts, most typically subordinating their precepts of the common good to the institutional and political agendas (Sager, 2009).

Whilst some practices (such as medicine or planning) are performed by formally trained practitioners, others have a more inclusive nature. A single practice of this kind can be the focal activity of an entire local community, as in the fishing village of Thorupstrand. Traditionally, many rural communities have been similarly organized around the practice of farming. Agriculture has therefore been a practice to which MacIntyre has often referred in illustrating the more general concept. Farming is a socially established human activity with particular standards of excellence. To be an excellent farmer, one must care for one's land and for the excellence of one's livestock and crops. Besides such "excellence of the products" particular or internal to any practice, there is a second kind of good internal to any particular practice. This is "the good of a certain kind of life," including moral and intellectual virtues necessary for the conduct both of such a life and, more generally, of civic life. This includes virtues such as fairness, perserverance, frugality, etc.

Here, we may note MacIntyre's difference from Aristotle about the relation of farming to the good life. For Aristotle (and for Arendt, 1958, 136–247), production is an activity based on technical skill (such as shipbuilding, shoemaking or even creating works of art) entirely different from action, which they limit to politics. Furthermore, in Aristotle's view engaging into productive activity is a form of cultivating intellectual virtue that does not, like action, contribute to the cultivation of moral virtue (Aristotle, 2014, 101: 1139b38-1140a24). Time, effort, and knowledge expended in production are, on this account, for the sake of the product, not of the human agent. MacIntyre, in contrast, does not distinguish between *praxis* and *poiesis*, calling both practices. In specifying that the excellence of products (or of performances, in the case of, e.g., sports) is typically accompanied by the "internal" goods of the way of life particular to these practices, he makes clear that he views productive practices as ethical activities pursuant of genuine goods. With the concept of practice as ethical activity, MacIntyre places productive work and workers at the centre of the ethical community from which Aristotle and many others have excluded them.

What is important for the cultivation of virtue on MacIntyre's account is that a person recognizes something beyond their present self as a good for the sake of which they should subject other desires to education and rational reordering. If someone desires to become an excellent farmer, capable of excelling in and extending farming's standards of production and practical reasoning, then they must subject their "own attitudes, choices, preferences and tastes" to the common goods and standards internal to farming as a shared practice (MacIntyre, 2007, 189–190; cf. MacIntyre, 1998b & 2016, 1–13). Only then will they become capable of exercising practical reasoning in overcoming new challenges and solving new problems.

3.4   Facilitating Practices and Virtue Communities in Contemporary Cities

3.4.1   Three Concerns for Public Space Development

We believe this conceptual apparatus of practices, institutions, and communities of virtue provides a promising approach to the development of urban public space and a feasible way to operationalize in the urban settings the Aristotelian conception of a good life as cultivating the virtues. In the following, we identify three concerns to be addressed in a public space development process: (i) identifying practices, (ii) mapping the involved goods, and (iii) facilitating communities of virtue. The concept of a practice offers a fine point of departure for public space development, since practices are constituted and identifiable by the goods internal to them and because they serve as schools of the virtues (MacIntyre, 2007 184–202, 227–228, 273–274; Knight, 2008b). In line with Aristotle's emphasis on the importance of direct political engagement and the exercise of practical reason for human flourishing, these concerns should always be pursued in dialogue with local practitioners and citizens.

(a) **Identifying local practices**: what practices can be facilitated/accommodated in a given public space?

Addressing this question is different from thinking about functions of public space, such as recreation or commercial services (Gehl, 2010), as we discussed in the previous section referring to MacIntyre (2007 184–202, 227–228, 273–274). Urban agriculture or horticulture, even pursued simply for ornamentation or relaxation, is an example of practice that can be facilitated in public space development. It can be advantageously accompanied by other practices co-existing in the same location—such as herbal medicine, carpentry, mindfulness, art, music, chess, cooking, or wine-making. Typically, the more practices we can facilitate in one space, the better—this makes a given space appealing for broad segments of users and provides more opportunities for development of civic friendship. The identification of practices should always be a participatory process, mapping both the needs of local stakeholders and place values. A variety of methodologies and methods may be used here (Brown et al., 2020). Both the accommodation of diversity of practices in one location and involvement of local stakeholders are in line with recommendations of placemaking community—advocating extensively tested, experience-based principles that can be used to transform public spaces into "community places" (Madden, 2018; see also Chap. 7).

(b) **Mapping the involved "goods"**: "external goods" of an institution vs. goods "internal" to practices. This stage of the process is very much about mapping the power dynamics at play, and anticipating possible conflicts.

Usually, the initiatives regarding public space development come from municipal actors or the private sector. At times, practices in urban spaces emerge spontaneously, as grassroot initiatives. These, however, are usually short-lived without any kind of institutional support (still, even a temporary, informal space for practice(s) can have numerous benefits in terms of *eudaimonia*, virtue, and political friendship). A practice that is to survive in urban public space in a long-term perspective typically needs to be systematically supported by an institution (such as a municipal office of city planning, a NGO, a private developer). In this context, it is important to remember that the goods of money, power, and status distributed by institutions are always in tension, if not conflict, with pursuit of the goods internal to particular practices, and therefore with the excellences internal to the way of life of practitioners. On this neo-Aristotelian view, it is important for the development of public space to create and sustain conditions conducive to the cooperative care for goods internal to practices, enabling them to resist the acquisitiveness of institutions and find ways to mitigate the potentially disastrous consequences of shifting power relations and political agendas.

Practices and institutions can be juxtaposed on multiple levels. For example, there is usually some need of self-organization within the local community of practitioners—taking care of such formalities as paying membership fees and safeguarding shared resources. Even with no need for formalities, leaders usually emerge. This may introduce into the community of practitioners the element of institutionalized external goods—seeking prestige, acknowledgement, or other forms of external gratification. The interplay of internal and external goods should therefore be under constant scrutiny.

(c) **Facilitating the development of communities of virtue** around selected practices.

We have described communities of virtue as localities that are socially consolidated by the identification of common goods internal to practices, upon which political activity might construct a more comprehensive common good. Facilitating communities of virtue in urban neighbourhoods requires providing conditions for collective self-organization through the cooperative coordination of different practices and raising the possibility of collective self-governance in actualizing such local autonomy. Public authorities, corporate powers, and more impersonal market forces can all obstruct such development and almost always do. What we propose is that public authorities, including planners, rather than regulate the organization of urban communities of practitioners, can and should concentrate upon regulating corporate power and doing their best to allow locals to secure whatever resources they require for cooperative projects and the cultivation of their shared, local practices (Fig. 3.1).

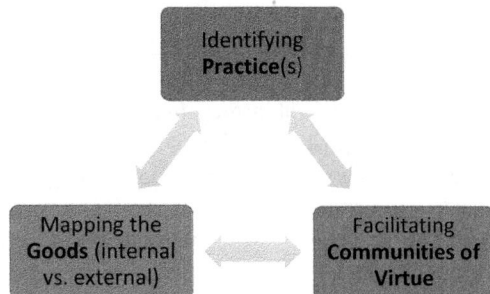

Fig. 3.1 Three concerns in public space development

Identifying **Practice**(s)

Mapping the **Goods** (internal vs. external)

Facilitating **Communities of Virtue**

3.4.2 The Example of Urban Agriculture

In the following we focus on urban agriculture as an example of a practice to be integrated in public space development. We propose that urban agriculture projects can function as locally based communities of virtue, that is, as arenas of social engagement that facilitate both the development of civic friendship and personal self-cultivation through the exercise of moral and intellectual virtues.

Urban agriculture remains a part of humans' ancient practice of farming, upon which the more institutional but scarcely less ancient process of civilization, the creation and sustaining of urban communities, has always depended. Nonetheless, the institutional context of urban agriculture differs markedly from its more traditional, rural settings. Water and land for cultivation are likely to be provided by public institutions or by private actors under public regulation, because in today's market realities, these are otherwise unobtainable through simple collective effort. Under these conditions, practitioners' shared reasoning is likely to be more often concerned with how to negotiate with such institutions and how to satisfy their requirements by mobilizing political support, than with such activity as the planting of turnips. Furthermore, particular activities such as cultivating specific crops are likely to be subject to more collective reasoning in urban agriculture than is traditional under rural conditions. It follows, however, that urban agriculture is likely to provide a more intensive education in the virtues (especially intellectual virtues) than the more traditional agricultural forms celebrated by such protagonists of the virtues as Hesiod, Jefferson, and MacIntyre. Apart from theoretical knowledge, practical reason, and skills, the practice of urban agriculture requires cultivation of justice, courage, and temperateness, as well as all of the moral virtues necessary for people to sustain their own and others' commitment and work toward a common good and shared goals.

Urban agriculture of the kind recorded, analysed, and championed in this book is a radically social and cooperative practice. Participants must learn how to work with others for a common good. Whilst that good can and should be understood as contributing to the wider, communal, and political good of their city, it is nonetheless likely that their fellow citizens, as well as the city's professional managers and politicians, will require constant persuasion that scarce resources of land and money should be made available to practitioners and that regulations should be interpreted or changed to facilitate their activity. The argument will always be met that, since food can be efficiently supplied from the countryside, cities should be ordered to providing more lucrative services. Under such conditions, urban farmers are likely to require even greater cultivation of moral and intellectual virtue (if perhaps a lesser range of technical skills) in resisting the corrupting power of institutions than is demanded of rural farmers in resisting market and regulatory pressures. The *telos*, the good and goal internal to the project and practice of urban farming, and common to its practitioners, will make significantly different demands upon them than are made upon rural farmers, but, insofar as their time, energy, and determination are similarly committed to it, the demands may prove no less difficult to meet than those pressing upon their rural relations. Indeed, given that the good they pursue is more marginal to the politics and economy of their locality, the corrupting power of their local institutions will feel all the greater.

For the goods and practice of agriculture to be pursued and sustained in an urban environment, kinds of local institution need to be created that differ greatly both from national farmers' unions and from such traditional, rural farming cooperatives as those identified by MacIntyre (2016) in Donegal, Ireland. Creating and sustaining the institutions necessary to organize and defend communities pursuing common goods is what MacIntyre calls politics in the Aristotelian sense. He cautions that such political practice must always be understood apart from the politics of the modern state: "All power tends to coopt and absolute power coopts absolutely" (MacIntyre, 2007, 109). Since organizational institutions necessarily deal in the currencies of money, power, and status, their very success and growth always tend to exacerbate the danger of corrupting or betraying their original purpose, as tasks of administration take their officials away from the task of production and into meeting and negotiating with external bureaucrats and executives. If the project of urban agriculture is to succeed, its administration must subserve its practical aim. In MacIntyre's Aristotelian terms, external goods must be used for the sake of the goods internal to the practice of urban agriculture. Insofar as this practice is sustained, it will sustain local communities of virtue in which all living beings may flourish in their various, specific ways.

3.5 Concluding Remarks

We conclude with a more general reflection on the relevance of the neo-Aristotelian perspective for contemporary planning discourse, particularly regarding the challenges related to urban sustainability.

The prevailing ethic in urban planning is that of a utilitarian concern with the efficient distribution of resources in pursuit of growth. For example, the European Commission frames social exclusion and environmental degradation as "obstacles to growth" (European Commission, 2009, 18), envisioning "an urbanised EU with cities driving growth and resource efficiency" (European Commission, 2014, 3). This approach is evident in extensive use of sustainability indicators and cost-benefit analyses.

Weaknesses of this conceptual framework emerge in several contexts. First, it pays too little attention to nonmaterial aspects of human well-being, including the social, cultural, and spiritual backgrounds of our lives. Numerous voices suggest that we need a different, more human-orientated and context-specific approach to sustainability (Williamson et al., 2003; Jackson, 2009; Demaria et al., 2013). Such an approach has been said to require a "new politics of the common good," "a more demanding idea of what it means to be a citizen, and … a more robust public discourse – one that engages more directly with moral and even spiritual questions" (Sandel, 2009).

Secondly, it gives a false appearance of value neutrality. Since the concepts of utility and effectiveness are far from being merely technical in nature, they are prone to ideological misuse. As MacIntyre (2007, 70) observes, too little attention is put on the essential difference between short-term and long-term effectiveness. Likewise, the utilitarian idea of the substitutability of different goods and the possibility of "summing" a variety of aims people value is highly questionable. To use these concepts as if they could provide us with a rational, value-neutral criterion "is indeed to resort to a fiction" (ibid.). In utilizing such a criterion, neoliberal policies implicitly promote a vision of individuals' lives that is in many respects inimical to their flourishing.

Thirdly, the utilitarian approach has failed to tackle the fundamental causes of our environmental predicaments. Whilst sustainability has remained on the agenda for nearly 40 years, neoliberal policies have failed to resolve cities' socio-economic and environmental problems. Arne Næss's original (1973) distinction between "shallow" and "deep" ecological purposes and values continues to be pertinent. The "shallow" approach stops before the ultimate level of fundamental change, often promoting short-term, technological fixes, whereas the "deep" approach, targeting the root causes of our environmental problems, involves rethinking our relationship to external nature in order to facilitate both its and our own flourishing. Our current policies are predominantly operating on the shallow level, hardly addressing the real causes of our environmental problems—the paradigm of growth and unsustainable lifestyles. In order to escape the current crisis, we need to go further than focus on resource efficiency and environmental impacts; we need to rethink our value frameworks and redefine the way we think about human prosperity (Jackson, 2009; Demaria et al., 2013).

Finally, neo-Aristotelian insight also requires a new approach to education in which students are provided with an opportunity to acquire experience and develop the character traits and abilities necessary to become fully ethical actors. As Russell (2013: 3) observes, students most "need, not a decision procedure from a text-book, but the practical wisdom to understand for themselves how to be people who take responsibility and why taking responsibility matters." The dominant models of education discourage such engagement. As one graduate reflects, "young people are not being educated to take their place in society. They are being trained – trained in a narrow body of knowledge and skills that is taught in isolation from larger and vital questions about who we are and what we might become" (Friedmann, 2002, 105).

The neo-Aristotelian perspective provides a viable basis for an alternative, "deep" approach to sustainability. Applied to planning and public space development, it demands incorporation of the human *telos*—a fulfilling individual and communal life—and an explicit normativity in planning and urban development strategies. Focusing on the excellence of human character and emphasizing such social virtues as solidarity and responsibility toward others, it should contribute to an alternative model of economic development and the inspiration of social change. It may also encourage a more respectful attitude toward natural environments and a limit to personal consumption, since an Aristotelian reflection on the virtues acknowledges non-human natural goods (MacIntyre, 1999: 11–85).

In sum, the concepts of the human flourishing, the common good of participative communities of practice and locality, and of particular virtues—including that of civic friendship—can all be applied in urban planning. In this book we try to illustrate this empirically with cases of urban agriculture—referring to the goods internal to the practice itself (such as food production), to the part that such shared participation and pursuit plays within the life of each practitioner, and to how it contributes toward society's wider common good, by, for example, distributing fresh local produce, disseminating nutrition and farming knowledge, and cultivating social and political activity befitting real citizenship. Understood in these terms, an Aristotelian case may be acknowledged, as well as endorsed, by urban planners concerned with the efficient allocation of limited institutional resources.

As we have now emphasized, the Aristotelian case against its normative, institutionalized rivals might also be taken further. To do so would involve politicizing and democratizing planning, so that it is no longer understood as primarily the domain of institutional experts but as the common concern of all those citizens whose neighbourhoods are being developed. In this, our neo-Aristotelian vision supports the "right to the city" perspective (Lefebvre, 1996) that emphasizes two principal rights for urban inhabitants: the right to participate in urban decision-making and the right to appropriate urban spaces, based on citizens' needs.

References

Aligica, P. D. (2014). *Institutional diversity and political economy: The Ostroms and beyond.* Oxford University Press.

Anscombe, G. E. M. (1958). Modern moral philosophy. *Philosophy, 33*(124), 1–19.

Arendt, H. (1958). *The human condition.* University of Chicago Press.

Arendt, H. (1968). *Between past and future: Eight exercises in political thought.* Viking.

Aristotle. (2014). *Nicomachean ethics* (C.D.C. Reeve, Trans.). Hackett.

Aristotle. (2017). *Politics: A new translation* (C.D.C. Reeve, Trans.). Hackett.

Brown, G., Reed, P., & Raymond, C. M. (2020). Mapping place values: 10 lessons from two decades of public participation GIS empirical research. *Applied Geography, 116*, 102–156.

Demaria, F., Schneider, F., Sekulova, F., & Martinez-Alier, J. (2013). What is degrowth? From an activist slogan to a social movement. *Environmental values, 22*(2), 191–215.

European Commission. (2009). *Promoting sustainable urban development in Europe: Achievements and opportunities.*

European Commission. (2014). *The urban dimension of EU policies: Key features of an EU urban agenda.*

Friedmann, J. (2002). *The Prospect of cities.* University of Minnesota Press.

Gehl, J. (2010). *Cities for people.* Pan American Copyright Conventions.

Hardin, G. (1968). The tragedy of the commons. *Science, 162*, 1243–1248.

Huta, V., & Waterman, A. S. (2014). Eudaimonia and its distinction from hedonia: Developing a classification and terminology for understanding conceptual and operational definitions. *Journal of happiness studies, 15*, 1425–1456.

Irwin, T. (2007–2009). *The development of ethics (3 volumes).* Oxford University Press.

Irwin, T. (2009). *The development of ethics: A historical and critical study, vol 3: From Kant to Rawls.* Oxford University Press.

Irwin, T. (2020). *Ethics through history: An introduction.* Oxford University Press.

Ivanhoe, P. (2013). Virtue ethics and the Chinese confucian tradition. In D. C. Russell (Ed.), *The Cambridge companion to virtue ethics*. Cambridge University Press.

Jackson, T. (2009). *Prosperity without growth? The transition to a sustainable economy*. Earthscan.

Knight, K. (2007). *Aristotelian philosophy: Ethics and politics from Aristotle to MacIntyre*. Polity Press.

Knight, K. (2008a). Practices: The Aristotelian concept. *Analyse & Kritik, 30*(2), 317–329.

Knight, K. (2008b). Goods. *Philosophy of Management, 7*(1), 107–122.

Knight, K. (2011). What's the good of post-analytic philosophy? *History of European Ideas, 37*(3), 304–314.

Knight, K. (2023). Social practices, institutions, and common goods. In T. Angier (Ed.), *MacIntyre's after virtue at 40*. Cambridge University Press.

Lefebvre, H. (1996). *Writings on cities*. Blackwell.

MacIntyre, A. (1998a). Politics, philosophy and the common good. In K. Knight (Ed.), *The MacIntyre reader*. Polity Press.

MacIntyre, A. (1998b). Plain persons and moral philosophy: Rules, virtues and goods. In K. Knight (Ed.), *The MacIntyre reader* (pp. 136–152). Polity Press.

MacIntyre, A. (1999). *Dependent rational animals: Why human beings need the virtues*. Duckworth.

MacIntyre, A. (2007). *After virtue: A study in moral theory* (3rd ed.). University of Notre Dame Press.

MacIntyre, A. (2008). What more needs to be said? A beginning, although only a beginning, at saying it. In K. Knight & P. Blackledge (Eds.), *Revolutionary aristotelianism: Ethics, resistance and utopia* (pp. 261–276). De Gruyter.

MacIntyre, A. (2016). *Ethics in the conflicts of modernity: An essay on desire, practical reasoning and narrative*. Cambridge University Press.

MacIntyre, A. (2020). Four – Or more? – Political Aristotles. In A. Bielskis, E. Leontsini, & K. Knight (Eds.), *Virtue ethics and contemporary aristotelianism: Modernity*. Conflict and Politics.

Madden, K. (2018). *How to turn a place around: A placemaking handbook*. Project for Public Spaces.

Næss, A. (1973). The shallow and the deep, long-range ecology movement: A summary. *Inquiry, 16*(1–4), 95–100.

Nussbaum, M. (1994). *The therapy of desire: Theory and practice in Hellenistic ethics*. Princeton University Press.

Nussbaum, M. (2000). Aristotle, Politics, and Human Capabilities: A Response to Antony, Arneson, Charlesworth, and Mulgan. *Ethics, 111*(1), 102–140.

Nussbaum, M. (2011). *Creating capabilities: The human development approach*. Belknap Press of Harvard.

Ostrom, E. (1990). *Governing the commons*. Cambridge University Press.

Parkinson, J. (2012). *Democracy and public space: The physical sites of democratic performance*. Oxford Academic.

Rawls, J. (1999a). Justice as fairness. In S. Freeman (Ed.), *John Rawls: Collected papers* (pp. 47–72). Harvard University Press.

Rawls, J. (1999b). *A theory of justice* (2nd ed.). Harvard University Press.

Russell, D. (2013). Introduction: Virtue ethics in modern moral philosophy. In D. C. Russell (Ed.), *The Cambridge companion to virtue ethics*. Cambridge University Press.

Ryan, R. M., & Deci, E. L. (2001). On happiness and human potentials: A review of research on hedonic and eudaimonic Well-being. *Annual Review of Psychology, 52*, 141–166.

Ryan, R. M., Huta, V., & Deci, E. L. (2008). Living well: A self-determination theory perspective on eudaimonia. *Journal of Happiness Studies, 9*(1), 139–170.

Sager, T. (2009). Planners' role: Torn between dialogical ideals and neo-liberal realities. *European Planning Studies, 17*(1), 65–84.

Sandel, M. (2009). *A new citizenship: The Reith lectures 2009*. British Broadcasting Corporation.

Schwarzenbach, S. (1996). On civic friendship. *Ethics, 107*(1), 97–128.

Strang, J. V. (1998). Ethics as politics: On Aristotelian ethics and its context. *The Paideia Archive: Twentieth World Congress of Philosophy, 3*, 274–285.

Vittersø, J. (Ed.). (2016). *Handbook of eudaimonic Well-being*. Springer International Publishing.

Weber, M. (1994). The profession and vocation of politics (R. Speirs, Trans.). In P. Lassman & R. Speirs (Eds.), *Weber: Political writings*. Cambridge University Press.

Williamson, T., Radford, A., & Bennetts, H. (2003). *Understanding sustainable architecture*. Spon Press.

Wittgenstein, L. (2009). *Philosophical investigations*. Wiley-Blackwell.

Part II
Public Urban Agriculture in Northern European Contexts

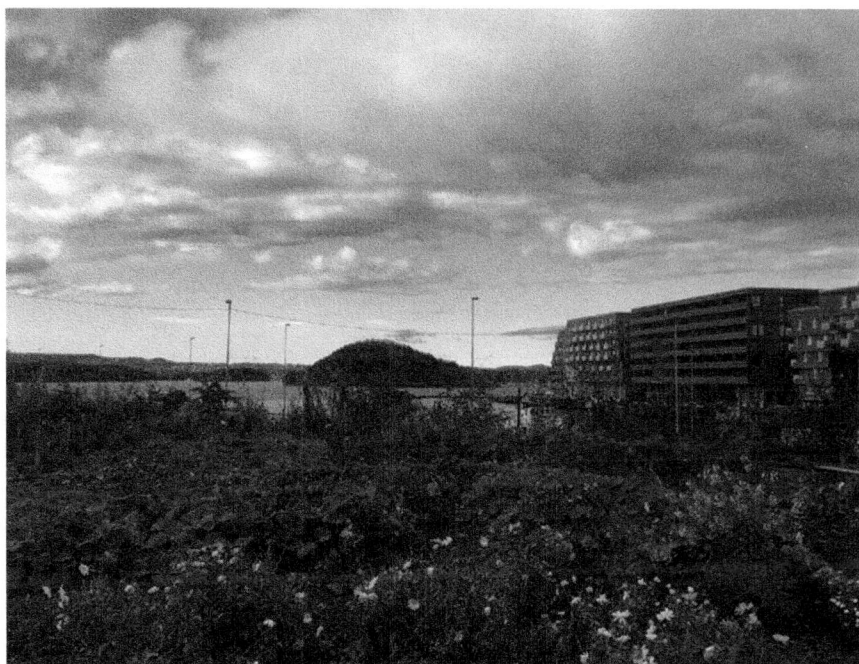

Chapter 4
Cultivating Publicness Through Urban Agriculture: Learning from Aarhus and Rotterdam

Melissa Anna Murphy and Pavel Grabalov

4.1 Introduction

In cities worldwide, urban agriculture – defined here strictly as food cultivation in publicly accessible outdoor urban spaces – is becoming increasingly popular both among urban agriculture actors and municipal authorities. Urban agriculture is believed to have multiple benefits, such as food security (Warren et al., 2015), community building (Audate et al., 2022), increased well-being (Kirby et al., 2021) and enhanced quality of life of citizens by contributing to a range of capabilities (see Chap. 2). In this paper, we focus on public benefits of urban agriculture which go beyond those offered to individuals. Integrating urban agriculture into public space can, however, breed both synergies as well as conflicts with the other pressing needs and uses of public space, which proves an especially relevant challenge for cities experiencing population growth and densification. Public space in this chapter refers to all urban spaces that are publicly accessible, regardless of ownership or maintenance responsibility.

In exploring synergies and conflicts between different urban agriculture benefits, it is useful to ask *to whom* these benefits are provided. In the "Cultivating Public Space" (CPS) research project, which formed the basis for this anthology, we followed the division of primary, secondary, and tertiary users suggested by Eason (1989). In the context of urban agriculture, we distinguished urban gardeners as primary users, local residents occasionally engaged in urban agriculture activities as secondary users, and

M. A. Murphy (✉)
Department of Culture, Religion, and Social Sciences, University of South-Eastern Norway, Drammen, Norway
e-mail: melissa.murphy@usn.no

P. Grabalov
Department of Urban and Regional Planning, Faculty of Landscape and Society, Norwegian University of Life Sciences, Ås, Norway

B. Sirowy, D. Ruggeri (eds.), *Urban Agriculture in Public Space*, GeoJournal Library 132, https://doi.org/10.1007/978-3-031-41550-0_4

the larger urban community as tertiary users. Benefits for one of these groups can be either advantageous or disturbing for other groups. To explore relations between different public benefits of urban agriculture, we engaged with scholarship on publicness (Tornaghi & Knierbein, 2014; Varna & Tiesdell, 2010), which can be captured through the magnitude of user groups attracted to urban space and tensions therein. This chapter looks at how different kinds of publicness can be cultivated through urban agriculture and examines how different municipalities facilitate urban agriculture and how that facilitation plays out in urban agriculture in public spaces.

For this chapter, we collected empirical material from two cities: Aarhus in Denmark and Rotterdam in the Netherlands, chosen due to contrasting approaches to facilitating urban agriculture. Both cities are active in urban agriculture and have contextual similarities to Norwegian cities, the focus of the CPS research project. Aarhus (municipal size: population 355,328; area 468 km^2) and Rotterdam (municipal size: population 651,157; area 324 km^2) are the second largest cities in their countries. They are situated in coastal areas in the Northern part of Europe. Both cities are governed using a parliamentary model with left-wing parties being in power during our fieldwork in 2018.

In both Aarhus and Rotterdam, we studied urban agriculture on two levels: the policy level of municipal facilitation and the ground level of specific urban agriculture initiatives. Our empirical material included urban agriculture-relevant policy documents, interviews, and field observations. At each site, we conducted formal and informal interviews with gardeners and visitors, making field notes, photographs, and maps. The analysis of the empirical material employed a people-centered, critical policy ethnography approach which highlights the interrelationship between the policy and ground levels (Dubois, 2015). This approach allowed us to consider the context specificity of each urban agriculture initiative as well as how the policy level plays out on the ground.

In this chapter, we offer an in-depth review of seven cases in Aarhus and Rotterdam that illustrate the variety of the ways urban agriculture initiatives can perform in public space. We selected these seven cases from a wider range of the initiatives in the two cities. In selecting them, we aimed for a diversity in types, organizational models, and design solutions. The exploratory nature of the early fieldwork activities, together with limitations due to informant availability and field visit length, provided a varying amount of data from each case. While we focus on the cases with most data, we find the inclusion of secondary cases useful for this chapter to illustrate the variety we have witnessed in these cities. The description of the cases is supplemented with photographs and, for some urban agriculture initiatives, with maps of the sites.

This chapter begins with an outline of our conceptual framework built around different aspects of publicness. A presentation of empirical material from Aarhus and Rotterdam covers both municipal policies and descriptions of specific urban agriculture initiatives. This information generates a cross-case discussion highlighting four trajectories for how urban agriculture can benefit different publics and contribute to the development of the capabilities of gardeners and the larger urban community. In the conclusion, we summarize our findings and identify the trade-offs between these trajectories.

4.2 Conceptual Framework: Publicness

The CPS research project wanted to explore the dynamic relationships between urban agriculture activities and the public spaces where these activities take place. Our theoretical foundation for this chapter's analysis ties together scholarship on publicness (Tornaghi & Knierbein, 2014; Varna & Tiesdell, 2010), theory of the commons (Eidelman & Safransky, 2021; Feinberg et al., 2021; McNutt, 2000), and the capabilities perspective as operationalized in Chap. 2. We also outlined our theoretical foundation in more details elsewhere (Murphy et al., 2022; Murphy et al., Unpublished manuscript).

Nussbaum's (2011) capabilities approach grounded this work in an understanding of the basic benefits (safety, education, food, recreation, contact with nature, exposure to diversity) which everyone should expect, so we can assess who gets which ones from public space. For Nussbaum (2003), capabilities are also vital to entitlement – giving back power to those (like women or minorities) whose agency has been undermined by past policies and practices. While the capabilities perspective focuses on the dimensions of individual well-being, the concept of publicness offers an understanding of the breadth of user groups public space can support and several areas where space may discourage use.

Acknowledging vivid scholarly debate on the meaning of the concept of publicness (see, e.g., Kohn (2004), Langstraat and Van Melik (2013), Madanipour, (1999), and Németh and Schmidt (2011)), we found it necessary to tie together different conceptualizations to address the many ways that urban agriculture can interact with people and public space. Following a relational, socio-material definition, publicness can describe interactions in and with physical space that link people (Tornaghi & Knierbein, 2014). Such a relational and inclusive definition allows us to analyze the built environment together with the social interactions that happen there and to understand its materiality as generative of potential social links between people and publics.

Analyzing the material aspects of urban agriculture in this approach is further supplemented with scholarship on public space. Design principles for supporting public use by urban designer Jan Gehl (2010) give a background for what kinds of materials and design moves can support different kinds of public uses in urban space. Varna and Tiesdell's (2010) "star model" of publicness further brings together aspects of design and spatial management that can limit or discourage use by a variety of groups and individuals.

To focus on the benefits urban agriculture provides, we looked at urban agriculture spaces from the public and club goods perspective connected to the theory of the commons (McNutt, 2000). According to Webster (2007), "public goods" are universally accessible benefits that people should not compete for (e.g., air, lighting, safety). Conversely, "club goods" favor a particular community – a club – to prevent competition between members. A goods-based model of publicness implies diversity of the benefits, while also highlighting possible synergies and conflicts between different activities in public space and groups.

Drawing from this conceptual background, we constructed a theory grounded in publicness dimensions refined in an iterative process with data collection throughout the study. Varna and Tiesdell's star model (Varna & Tiesdell, 2010) points to five dimensions of publicness: ownership, control, civility, physical configuration, and animation. These focus on what is happening in an urban space itself, who can access it, how different activities are supported, and who feels welcome to use it. We summarized the publicness described by the star model as "Access and Animation" (Varna & Tiesdell, 2010: 585) to include public space aspects that draw users and maintain high levels of activity. In considering the goods that can be produced in public space and how they can relationally link people, we add three dimensions specific to urban agriculture in public space: community, food, and knowledge. These dimensions allowed us to see the benefits of urban agriculture for broader publics rather than limiting them to the people who physically visit the sites. The resulting model enables comparative descriptive analysis of publicness of urban agriculture initiatives of different scales, typologies, and organizational modes.

This conceptualization was further refined through findings in our data collection, allowing us to identify four trajectories through which urban agriculture supports publicness:

- **Access and animation: increasing accessibility and vitality in public space**
  Urban agriculture initiatives affect who controls public space and how. Control can both decrease access and animation by having restrictive regulations as well as increase it by adding safety when gardeners are present in public space. Among our cases, there were several which were fenced because their functioning was dependent on production and selling of the harvest. Urban agriculture initiatives can increase animation by creating a comfortable, welcoming, and aesthetically pleasant environment. Urban agriculture, however, can also challenge access and animation by reducing diversity of user groups and comfort because of, for example, neglect.
  Access and animation impacts depend largely on the spatial context of urban agriculture initiatives and how the space works with its surroundings. For example, we found that urban agriculture can increase accessibility and publicness of neglected and peripherical spaces. For more central and well-connected areas, urban agriculture can in fact decrease this type of publicness by privatizing space. Urban agriculture can either be an attraction which works as a magnet for new users, or an obstacle to publicness in urban fabric.
- **Community: contributing to social services**
  When people like urban agriculture actors engage in a specific public space, they have the potential to use it and generate activity to welcome others in. We see urban agriculture serving school groups and collaborating with welfare organizations to provide a variety of therapy, job, and social training.
- **Food: producing and distributing food**
  By its nature urban agriculture can contribute to food production; to increase publicness this food should benefit the public and be distributed broadly, such as in examples we have seen that collaborate with food pantries for the disadvan-

taged. However, cultivation can also put additional pressures on the issues of control and setting limits to physical access.

- **Knowledge: building communities to spread cultivation knowledge**
  Urban agriculture activities have the potential to provide benefits to the public by disseminating cultivation awareness and skills – shared public goods for which different user groups do not have to compete. Such knowledge can include not only food cultivation per se but also cooking, nutrition, health, and management of an urban agriculture initiative.
  Urban agriculture can help different communities emerge and take shape: not only communities of gardeners but also more heterogeneous communities of passers-by, neighbors, and consumers. To what extent gardeners' community should be inclusive in order to increase publicness of space and grow food is an open question.

The discussion presents a detailed description of these trajectories and how they interact, linked to the capabilities operationalized within the CPS project (see Chap. 2). The next two sections will present urban agriculture of Aarhus and Rotterdam: both how the municipalities enable and regulate it and how urban agriculture initiatives play out on the ground. For each of the seven described initiatives, we provide their ranking with regard to the four publicness trajectories highlighted above.

4.3 Aarhus: Urban Agriculture as a Tool for Citizen Engagement

In Aarhus, urban agriculture facilitation is placed in the context of co-creation and active citizenship (similar to Trondheim in Norway; see Chap. 11). Here, the municipality's efforts to promote urban agriculture are channeled through a citizen engagement team. This team belongs to the technical department but works across administration silos. Our informant from the technical department suggested that by creating this team the municipality wanted to move away from the new public management agenda, to make citizens more active and engaged, and to shorten the distance between the municipality and citizens. The citizen engagement team is tasked with supporting co-creation with citizens. The team also actively collaborates with other municipal agencies and educates them regarding the importance of citizen involvement in decision-making.

The program "Taste Aarhus" (*Smag på Aarhus*[1]) is one of the primary projects of the team. It was initiated in 2014 to engage citizens and prioritize high-quality, edible green spaces. The idea came from the citizens themselves and was later supported by the municipality and funded by a philanthropic foundation for the first five years of the project. The program team includes people with different backgrounds, among them a planner, a gardener, and an architect working with citizen

---

[1] http://smagpaaaarhus.dk/

engagement. They provide detailed advice on projects; help citizens to navigate planning issues, infrastructure, and pollution; and facilitate possible conflicts and accessibility challenges. In that sense, the citizen engagement team is not a controlling authority but an advisory agency that, when asked, can provide tools and knowledge. They also facilitate networking across urban agriculture groups and disseminate information.

Within the program, a contract for using municipal land was formalized and a minimum set of rules for the initiatives was imposed. Membership to urban agriculture initiatives must be open to all residents, not just one particular group. The urban agriculture initiatives are to be registered as organizations with a five-member board, provide public access to the gardens, give the public opportunities to harvest part of the produce, and clean the land upon termination of the lease. The organizations themselves can define how public access is maintained and how much of harvest can be shared with the public. They must also host biannual public events and report their activities to the municipality yearly.

Two major challenges with urban agriculture facilitation in Aarhus became clear from our municipal informants. First, public perception of the quality of urban soil challenged early recruitment to the program. The citizen engagement team worked hard to communicate clearly and convincingly that it was safe to grow food in the soil within the city. They asked a researcher to test city soils and hold public sessions disseminating the results (only soils around petrol stations were found contaminated). Second, the temporality of lease contracts for land is seen by some as deterrent for long-term initiative investments. The municipality's main challenge with granting longer-term permissions is in cases when initiatives use land slated for future redevelopment.

The citizen engagement team both facilitates citizens' projects and implements municipal projects. The team is directly involved in urban agriculture projects connected to kindergartens, schools, hospitals, elderly homes, social housing, and prisons. In order to secure ongoing funding from the municipality, the urban agriculture projects need to demonstrate how their benefits align with the existing goals of the city authorities, for example, public health, education, and integration. An informant explained in a following way:

> So, when they talk a lot about health then I talk about getting people to move a lot. If people walk outside to get apples one day, they can walk five kilometers collecting apples. Then I can refer to the health agenda and raise funding money from there. Or education, we can make school gardens, for social agendas, we can pick up integration… There is really nothing this project cannot speak to because it is about food, meals together, community, education. [an informant from the municipality of Aarhus].

"Taste Aarhus" is regarded as a success by the municipality. According to an informant from an urban agriculture initiative we visited, this project helped the initiative to navigate within the bureaucratic system. Our informants in the city suggested that the main motivation for the municipality to promote urban agriculture is primarily the re-engagement of citizens in decision-making and taking responsibility for public spaces, being less reliant on authorities to take action. In that sense, on the municipal level, urban agriculture is appreciated not for its food production capacity but for other functions which can improve quality of life of Aarhus residents. Such functions include getting people to be more active, facilitating socialization and recreation, and beautifying the urban environment. Our respondents further suggested that for the city administration, labeling green spaces in new redevelopment areas as "edible areas" helps to secure budget and a level of quality for these spaces, as people can easily relate to this purpose: "being pretty is not enough" (an informant from the municipality of Aarhus).

Three initiatives (Fig. 4.1) were chosen to present public benefits of urban agriculture in Aarhus: *PIER2 Haven*, "edible pathways" project, and *Gallo Gartneriet*. These initiatives are different in scope and level of municipal involvement, demonstrating the span of urban agriculture that can be found in Aarhus.

1. PIER2 Haven: Waterfront cultivating and culture[a]

Increasing access and animation in public space	Contributing to social services	Producing and distributing food	Building communities to spread cultivation knowledge
●	○	◑	●
Significantly present, reaching a large public	Not present or reaching beyond members	Present, smaller public	Significantly present, reaching a large public

[a]https://www.pier2haven.dk/

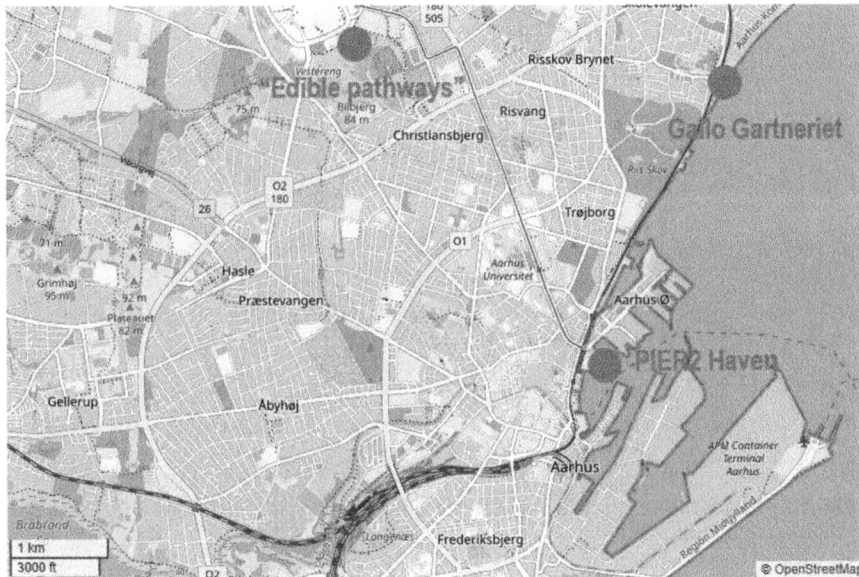

Fig. 4.1 Location of the studied urban agriculture initiatives in Aarhus. (Basemap: OpenStreetMap)

Location and Connectivity A raised-bed garden initiative (Figs. 4.2, 4.3, 4.4, and 4.5) started in 2017 on a 1390 m² site along the waterfront of Aarhus, 8 minutes by bike from the central railway station. The whole waterfront is part of a redevelopment process, changing it from an industrial area into a multifunctional urban district. The garden is situated on a peninsula with no through traffic. There are no fences except one bordering a nearby construction site. The whole area is open visually from all sides. The initiative collaborates closely with two neighboring organizations: the Dome of Visions[2] (a cultural institution and a café) and *Fra grums*

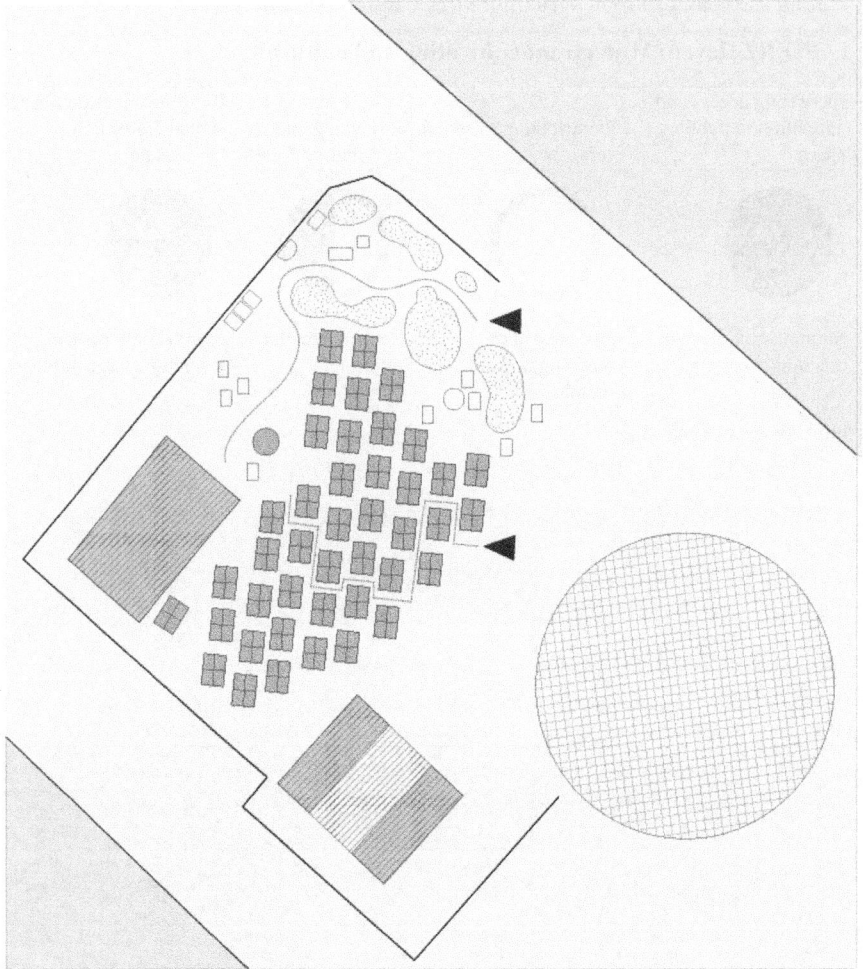

Fig. 4.2 Map of PIER2 Haven in Aarhus with entrances (red arrows) and paths (red dash line). (Map design: Kristin Sunde)

---

[2] https://domeofvisions.dk/

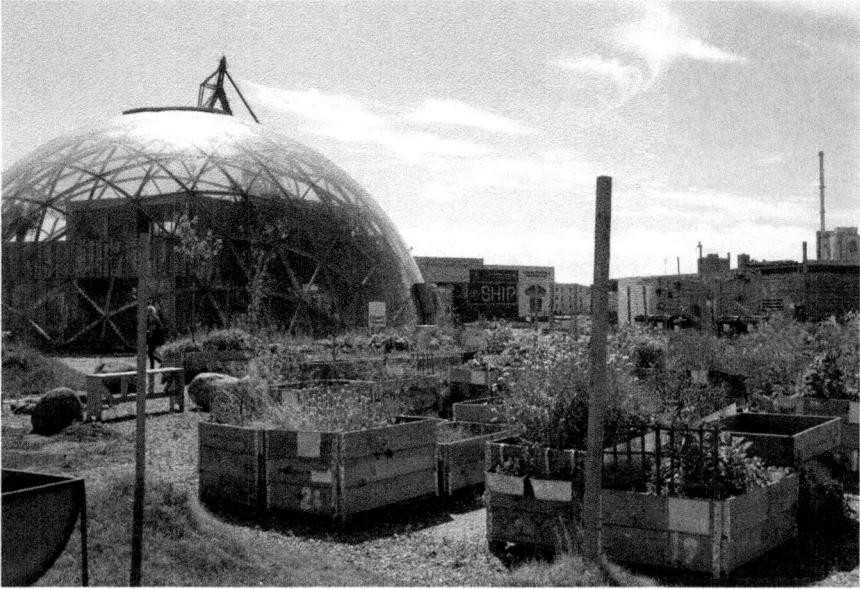

Fig. 4.3 The pallet boxes of PIER2 Haven in Aarhus. (Photo: authors)

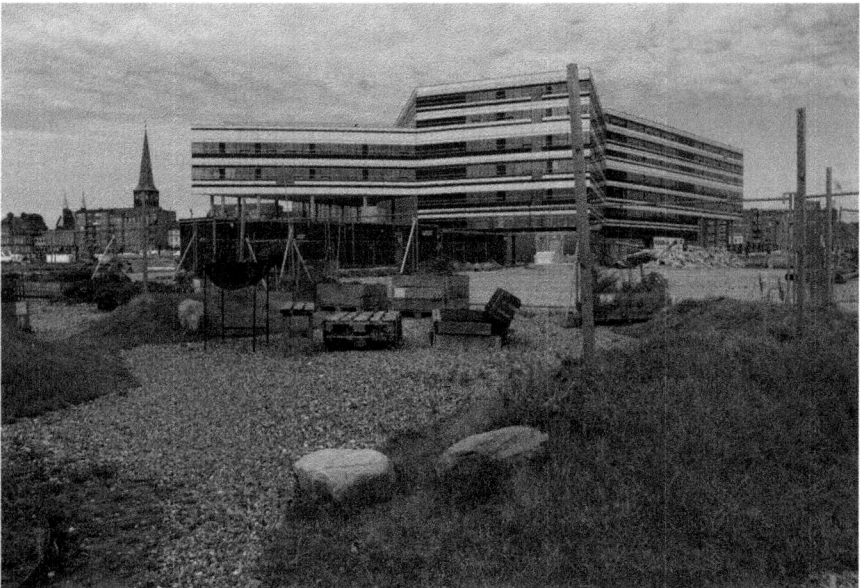

Fig. 4.4 The grill zone at PIER2 Haven with both formal and informal sitting opportunities. (Photo: authors)

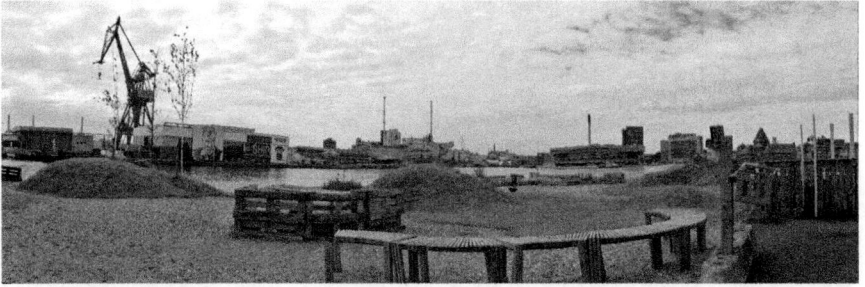

Fig. 4.5 Views from the siting area next to PIER2 Haven. (Photo: authors)

til gourmet[3] (an entrepreneur growing mushrooms on used coffee grinds). Some crew of both the Dome of Visions and *Fra grums til gourmet* are members of the initiative's foundation and facilitate collaboration as they have similar visions: "Dome of Visions and some of the community wanted a green park in the area close to the sea. So we have gotten together and are forming a dialogue about it. Many people have dreams about the space, like more gardens and boat access…" (an informant from the urban agriculture initiative).

Management and Funding Mechanism The garden was initiated by a group of residents who came together to establish a garden community and got help from the municipality to find a space for it. The initiative is run by a foundation the group started, with an annually elected board. According to our informants, it attracted people who had small apartments with no green spaces and wanted to have a yard, as well as those who wanted to be a part of a community in addition to having a garden. Middle-aged women were reported to be the most active members of the board of the urban agriculture initiative. Three groups are actively involved, including a garden construction group, a workday organizing group, and a communication team. According to our informants, the structure is flexible, and anyone can get involved in the groups' work without any special permission from the board. The foundation uses social media to attract new members and to invite visitors to come on Sunday picnics. The municipality owns the land and leases it for free to the garden community, but at the time of our fieldwork, the plot was likely to be sold for development. The "Taste Aarhus" program provided materials and financing for the first year of the initiative. Beyond that, the garden has been run on financial contributions from the members and supporters.

Design and Amenities The garden consists of 45 pallet boxes, mostly kept by individuals, but some are reserved for public harvest according to the rules stipulated by the Aarhus municipality. The garden's rules and information presented on site aim

---

[3] https://www.facebook.com/fragrumstilgourmet

to distinguish between private boxes and boxes for the public. Initially, an architect suggested building an integrated, designed garden, but this option seemed to be too expensive, given the unknown future, and was not realized. *PIER2 Haven* instead appears as a tidy, well-kept series of pallet boxes with some low-threshold DIY berms and decorations. Empty space around the garden allows some flexibility, and the garden can often be adapted and transformed. There are both formal (benches, pallet deck chairs) and informal (grass mounds, large rocks, etc.) seating opportunities at the grill and fire pit, all built by the gardeners themselves.

Activities   The initiative grows fruits, vegetables, and herbs. Everybody can come to the garden, sit, and enjoy coffee from the nearby Dome of Visions. During our visits, there were many visitors there, many attracted by the fresh air and by nearness to the water: young people, students, locals from downtown, and young families with children. The initiative organizes pancake dinners and concerts, plus days of collective voluntary work. The site facilitates interaction between the garden community and different groups that visit the Dome of Visions. Together they offer a variety of outdoor and indoor open space for larger events as well as for retreating to more intimate spaces.

Relations to the Municipal Authorities and Policies   The garden was originally established under the municipal program "Taste Aarhus." This case demonstrates the typical support "Taste Aarhus" gives to new urban agriculture initiatives: helping with the first steps and establishment of the foundation, finding land, providing a 1-year lease contract and initial funding. The contract is up for renewal annually. Our informants reported satisfaction with the relationship with the municipality as they felt the rules were not strict. The garden community became engaged in the area's development and wanted to be included in future plans. The garden aims to showcase to politicians its value and the importance of having accessible green spaces. Among the challenges the initiative faces are funding ongoing maintenance and predictability in the length of lease.

2. "Edible pathways": traffic interventions[a]

Increasing access and animation in public space	Contributing to social services	Producing and distributing food	Building communities to spread cultivation knowledge
Present, smaller public	Not present or reaching beyond members	Significantly present, reaching a large public	Present, smaller public

[a] http://smagpaaaarhus.dk/byhave/danmarks-maaske-laengste-jordbaerbed/

Location and Connectivity Under the "Edible pathways" project, we collect several urban agriculture initiatives (see Figs. 4.6, 4.7, and 4.8) – or interventions – aimed to complement bicycle and pedestrian paths through edible edges and zones. These are multi-departmental municipal projects along existing paths which lead out of the city toward residential areas and suburbs. They include both commute routes, where riders were cycling faster than the municipality wanted, and walking paths the municipality hoped to activate further. Edible edges together with recreation areas were supposed to slow the cyclists. As "surprise elements," they could cause the cyclists to slow down and make walkers more observant of the natural surroundings.

Management and Funding Mechanism This urban agriculture initiative is an example of top-down projects realized by the municipality, without local grassroots involvement. The interventions are facilitated by the citizen engagement team and maintained by the technical department. The team worked with the forestry department to thin the forest along bicycle paths in order to allow sun, slow bicycle traffic, and make public berry cultivation possible. The role of the citizen engagement team as facilitator of this top-down project might be seen surprising. However, the team's mandate includes not only supporting citizens' initiatives but also working across sectors and reaching out to the people. By connecting the "Edible pathways" to the "Taste Aarhus," the team could stimulate citizen awareness of edible food in the city.

Fig. 4.6 Bike lanes along fruits trees in Aarhus. (Photo: authors)

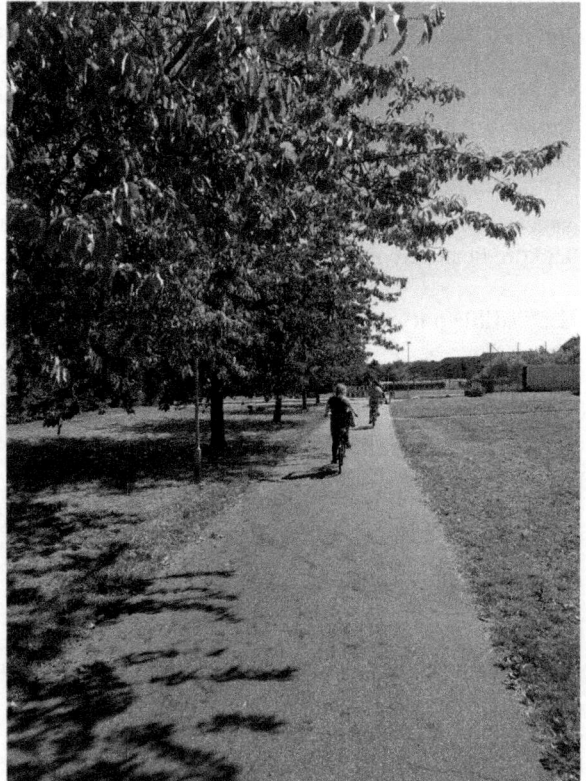

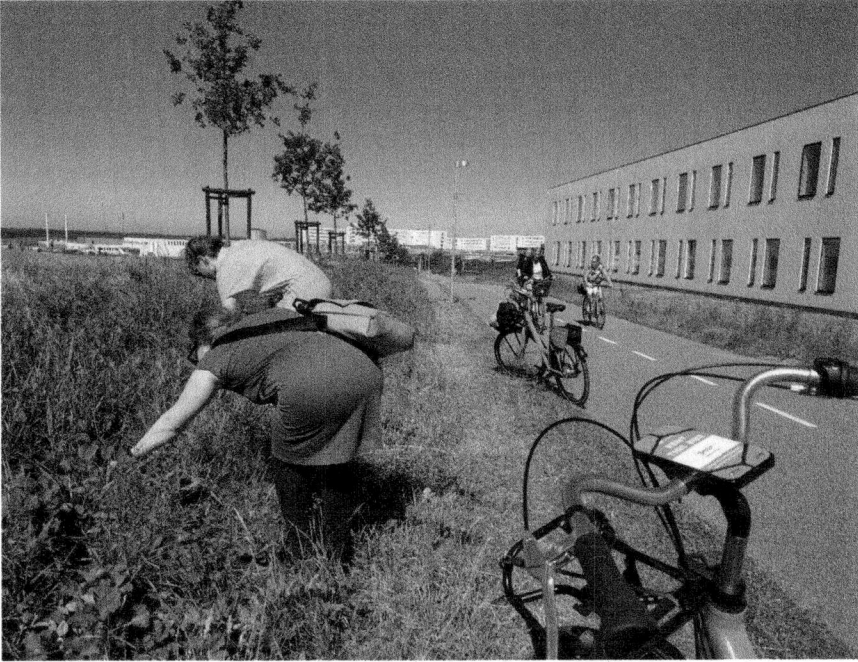

Fig. 4.7 Picking berries along the bike lane in Aarhus. (Photo: authors)

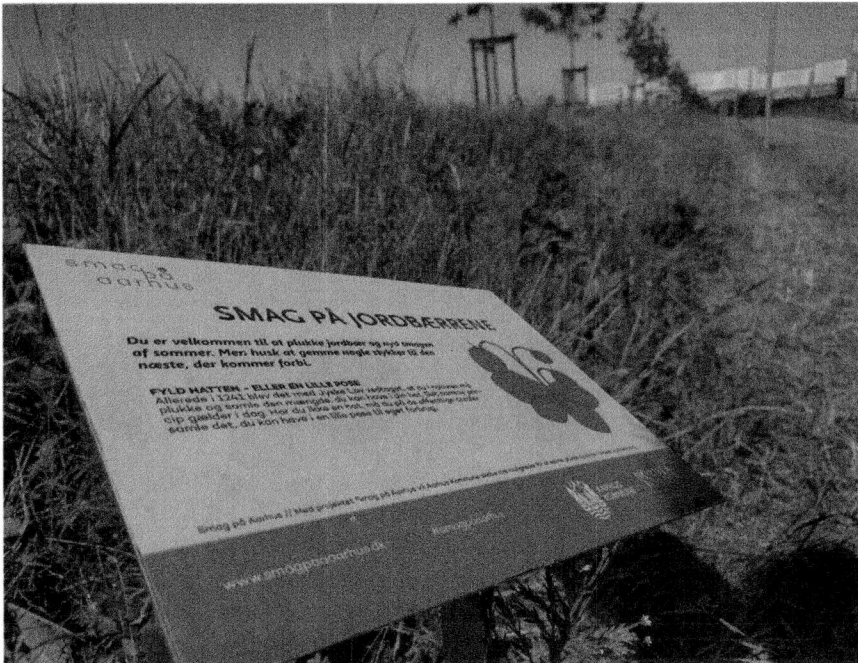

Fig. 4.8 An information board with a revised old Danish law regarding harvesting in nature. (Photo: authors)

Design and Amenities Designed by the municipality's technical department, the initiatives follow a high level of material quality. They rely on native species and plants that thrive in the wild with little maintenance. Vegetation is used both decoratively and to blend in with its surroundings, introducing or promoting edible plants corresponding to natural growth patterns. One of the interventions included a 600 m stretch of strawberries and fruit trees along a new bike path to the hospital. This edible edge was supplemented with circular planting beds with recognizable flowers and herbs. Recreational interventions alongside the path introduced a fireplace with a grill, benches, and picnic tables.

Activities The edible paths have signage to provide information to the public regarding the interventions and let people know when they can pick berries and fruits. This information includes guidelines for how much it is reasonable to harvest – an old Danish law about filling your hat is today revised to suggest you can fill a small bag with what you harvest, leaving enough for others to enjoy (see Fig. 4.8). When we were sampling the strawberries during our fieldwork, we met some friendly locals who stopped to chat while also picking berries. Some other cyclists stopped to taste the strawberries as well, and then a local school group walked across the path to use the picnic area. The bicyclists who did not stop slowed down to see what everyone was doing, showing the project's intentions at work.

Relations to the Municipal Authorities and Policies These initiatives demonstrate synergies from the combination of urban agriculture with municipal budgets aimed for other purposes – in this case bicycle safety – to create edible and multifunctional spaces. Such initiatives provide an alternative to more typical member-driven urban agriculture projects. Besides being transport corridors, the various elements of the edible paths serve as safety and social, as well as edible features in the landscape.

3. Gallo Gartneriet: Therapy through urban agriculture[a]

Increasing access and animation in public space	Contributing to social services	Producing and distributing food	Building communities to spread cultivation knowledge
●	●	●	◑
Significantly present, reaching a large public	Significantly present, reaching a large public	Significantly present, reaching a large public	Present, smaller public

[a]https://www.gallogartneriet.dk/

Location and Connectivity The garden *Gallo Gartneriet* (3531 m^2) is situated in a northern suburb of the city, next to an old train line which may soon be reactivated (Fig. 4.9). The garden is open to the public during the daytime of the growing sea-

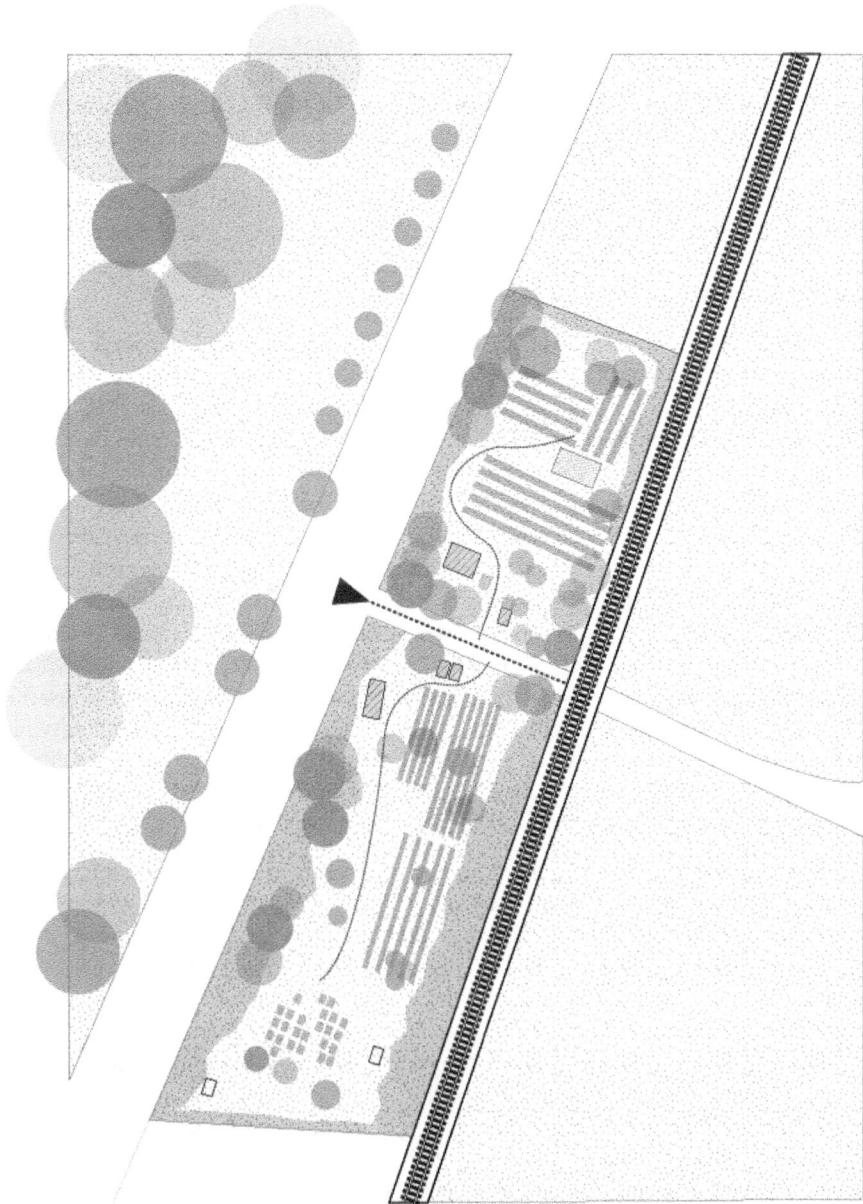

Fig. 4.9 Map of Gallo Gartneriet in Aarhus with entrances (red arrows) and paths (red dash line). (Map design: Kristin Sunde)

son, when members of the gardening community are there. It is closed at night and through the winter in order to protect tools and harvest. Some passers-by use the garden just to cross to the adjacent park or beach (see Fig. 4.12).

Management and Funding Mechanism The garden was established in 1990, originally as a part of the local psychiatric hospital to serve as a pilot project for garden therapy. At the time of our fieldwork, the hospital had moved and transferred the garden to the county, which owned it and leased it for free to the gardeners. The garden today is both a therapeutic and community garden, maintaining a portion of social program-funded volunteers and a waged coordinator to aid in reintegration and job-training skills on site. A member describes the garden as "the only place in Aarhus where people work as a community." The initiative is connected to a larger foundation with an art gallery among other things. The foundation's board is well established and meets six to eight times a year.

Around 70 people are involved in gardening activities over the season (from April to November) and 12–15 daily. The community is open for anyone to join and has different levels of membership to share produce and access. Half of the volunteers are members of the community and pay small annual membership fees which also allows them to get a 20% rebate off the garden's produce. The paid part-time coordinator position is unique to this garden and external to the "Taste Aarhus" program, funded rather by a social welfare department of the municipality. The coordinator facilitates, organizes, and helps people to collaborate, inspects the garden daily in order to check what needs to be done, hosts morning meetings, and allocates tasks. According to the informants, the salary helps to ensure continuity and consistency in leadership, though the tasks are distributed democratically among those present each day. People choose what interests them from the task list depending on skill and strength or energy required. The gardening community has a roadside kiosk where they sell their produce at affordable prices. The profits go entirely back to the operations. That is why it is so important to protect the harvests as they are vital for the financial sustainability of the garden.

Design and Amenities The garden has predominantly raised cultivation beds with hedges and fruit trees (see Figs. 4.10 and 4.11). It is a well-designed and comfortable space, even if aging and built in several phases in a DIY fashion. The whole garden has a feeling of having evolved over time with different interests represented. There is a lot of moveable seating and flexibility, making it a peaceful and comfortable place for relaxation and interaction with others. The garden also has greenhouses, toilets, and beehives run by the urban beekeepers' community *BiStad*.

Activities This garden was the only urban agriculture initiative we visited in Aarhus where food was cultivated communally by the gardeners (since 2016 there have been a limited number of individual boxes). They cultivate fruits, vegetables, herbs, and flowers in an ecological manner. The garden involves the unemployed and offers programs for youth struggling with education. The members of the community we talked to described the garden as "the best doctor" – relieving stress – and explained that the gardeners together form a warm and welcoming community. The members are helpful to provide information to the visitors, offering tours and coffee. The community hosts an open garden event a couple of times during the summer since joining the "Taste Aarhus" network. The garden facilitates socialization both between the members of the community and between the members and passers-by.

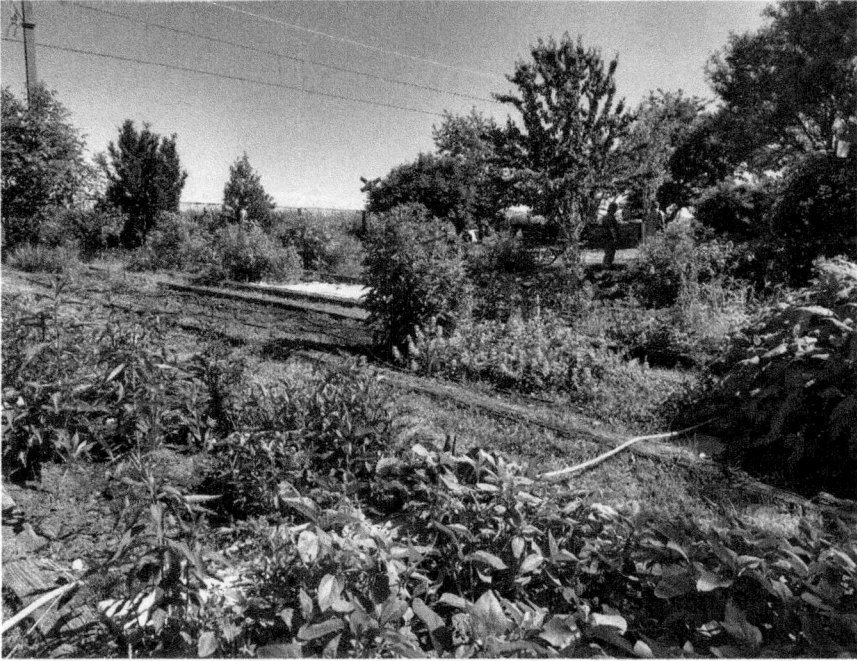

Fig. 4.10 Gallo Gartneriet initiatives in Aarhus: polyculture cultivation beds, grass paths, and a seating area under a shady cherry tree. (Photo: authors)

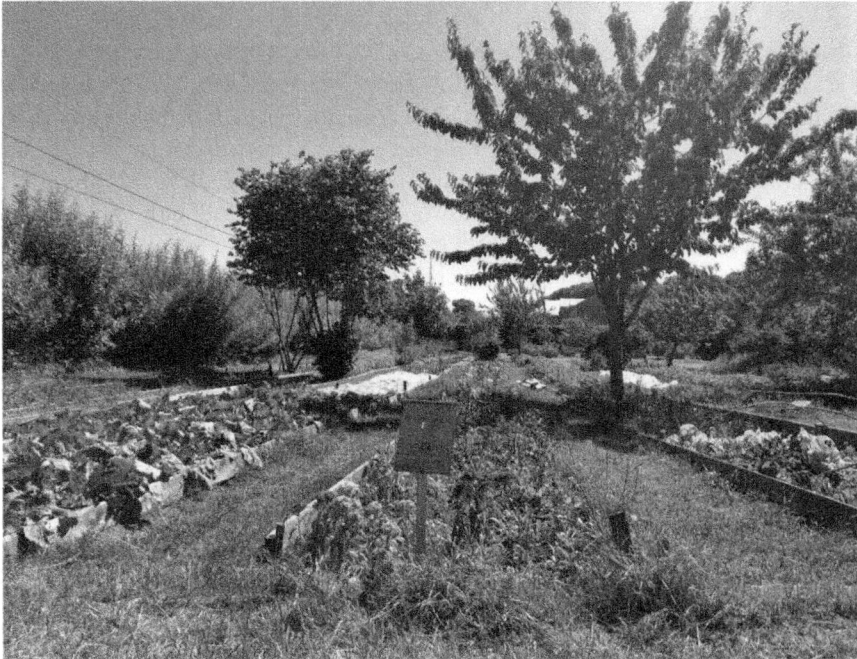

Fig. 4.11 Well-maintained cultivation beds in Gallo Gartneriet in Aarhus. (Photo: authors)

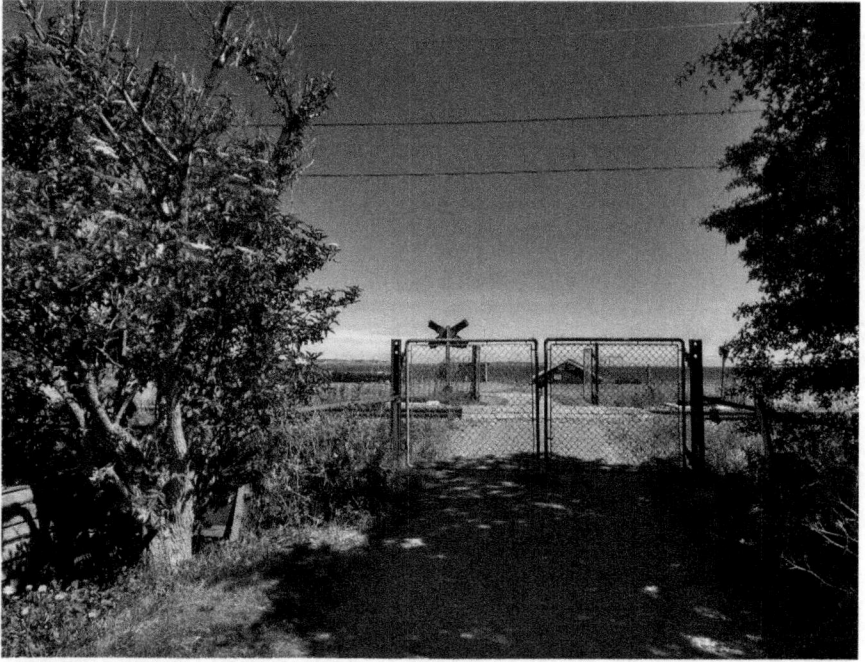

Fig. 4.12 A path from the garden to the beach through a train line. (Photo: authors)

Relations to the Municipal Authorities and Policies This garden with a 30-year history only recently joined the "Taste Aarhus" network and did not receive any financial support from them as it was not a new initiative. Other municipal departments, however, support the garden through welfare and disability funding and financing some of the volunteers. "Taste Aarhus" assists the garden with visibility and event promotion. During our fieldwork, this garden faced an uncertain future because of the pressure for land development in the area. No longer owned by the hospital, the land could be highly valuable for development due to its location. Our informants hope that the local government will help them to secure the land and provide funding to upgrade their aging toilets and equipment.

4.4 Rotterdam: Different Budgets, Different Benefits

Rotterdam has been early engaged in urban agriculture and alternative food systems movements. The municipality drafted an urban agriculture policy already in 2012 to make the city greener, but because of political change and financial difficulties, the policy has not been adopted. Urban agriculture in the city at the time of this study relied on bottom-up initiatives, was supported by different departments on a case-by-case basis, and was not covered by a specific policy or program like in Aarhus.

Our informants name several departments as particularly significant for supporting urban agriculture initiatives: city planning (land use policies), city maintenance (maintenance of public spaces), community services (well-being and social cohesion), and social affairs (employment and welfare policies). Funding of initiatives is always tied to specific outcomes (especially related to health and job creation) and requires specific reporting. On top of that, there are citywide support measures for community-based initiatives in public space[4]. The city district authorities can also support urban agriculture as part of urban renewal projects. The informants point out that the lack of coordinated activities between the departments (often run by different political parties) – coupled with a slow bureaucratic process – is a barrier to urban agriculture initiatives in the city: urban agriculture facilitation remains fragmented and inconsistent.

Urban agriculture initiatives in Rotterdam must register as foundations. These foundations then get approval from the city to use public land or land reserved for redevelopment. The municipality of Rotterdam has a policy[5] for the adoption of green spaces which gives a framework for providing land for urban agriculture initiatives. This policy outlines opportunities, rules, and available guidance. It seeks to promote voluntary maintenance of outdoor space which should, nevertheless, maintain public character and public access. The municipality keeps minimal regulations but focuses on safety, accessibility, and aesthetic qualities. According to the policy, the municipal authorities accept initiatives, including urban agriculture initiatives, in public land if they are found to be appropriate: easy to manage, have support among local residents, and are reconciled with other existing functions of the space. The policy stipulates that "in the main district structure, private initiatives that change the layout are in principle not desirable, unless they join (in image, use, material use and management) the prescribed structures" (our translation).

At the time of our fieldwork in Rotterdam, the maximum land lease time for urban agriculture initiatives was five years, which was considered not enough for serious investments. As a result, "most initiatives are not living up to their full potential" (a local researcher/urban agriculture activist). Development pressure and uncertainty regarding the future of land contracts affect how the initiatives are run and how much money and labor they invest. In the case when urban agriculture land is up for redevelopment, the municipality does not always provide a replacement plot to the initiative affected. If new land is provided, it can be of a smaller size or in a very different location.

The urban agriculture initiatives in Rotterdam we visited relied primarily on their own fundraising and membership fees. Other financial sources included social housing providers, philanthropic foundations, commercial companies, and regional banks. Social housing providers see the benefits of urban agriculture in enhancing the feeling of ownership and care important for the local residents, reducing crime,

---

[4] One relevant example is CityLab010, a support program for residents, entrepreneurs and organizations that provide a solution for social challenges in Rotterdam: https://citylab010.nl/

[5] Municipality of Rotterdam. "Bewonersinitiatieven en zelfbeheer in de buitenruimte: aanbod, spelregels en advise"

and lowering maintenance expenditures for public spaces. The municipal authorities are not so active in providing funding for urban agriculture but can support the initiatives through sources related to other municipal objectives, including welfare, integration, social inclusion, landscaping, and green space management. Our informants point out that it was easier to find funding from sources indirectly connected to urban agriculture. Hands-on support is provided by civil servants tasked with facilitating residents and social entrepreneurs. The maintenance department employs a city gardener that gives gardening advice and helps with maintenance work. It is also possible to borrow tools and equipment from the municipality.

We chose to describe four of the urban agriculture initiatives (Fig. 4.13) we studied in Rotterdam: *Tuin op de Pier*, *Rotterdamse Munt*, *Hotspot Hutspot Krootwijk*, and *Voedseltuin Rotterdam*. They do not represent all the variety of typologies of urban agriculture in the city but illustrate the span of different trajectories in how it can benefit the general public.

4. Tuin op de Pier: waterfront permaculture[a]

Increasing access and animation in public space	Contributing to social services	Producing and distributing food	Building communities to spread cultivation knowledge
●	◑	◑	◑
Significantly present, reaching a large public	Present, smaller public	Present, smaller public	Present, smaller public

[a]http://www.tuinopdepier.nl/

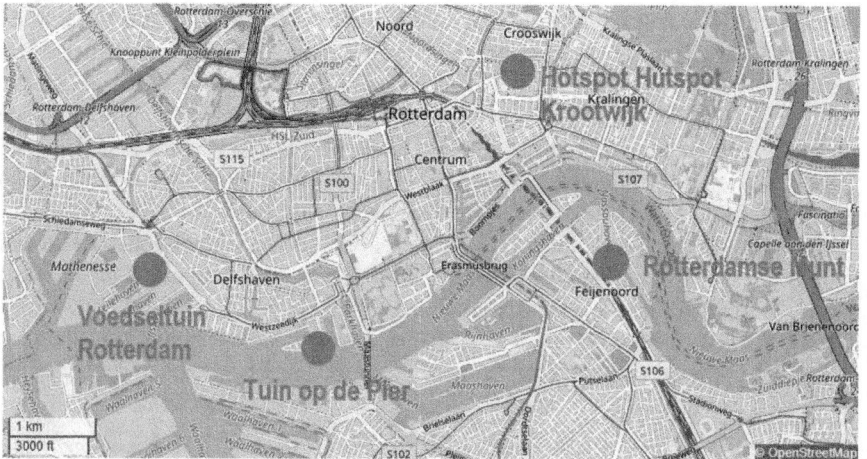

Fig. 4.13 Location of the studied urban agriculture initiatives in Rotterdam. (Basemap: OpenStreetMap)

Location and Connectivity The initiative began as a collective garden in 2011 and in June 2018 occupied a site (4500 m²) designated for future residential development (delayed due to the economic crisis) at Rotterdam's waterfront. After 2018 this urban agriculture initiative moved to another site, but the description here captures the situation during our fieldwork (see Figs. 4.14, 4.15, 4.16, and 4.17). The site was surrounded by recent residential and office buildings, a parking lot, and green space. The area was characterized by low traffic and oriented toward walking and cycling. Our informants described typical residents of the area as white and affluent. The site we visited had open access and partial fencing but no gates, thereby both visually and physically permeable for the public. The garden itself provided great views over the harbor. Together with the adjacent green space and playground, the garden was part of a bigger multifunctional area with a variety of recreational activities.

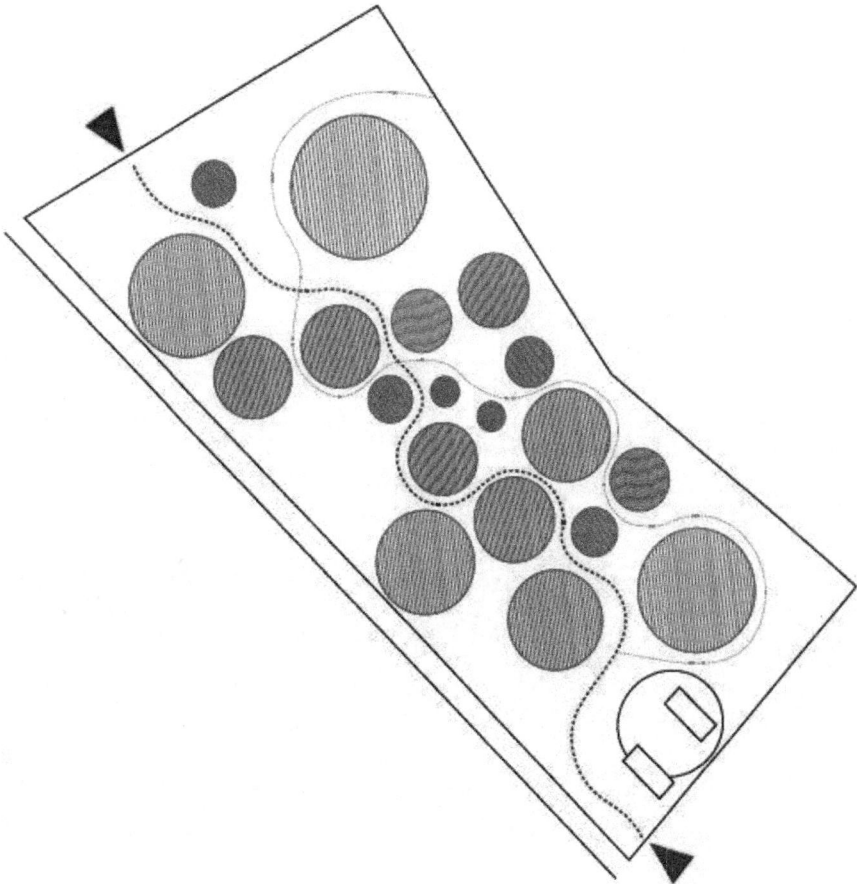

Fig. 4.14 Map of Tuin op de Pier in Rotterdam with entrances (red arrows) and paths (red dash line). (Map design: Kristin Sunde)

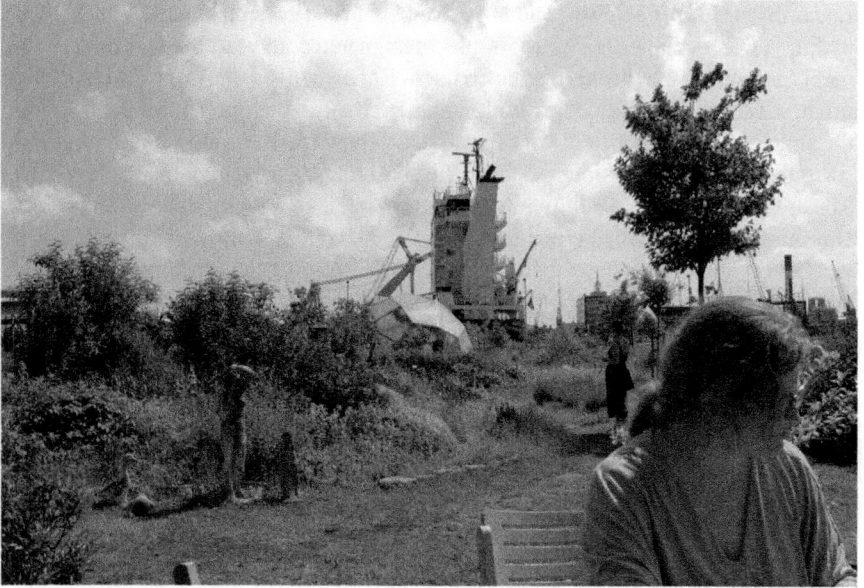

Fig. 4.15 Tuin op de Pier in Rotterdam has a variety of plants in their cultivation beds of a circular form. Surprise elements like sculptures and curiosities can be found throughout. (Photo: authors)

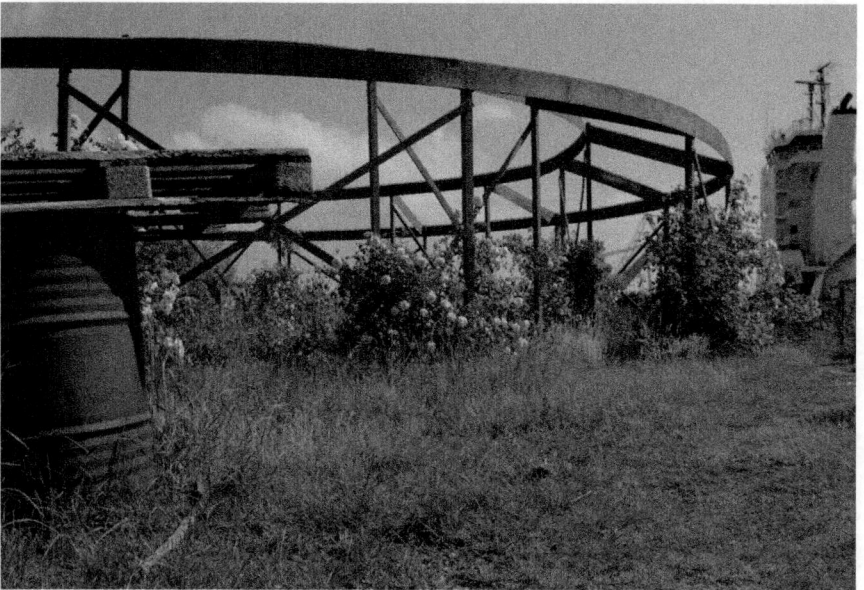

Fig. 4.16 Design elements of Tuin op de Pier in Rotterdam. (Photo: authors)

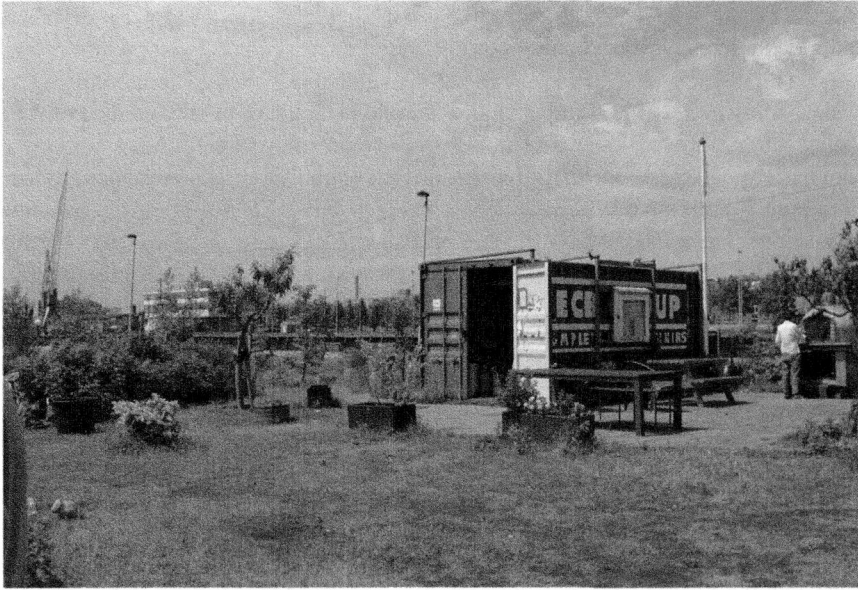

Fig. 4.17 Tuin op de Pier in Rotterdam: minimal protection from bad weather, a storage, and a pizza oven. (Photo: authors)

Management and Funding Mechanism The garden was run as a communal one – without individual allotments, with tasks shared by the 10–15 members of the urban agriculture initiative. It was managed by a foundation, whose board were residents of the neighboring high-rise (marked by above-average market prices). The land was owned by the municipal authorities, which gave permission for use through a 7-year rent-free lease contract, while the plot was awaiting development. In 2018, the site was slated for development, and the garden was preparing for relocation to a smaller (750 m²) spot nearby when we visited. The urban agriculture initiative was established through the voluntary work of members with a financial grant from a bank along with help with material and equipment loaning from the regional and municipal authorities. Maintenance was covered by membership fees and supporting business: each donated around 25€ per year in exchange for their name on the garden sign.

Design and Amenities The initiative was a designed garden focused on permaculture – an alternative to the industrial agriculture movement emphasizing eco-design principles, site specificity, and the importance of agroecological configuration (Ferguson & Lovell, 2014). The garden was designed by a member of the initiative who happened to be a landscape architect and consisted of permaculture beds, a greenhouse, sheds for storage of tools, and a pizza/bread oven. It also had a limited number of picnic tables and benches. The site lacked any lighting but was lit from the nearby areas. The design of the garden allowed the presence of loose, adaptable, and unrestricted areas that could evolve over time. Between the growing areas, there was significant space that allowed movement.

Activities Active participation in the gardening was limited to the members, although anyone was welcome to join gardening occasionally. The members grew vegetables, herbs, and flowers and took care of the garden. There were regular weekend meetings followed by joint work and socializing. A few members of the urban agriculture harvested and stored food for others to pick up when some were not available. According to our informants, the initiative facilitated socializing and community building by allowing people to get to know each other and develop relationships: "It's a place where people meet and BBQ together" (a member of the initiative). The initiative also engaged with people outside of their community. The garden held two major events per year (in December and July), attracting up to 100 visitors, and invited groups from local schools to pick strawberries. The initiative tried to reach nearby disadvantaged communities but attracted few new members, as many wanted individual plots, which the garden did not offer. The gardeners also experienced homeless labor migrants loitering and stealing harvest, despite being invited to share in the work and harvest in shorter periods.

Relations to the Municipal Authorities and Policies As mentioned by several of our informants, this initiative helped the municipality of Rotterdam to transform an earlier dumping ground associated with drug dealing and prostitution into a safe and clean area ready for redevelopment. The municipality assisted with initial soil remediation and provided access to water, but the foundation itself brought in additional soil, suitable for gardening, from local farms. The municipal authorities were not involved in the management of the initiative, except for establishing some standards for aesthetics and maintenance and sending occasional complaints if these standards were not met. As mentioned by one of the gardeners, they wanted as little involvement from the municipality as possible. In general, the initiative had a good working relationship with the municipal authorities. The initiative was a part of the "Green connection"[6] – a city walking tour used in public health and tourism promotion of Rotterdam.

5. Rotterdamse Munt: commercial herb garden[a]

Increasing access and animation in public space	Contributing to social services	Producing and distributing food	Building communities to spread cultivation knowledge
Present, smaller public	Significantly present, reaching a large public	Present, smaller public	Present, smaller public

[a]https://www.rotterdamsemunt.nl/

[6] de Groene Connectie: https://degroeneconnectie.nl/

Location and Connectivity The initiative *Rotterdamse Munt* (see Figs. 4.18, 4.19, 4.20, and 4.21) started in 2014 and occupied a spot of 4600 m² reserved for future development in a socially disadvantaged neighborhood characterized by ethnic diversity of the residents. The urban agriculture initiative moved after our visit, but in 2018, its site was surrounded by two roads with car traffic as well as bicycle paths. It was enclosed by transparent fences with barbed wire. An informant from the garden explained this decision due to a lot of vandalism and theft at a nearby allotment garden. There were only two entrances, not otherwise connected to main paths or other activities. The garden was open to the public during the afternoons a few days a week, but as pointed out by the initiative leader, few people came despite open gates and welcome signs.

Management and Funding Mechanism The garden was initiated by a social entrepreneur who gathered partners and secured funding from the authorities (on the city, regional, and national scales) and private entities, such as a bank. The garden was started as a private social enterprise managed as a foundation with one main manager. The foundation per requirements was managed by a board and paid a partial salary to one coordinator also working in the shop/café. The land was owned by the Rotterdam municipality and provided on a temporary basis. The initiative managed to negotiate a permanent contract for a larger amount of land situated nearby and positioned over a metro line that stops it from future development and moved after our visit in 2018. The garden was run on the labor of volunteers who were mainly nearby residents or social clients from the municipality. The urban agriculture initiative was envisioned as a business that sells both products produced by the garden itself and local and sustainable products from other sources. The goal of the initiative was to become self-sufficient and cover the salary for its management along with material needs (the goal had not been reached at the time of our fieldwork). The initiative also invited sponsors and had signage with sponsors' names, both public and corporate. The initiative had around 40 volunteers with

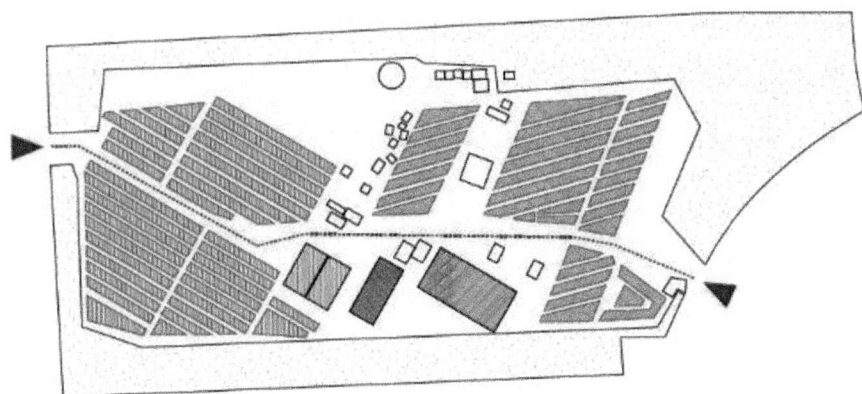

Fig. 4.18 Map of Rotterdamse Munt in Rotterdam with entrances (red arrows) and paths (red dash line). (Map design: Kristin Sunde)

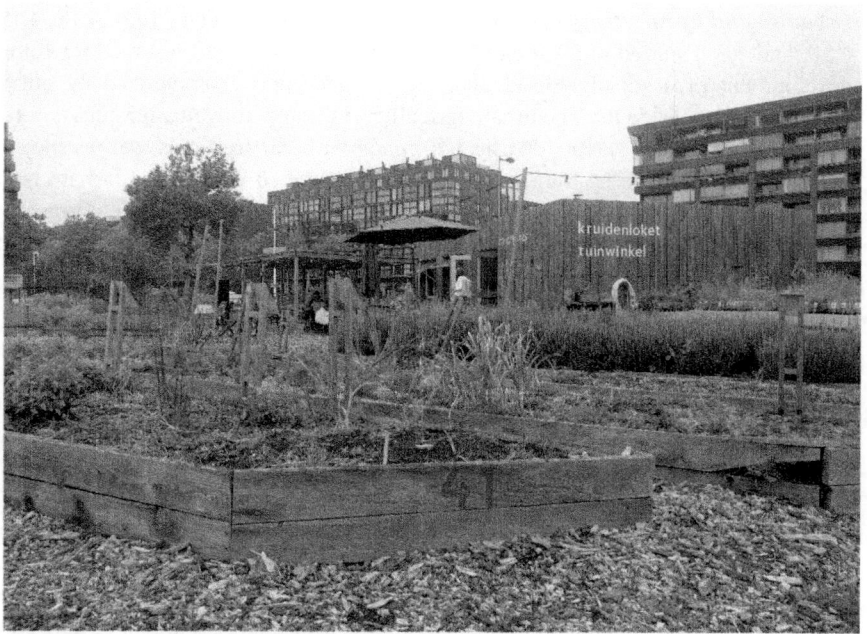

Fig. 4.19 Cultivation beds in Rotterdamse Munt in Rotterdam with a permanent shelter and a cafe/shop in the background. (Photo: authors)

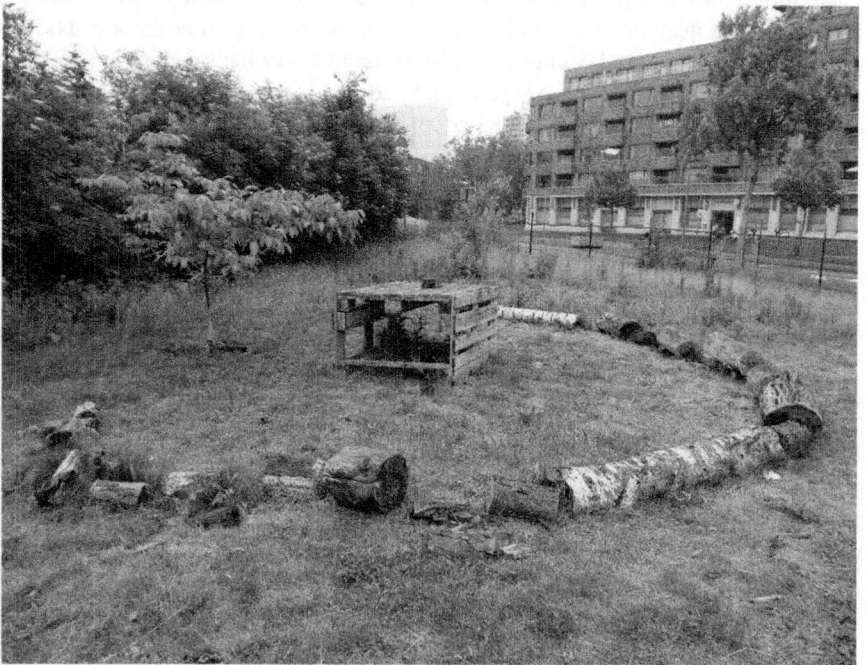

Fig. 4.20 Informal open-space seating area in Rotterdamse Munt in Rotterdam. (Photo: authors)

Fig. 4.21 An insect hotel in Rotterdamse Munt in Rotterdam. (Photo: authors)

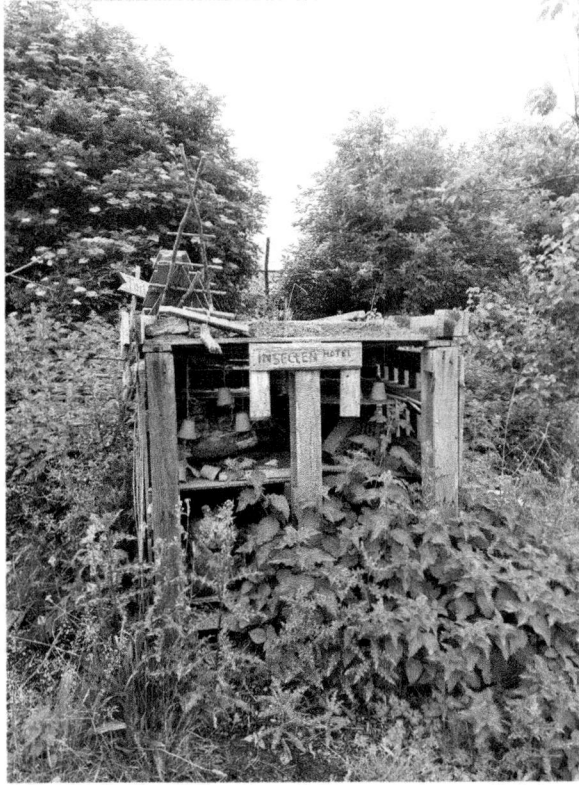

diverse backgrounds and life situations; some of them were sent for support in integrating into work life. Volunteers spent different amounts of time in the garden and usually stayed for a year each. All volunteers went through a process to become involved, including an introduction meeting, communication of expectations, and mentoring with someone more experienced.

Design and Amenities The garden was well maintained and beautifully designed with attractive solutions like clearly laid out raised beds with signage about each plant and windscreens over shipping containers. This garden demonstrated one of the ways to practice urban agriculture in an aesthetically pleasing and well-kept place. On the site, there were nicely designed beehives, greenhouses, and a shop/café with outdoor seating. The greenhouses function as space for education, plant production, and storage. There was also a sheltered gathering place for storytelling or group sessions. The visual identity was consistent in all the building cladding, down to the branding of the produce. At the same time, the space was the most controlled among all we visited during fieldwork and was strictly functionally planned. The space itself did not facilitate spontaneous interactions: it did not feel comfortable to just come in and sit in the garden without being a member or customer. There were no dedicated places for recreation aside from the gathering place and area near the café.

Activities The garden produced herbs and honey from their own beehives and sold a range of sustainable products and gardening tools. Visitors could come to clip and buy herbs or purchase dried teas and herb mixes. However, the main mission of the garden was stated as connecting people with nature, with food (by developing people's tastes), and with each other. The initiative organized events, at least two festivals a year. The initiative also held a variety of educational and social activities: they collaborated with nearby schools, organizing school visits that help to connect children to food cultivation.

Relations to the Municipal Authorities and Policies The initiative relied on the good relationship with the Rotterdam municipality for their land and some of their funding. It also worked as a provider for the city in terms of school and reintegration services. According to our informant, some volunteers were paid by the authorities (through the municipality or the Dutch employee insurance agency) for their work from reintegration or social care budgets. Our respondents reported that the garden helped to rebuild people's self-esteem and confidence: volunteers were successfully finding their jobs somewhere else after working in the garden. However, according to the manager of the garden, in municipal funding, the value of such things as rebuilding of confidence of people looking for jobs was underestimated as concrete results were difficult to report. The garden had to develop a cost-benefit analysis to demonstrate to the authorities the value of their job reintegration services.

6. Hotspot Hutspot Krootwijk: social housing enterprise[a]

Increasing access and animation in public space	Contributing to social services	Producing and distributing food	Building communities to spread cultivation knowledge
◗	●	●	●
Present, smaller public	Significantly present, reaching a large public	Significantly present, reaching a large public	Significantly present, reaching a large public

[a]https://www.hotspothutspot.nl/hotspot-hutspot-krootwijk/

Location and Connectivity The initiative started in 2017 as a common garden built in the yard of a social housing complex (see Fig. 4.22) in a marginalized neighborhood. The garden is not fenced, which was a conscious decision of the initiative even though they experience cases of vandalism and theft. The project coordinator explains: "These kids are so poor. So, if they're stealing vegetables for their families, then that's actually great."

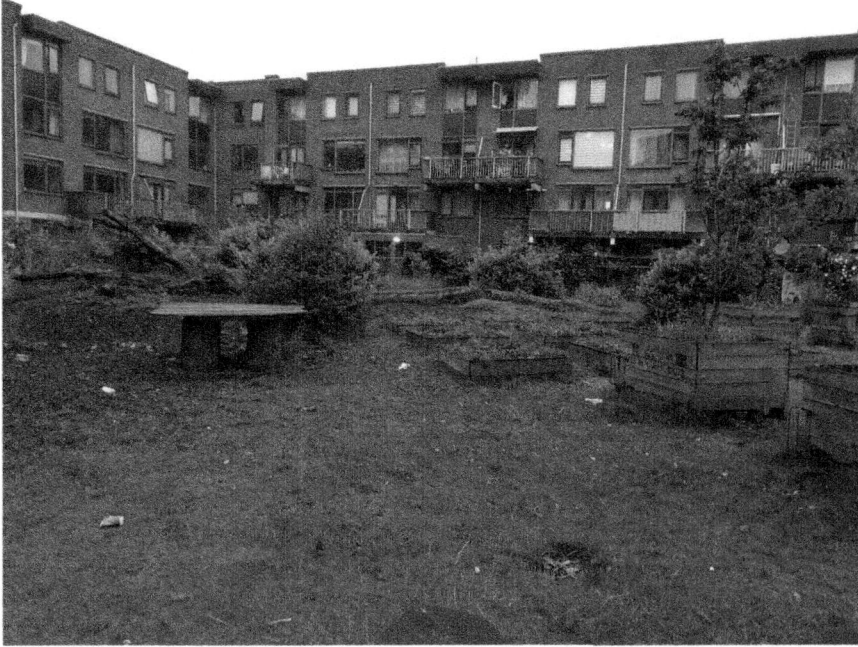

Fig. 4.22 Hotspot Hutspot Krootwijk in Rotterdam is situated in the courtyard of social housing. (Photo: authors)

Management and Funding Mechanism This initiative is one of several social enterprises in Rotterdam which combine urban agriculture with the provision of social services. It was established by an artist-activist. The initiative is financed by a variety of actors. The coordinator's salary is paid by a subsidy from the municipality's housing department, while other costs are covered by a grant given by a philanthropic organization to enhance social cohesion and participation. At the time of our fieldwork, the garden was primarily run by the project coordinator, who was also a chef in the subsidized café on the housing site. He has experience working with challenged youth and adults and engages local residents and their children in work both in the garden and in the café.

Activities This garden and café together work toward combating local social issues. The café uses produce from the garden, a nearby farm, and grocery store discards. They provide affordable warm meals for any visitor and those who cannot afford to pay eat for free. Children from the neighborhood volunteer to wait tables and help with cooking as well as gardening and learning food-related skills. The café further hosts a free library of donated books and runs different activities in the neighborhood.

7. Voedseltuin Rotterdam: the food garden[a]

Increasing access and animation in public space	Contributing to social services	Producing and distributing food	Building communities to spread cultivation knowledge
◑	●	●	●
Present, smaller public	Significantly present, reaching a large public	Significantly present, reaching a large public	Significantly present, reaching a large public

[a]https://voedseltuin.com/

Location and Connectivity The initiative started in 2010 and is the largest garden among those visited in Rotterdam. The garden (see Figs. 4.23, 4.24, and 4.25) occupies a previously vacant spot in a not-very-central area.

Management and Funding Mechanism The garden is run by a group of 45 volunteers. According to the garden's website, the initiative is both environmentally sustainable but also economically viable. The initiative invites different sponsors, listed on their website.

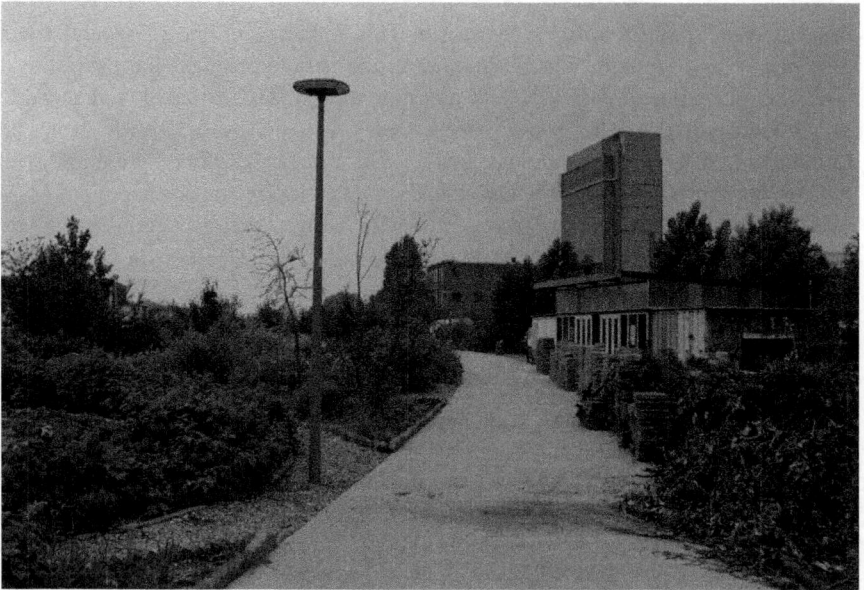

Fig. 4.23 Main path in Voedseltuin Rotterdam. (Photo: authors)

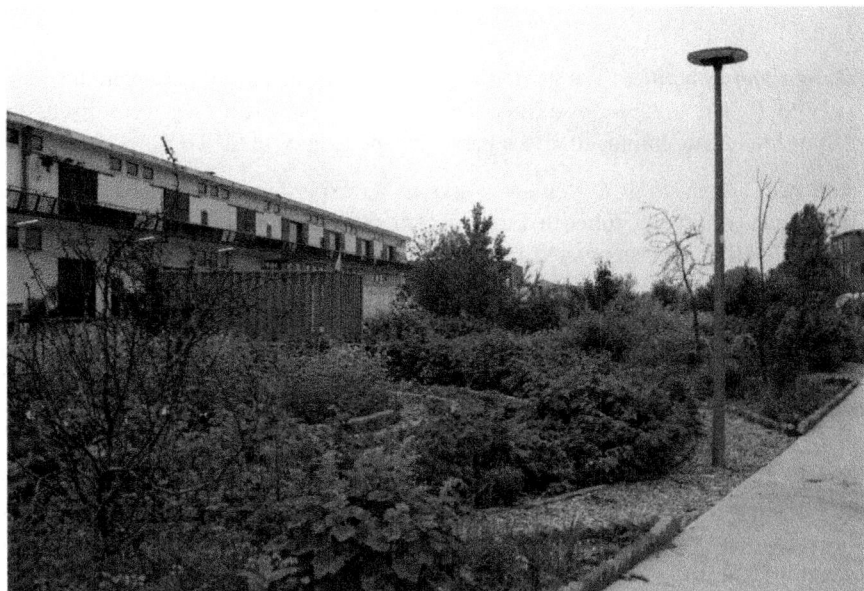

Fig. 4.24 Vegetation in Voedseltuin Rotterdam. (Photo: authors)

Figure 4.25 A seating area in Voedseltuin Rotterdam. (Photo: authors)

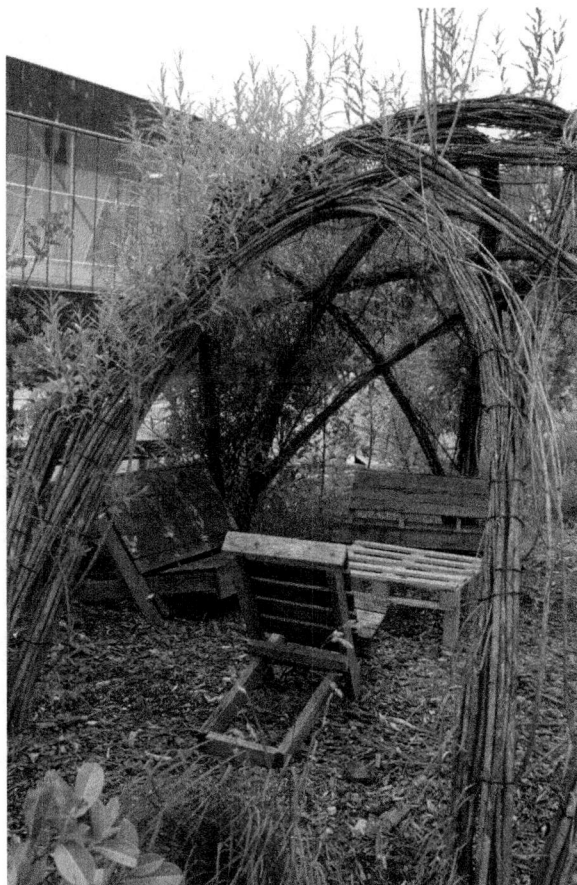

Design and Amenities The garden was run using principles of permaculture, similarly to *Tuin op de Pier* described above. During our visit, they were discussing expansion and ambitions to give a park-like appearance to the area.

Activities *Voedseltuin Rotterdam* works as an experimental space where experiments can be directly connected to new forms of gardening and food cultivation as well as welfare projects focused on the reintegration of people into work life. The garden produces fresh fruits, vegetables, and herbs for Food Bank Rotterdam,[7] which delivers free food packages to low-income households. The volunteers working in the garden were involved in construction work and growing, as well as the communication and marketing of the initiative. The initiative is also occupied with contributing to bettering the neighborhood's development.

Relations to the Municipal Authorities and Policies The initiative aims to make Rotterdam a healthy city: "We support a sustainable urban society with healthy food for everybody; without poverty and social exclusion. Working towards people who actively shape their personal lives and take responsibility for each other and for their environment" (our translation from the initiative's webpage).

4.5   Discussion: The Four Publicness Trajectories of Urban Agriculture in the City

The urban agriculture policies and initiatives described in the two previous sections show that great variation exists even in how the same municipal facilitation plays out on the ground. We saw that the Aarhus municipality developed a cohesive program focused on urban agriculture and aided gardeners by promoting existing initiatives, supporting new initiatives with funds and land negotiation, and initiating their own, top-down, urban agriculture-related projects. The initiatives described in Sect. 4.3, illustrate a variety of benefits to different publics provided by the urban agriculture – with or without municipal support. The municipality of Rotterdam lacked a cohesive urban agriculture policy but supported initiatives through land negotiation and through a variety of budgets for integrating, welfare, or green space management services. The initiatives presented in Sect. 4.4, differ in scale, organization, design, and which publics they serve.

This chapter critically examines the possibilities and trade-offs gained from integrating urban agriculture into public space, rather than providing a normative guide for how to facilitate urban agriculture. We discuss this across the cases through the four publicness trajectories identified at the beginning of this chapter: increasing access and animation in public space, contributing to social services, producing and distributing food, and building communities to spread cultivation knowledge.

---

[7] Voedselbank Rotterdam: https://voedselbank.nl/

A. **Access and animation: increasing access and animation in public space**

For Varna and Tiesdell (2010), animation "involves the degree to which the design of the place supports and meets human needs in public space, and whether it is actively used and shared by different individuals and groups" (p. 585). This trajectory of publicness is largely restricted to the people who can pass through the borders of the urban agriculture's plot and the associated public space surrounding it. The urban agriculture initiatives we studied in Aarhus and Rotterdam demonstrate a range of ways that positively affect access to, and animation in, the space they are situated. These include the following: making physical access easier for passers-by (*PIER2 Haven*), creating visually welcoming and aesthetically pleasant space (*Gallo Gartneriet, Tuin op de Pier*; see Fig. 4.26), organizing events, attracting new visitors (*Rotterdamse Munt, Tuin op de Pier*), increasing safety through regular gardener presence (*PIER2 Haven*), encouraging spontaneous interactions (*Gallo Gartneriet, "Edible pathways"*), and providing social opportunities (all).

Urban agriculture's potential to increase animation and access is especially visible in places under redevelopment, like in the cases of *PIER2 Haven* in Aarhus and *Tuin op de Pier* in Rotterdam. These qualities basically did not exist in these places before the urban agriculture initiatives activated them. As noticed by Larson (2006), urban agriculture has a potential to create sustainable communities by being a part of brownfield redevelopment processes. However, using urban agriculture as a tool in redevelopment is not unproblematic, as it can lead to gentrification in the long term, as suggested by literature devoted to green gentrification (see, e.g., Maantay and Maroko (2018)). *PIER2 Haven* and *Tuin op de Pier* can be seen as drivers and

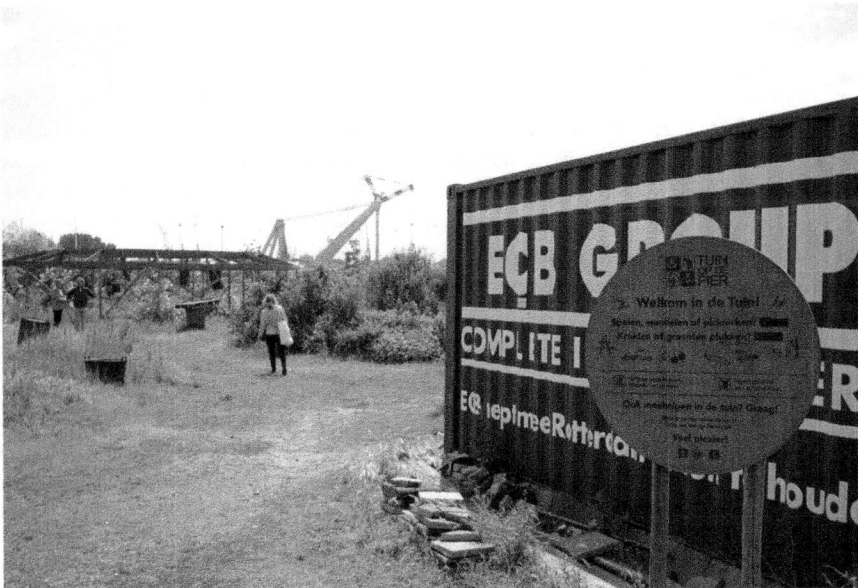

Fig. 4.26 Welcome sign and open access in Tuin op de Pier in Rotterdam. (Photo: authors)

products of gentrification, as they help attract market-rate or higher development and draw resource-strong users to previously working-class and industrial areas. Urban agriculture, nevertheless, can be both a contributor and a resistor to green gentrification (McClintock, 2018). As Sbicca (2019) reminds us, if urban agriculture supports or resists green gentrification depends on the conditions where it is realized, including the role of the municipal authorities. Here we see municipal provisions in both Aarhus and Rotterdam for urban agriculture to maintain an amount of access for all – no matter who the gardeners are. In this manner, the initiatives are prevented from fully restricting access to public space, even if the animation sparked in some initiatives may draw narrower publics than others.

B. Community: contributing to social services
In our empirical material from Aarhus and Rotterdam, we see that delivering social services, like educational and reintegration programs, is both a source of funding for urban agriculture initiatives and an argument for the municipalities to justify urban agriculture support. The provision of social services is especially vital for the survival of urban agriculture in Rotterdam, where a lack of urban agriculture-focused policy leaves financing to the creativity of initiative coordinators. In return, we see the initiatives strongest in this trajectory of publicness manage to reach a broad sector of society, including people with a variety of needs – well beyond local residents and gardeners. In this manner, the urban agriculture becomes a "public thing" – a matter of common concern, through which parts of our welfare system are exercised (Honig, 2017). This trajectory is fundamental for the essence of many – but not all – urban agriculture communities that strive to make the world a better place and frame themselves as an alternative path for societal transformation (McClintock, 2014).

Realizing urban agriculture as an agent of social services can meet some challenges, as the case of *Tuin op de Pier* in Rotterdam shows in their struggle to engage the homeless outside of a municipal mandate or funding. Additional resources, especially human resources, and comprehensive facilitation can, however, make this task more feasible, as we see in the other Rotterdam initiatives. *Rotterdamse Munt* leans heavily upon government-supported organized volunteer work for job reintegration and skill training. *Hotspot Hutspot krootwijk* was established to deal with social problems on the very local scale of the neighborhood, with assistance from the municipal housing department. *Gallo Gartneriet* in Aarhus is also interesting in this publicness trajectory because it was originally created as a therapeutic garden for people with mental challenges and has continued to provide welfare services with financial support while opening access to others interested in gardening (trajectory "Access and Animation"). Similar to findings from Oslo (see Chap. 6), the paid position of a coordinator seems to be vital for both longevity of urban agriculture and their ability to provide social services that reach a broader, city-wide public.

C. Food: producing and distributing food
Food production may be the most theorized area of municipal facilitation of urban agriculture (see, e.g., Meenar et al. (2017), Stanko ad Naylor (2018), and Thibert (2012)), but we see that it can also become a public good when the food is

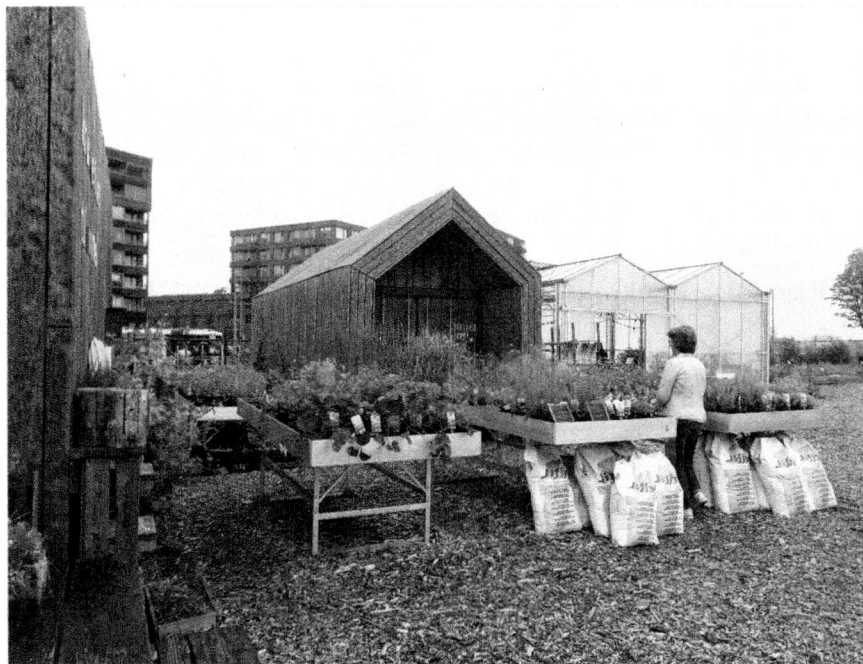

Fig. 4.27 Shop in Rotterdamse Munt. (Photo: authors)

distributed beyond the garden. The food serves as a physical but mobile link between the area of the garden, the gardeners, and the people who receive what has been produced there – extending a public beyond the physical border of the garden and broader than the group of gardeners involved in production. We see that both the Aarhus and Rotterdam municipalities view food as a by-product of urban agriculture and not as an end unto itself, as they favor other benefits. For example, the primary aim of Aarhus's *"Edible pathways"* intervention is to slow cyclists rather than strawberry production. For many urban agriculture initiatives, in contrast, food is the main motivation – *Rotterdamse Munt* is attempting to sustain itself as a commercial garden; *Gallo Gartneriet*'s produce is sold at a roadside kiosk to cover operations costs; *Voedseltuin Rotterdam* and *Hotspot Hutspot Krootwijk* began with the goal of distributing food to the poor (Fig. 4.27).

Food is a limited resource; therefore the question of distribution is crucial to assess its public benefit. Horst et al. (2017) suggest "caution in automatically conflating urban agriculture's social benefits with the goals of food justice" because "urban agriculture may reinforce and deepen societal inequities by benefitting better resourced organizations and the propertied class" (p. 277). We see this where initiatives in Aarhus largely have private boxes and produce remains within the gardening community. However, the municipality's guideline to provide publicly harvestable produce is a measure in the trajectory to increasing the public that can enjoy the produce.

We see that urban agriculture initiatives vary greatly in both the amounts of food grown and how broadly it is distributed. The initiatives that produced food beyond the gardening community clearly stand out as extending their public reach in this dimension (*Voedseltuin Rotterdam, Hotspot Hutspot Krootwijk, Gallo Gartneriet, Rotterdamse Munt*). Further, providing the produce for free or at subsidized prices appears to ensure a broader diversity of potential end users, whereas selling produce for profit narrows the potential pubic reached in this dimension (*Rotterdamse Munt*).

D. Knowledge: building communities to spread cultivation knowledge

While food itself is a limited resource, knowledge about food and cultivation can benefit an infinite number of people – reaching the broadest public out of these publicness trajectories. All initiatives we visited in Aarhus and Rotterdam contributed to disseminating cultivation knowledge in different forms, both on-site and through potentially far-reaching internet resources. For example, at *Rotterdamse Munt*, each planter box had a sign with information about plants, and their website has a shop where shipping of products is possible within all of the Netherlands. In *Tuin op de Pier* in Rotterdam, the gardeners promote permaculture by creating a special gardening place, explaining their principles online, and inviting to seasonal events. Because of the design, just being in the garden increases awareness regarding alternative ways of agriculture. Aarhus has built this dimension of publicness into their urban agriculture program, requiring all supported initiatives to host two events a year. They further support this by hosting an umbrella web resource[8] that connects all the initiatives and provides information as well as cultivation resources open to all. Even if food production has not been central, the knowledge of food cultivation is lifted as an arena to tie other qualities together and make public space with urban agriculture a matter of public concern.

4.6   The Publicness Trajectories and Capabilities

By briefly relating these four trajectories of publicness to the operationalization of Nussbaum's (2011) capabilities (see Chap. 2), we can see that the two conceptual frameworks are intertwined in attempting to define differing extents people are able to lead fulfilling lives through the use of public space in cities. Publicness here has offered us a way of framing the extent and recipients of benefit from a given public space through an urban agriculture initiative. We see that the different trajectories may reach differing extents in both breadth and number of people but also correspond to slightly different capabilities that can be offered to the public included.

The publicness trajectory "Access and Animation" is essential for publicness of urban spaces and contributes to several capabilities operationalized in the context of urban agriculture in Chap. 2: Life and Bodily Integrity (safety), Bodily Health

---

[8] http://smagpaaaarhus.dk/

(access to green spaces, good quality of outdoor areas), Senses, Imagination, Thought (qualities of design), Other Species (access to nature), and Play (cultural activities). While there are many capabilities that can be supported here, they are relatively restricted to a local presence in a specific space and specific interactions, which demand more of the details of the design and activity program of urban agriculture initiatives. The concept of access further can come into clear conflict with that of food production, where attempting to offer the capabilities connected with the trajectory "Food" may require lessening access in trajectory "Access and Animation."

Dealing with social challenges and providing social services are crucial for approaching human flourishing (see Chap. 2) and the publicness trajectory "Community" contributes to such capabilities as Bodily Integrity (crime prevention), Senses, Imagination, Thought (freedom of expression, opportunities for creativity, experience of well-being), Emotions (support of mental health, facilitation of meaningful relations with others, protecting from anxieties and fear), Practical Reason (opportunities for political engagement), and Affiliation (social inclusion, opportunities of various forms of social interactions). The social services we found approached in many urban agriculture projects presented here broaden the reach beyond one plot or demographic group, as can be a limitation among many gardening groups (Christensen et al., 2019). As we saw both in Aarhus and Rotterdam, urban agriculture initiatives can empower people and communities by enhancing their capabilities – thus contributing to social entitlements in Nussbaum's (2003) terms.

Producing and distributing food (trajectory "Food") can be identified within such capabilities in the context of urban agriculture as Bodily Health (access to local organic food), Practical Reason (bottom-up processes), and Other Species (involvement in growing food). The regulations around food production for distribution and the practicalities of food production in quantity can limit how accessible these are, defining one of the major tensions we find in urban agriculture in public space.

The publicness trajectory "Knowledge" supports several capabilities, including Senses, Imaginations, Thoughts (political activism, opportunities for creativity), Practical Reason (bottom-up processes, citizens' participation), Other Species (relation to nature), and Control over One's Environment (influence on physical settings). Here, urban agriculture initiatives can have much broader impacts, even to international publics from the activities they have in a singular, localized space.

Urban agriculture in public space becomes a resource for supporting these capabilities to different publics that can participate. This chapter clearly illustrates that the capabilities cannot be taken for granted as automatically growing from including urban agriculture in public space. They are possibilities for some that in certain situations exclude other people and possibilities. Both the organization and ground operations of each initiative and facilitation and regulation by municipal agencies must work together to maximize benefits to the majority, if not all users.

4.7 Concluding Remarks: Publicness Trade-Offs

In our research, we found that urban agriculture can contribute to a vast variety of benefits to different publics, reaching well beyond the boundaries of the garden. With urban agriculture, public spaces can engage in municipal and even international goals offering capabilities to both gardeners and more extensive publics. However, the different ways that urban agriculture can benefit external secondary and tertiary users (Eason, 1989) can come into conflict with its primary users – urban gardeners. In the urban agriculture contexts of Aarhus and Rotterdam, we identify both trade-offs and synergies between different urban agriculture benefits, as well as the extent benefits from one urban agriculture site may reach. We see that both food production and social services can lead to reducing access and animation within urban agriculture, as they produce particular needs for controlling access.

High levels of animation and easy and welcoming access are the starting point for most literature and normative goals for public space. We see that while they may come at the cost of what the space can produce, these qualities do contribute to the number of people exposed to cultivation knowledge – even without becoming active gardeners. This chapter offers a variety of trajectories for understanding what publicness can mean in urban space, allowing that inaccessible spaces may also provide public benefits. Retaining a balance and variety of publics served by urban spaces appears to be key for urban agriculture to contribute to a wide range of capabilities in a city.

Further study could attempt to understand the trade-offs between internal benefits, like the sense of community and personal growth and health, against the wider public benefits that this study has sought to bring forward. One may begin with a hypothesis acknowledged in public space literature (see, e.g., Hajer and Reijndorp (2001)), that the less intimate the space, the harder it may be to establish close and tight connections – highly animated urban agriculture projects may also struggle with supporting community and personal benefits.

How urban agriculture initiatives function in public space is complex, context-dependent, and defies simple normative or policy solutions. This anthology starts to point at a handful of potentially beneficial policy measures. To support human flourishing on the individual and community levels (see Chap. 2), cities need a variety of public spaces and urban agriculture initiatives that can alternately support internal relationships and reach out with a variety of public benefits. Not every urban agriculture project needs to be a physically accessible and inviting public space in order to benefit local society and support capabilities at personal, interpersonal, and societal levels. There are multiple ways that urban agriculture in public spaces can reach out to different publics, demonstrating that there are paths to publicness and capability building that can include physical fences and locks.

Acknowledgments This chapter acknowledges research assistants Abel Crawford and Kristin Sunde for their participation in fieldwork and data analysis. Co-authors of other project articles that helped develop some of the thoughts presented here are Peter Parker, Margot Hermus, Inger-Lise Saglie, and Beata Sirowy.

References

Audate, P. P., Cloutier, G., & Lebel, A. (2022). Role of urban agriculture in the space-to-place transformation: Case study in two deprived neighborhoods, Haiti. *Cities, 127*, 103726. https://doi.org/10.1016/j.cities.2022.103726

Christensen, S., Malberg Dyg, P., & Allenberg, K. (2019). Urban community gardening, social capital, and "integration"–a mixed method exploration of urban "integration-gardening" in Copenhagen, Denmark. *Local Environment, 24*(3), 231–248.

Dubois, V. (2015). Critical policy ethnography. In F. Fischer, D. Torgerson, A. Durnová, & M. Orsini (Eds.), *Handbook of critical policy studies* (pp. 462–480). Edward Elgar.

Eason, K. D. (1989). *Information technology and organisational change*. CRC Press.

Eidelman, T. A., & Safransky, S. (2021). The urban commons: A keyword essay. *Urban Geography, 42*(6), 792–811. https://doi.org/10.1080/02723638.2020.1742466

Feinberg, A., Ghorbani, A., & Herder, P. (2021). Diversity and challenges of the urban commons: A comprehensive review. *International Journal of the Commons, 15*(1), 1–20. https://doi.org/10.5334/ijc.1033

Ferguson, R. S., & Lovell, S. T. (2014). Permaculture for agroecology: Design, movement, practice, and worldview. A review. *Agronomy for Sustainable Development, 34*(2), 251–274. https://doi.org/10.1007/s13593-013-0181-6

Gehl, J. (2010). *Cities for people*. Island Press.

Hajer, M. A., & Reijndorp, A. (2001). *In search of new public domain: Analysis and strategy*. NAi Publishers.

Honig, B. (2017). *Public things: Democracy in disrepair*. Fordham University Press.

Horst, M., McClintock, N., & Hoey, L. (2017). The intersection of planning, urban agriculture, and food justice: A review of the literature. *Journal of the American Planning Association, 83*(3), 277–295. https://doi.org/10.1080/01944363.2017.1322914

Kirby, C. K., Specht, K., Fox-Kämper, R., Hawes, J. K., Cohen, N., Caputo, S., Ilieva, R. T., Lelièvre, A., Poniży, L., & Schoen, V. (2021). Differences in motivations and social impacts across urban agriculture types: Case studies in Europe and the US. *Landscape and Urban Planning, 212*, 104110. https://doi.org/10.1016/j.landurbplan.2021.104110

Kohn, M. (2004). *Brave new neighborhoods: The privatization of public space*. Routledge.

Langstraat, F., & Van Melik, R. (2013). Challenging the 'end of public space': A comparative analysis of publicness in British and Dutch urban spaces. *Journal of Urban Design, 18*(3), 429–448. https://doi.org/10.1080/13574809.2013.800451

Larson, J. T. (2006). A comparative study of community garden systems in Germany and the United States and their role in creating sustainable communities. *Arboricultural Journal, 29*(2), 121–141. https://doi.org/10.1080/03071375.2006.9747450

Maantay, J. A., & Maroko, A. R. (2018). Brownfields to greenfields: Environmental justice versus environmental gentrification. *International Journal of Environmental Research and Public Health, 15*(10), 2233. https://doi.org/10.3390/ijerph15102233

Madanipour, A. (1999). Why are the design and development of public spaces significant for cities? *Environment and planning B: Planning and Design, 26*(6), 879–891. https://doi.org/10.1068/b260879

McClintock, N. (2014). Radical, reformist, and garden-variety neoliberal: Coming to terms with urban agriculture's contradictions. *Local Environment, 19*(2), 147–171. https://doi.org/10.1080/13549839.2012.752797

McClintock, N. (2018). Cultivating (a) sustainability capital: Urban agriculture, ecogentrification, and the uneven valorization of social reproduction. *Annals of the American Association of Geographers, 108*(2), 579–590. https://doi.org/10.1080/24694452.2017.1365582

McNutt, P. (2000). Public goods and club goods. In B. Bouckaert & G. de Geest (Eds.), *Encyclopedia of law and economics* (Vol. 1, pp. 927–951). Edward Elgar.

Meenar, M., Morales, A., & Bonarek, L. (2017). Regulatory practices of urban agriculture: A connection to planning and policy. *Journal of the American Planning Association, 83*(4), 389–403. https://doi.org/10.1080/01944363.2017.1369359

Murphy, M. A., Parker, P., & Hermus, M. (2022). Cultivating inclusive public space with urban gardens. *Local Environment, 28*(1), 99–116. https://doi.org/10.1080/13549839.2022.2120461

Murphy, M. A., Sirowy, B., & Saglie, I.-L. (Unpublished manuscript). *Urban agriculture and the political publicness of urban space.*

Németh, J., & Schmidt, S. (2011). The privatization of public space: Modeling and measuring publicness. *Environment and planning B: Planning and Design, 38*(1), 5–23. https://doi.org/10.1068/b36057

Nussbaum, M. (2003). Capabilities as fundamental entitlements: Sen and social justice. *Feminist Economics, 9*(2–3), 33–59. https://doi.org/10.1080/1354570022000077926

Nussbaum, M. C. (2011). *Creating capabilities.* Harvard University Press.

Sbicca, J. (2019). Urban agriculture, revalorization, and green gentrification in Denver, Colorado. *Research in Political Sociology, 26*(The Politics of Land), 149–170. https://doi.org/10.1108/S0895-993520190000026011

Stanko, H., & Naylor, L. (2018). Facilitating (?) urban agriculture in Philadelphia: Sustainability narratives in the inequitable city. *Local Environment, 23*(4), 468–484. https://doi.org/10.1080/13549839.2018.1431615

Thibert, J. (2012). Making local planning work for urban agriculture in the North American context: A view from the ground. *Journal of Planning Education and Research, 32*(3), 349–357. https://doi.org/10.1177/0739456X11431692

Tornaghi, C., & Knierbein, S. (2014). *Public space and relational perspectives.* Taylor & Francis.

Varna, G., & Tiesdell, S. (2010). Assessing the publicness of public space: The star model of publicness. *Journal of Urban Design, 15*(4), 575–598. https://doi.org/10.1080/13574809.2010.502350

Warren, E., Hawkesworth, S., & Knai, C. (2015). Investigating the association between urban agriculture and food security, dietary diversity, and nutritional status: A systematic literature review. *Food Policy, 53*, 54–66. https://doi.org/10.1016/j.foodpol.2015.03.004

Webster, C. (2007). Property rights, public space and urban design. *The Town Planning Review, 78*(1), 81–101. https://doi.org/10.3828/tpr.78.1.6

Chapter 5
The Rise and Fall of Public Urban Gardens: Four Cases from in and around Copenhagen

Bettina Lamm and Anne Tietjen

5.1 Introduction

Over the last 15 years, a great number of urban gardens have emerged in Copenhagen and other cities in Denmark. These gardens have introduced into the city fabric new spatial aesthetics and social practices around the process of vegetable production. The main components of these spaces are plants and soil in raised planters built from recycled euro pallets, seating, compost bins, and toolsheds.

In the Western world, urban gardens and other temporary urban spatial projects have become a visually recognisable typology across urban areas (Skytt-Larsen et al., 2022). Urban gardens have often sprung up on vacant lots and cracks in the urban fabric and have given room to a style of management and maintenance that differs radically from those used in traditional urban open spaces. In addition to aesthetics and materiality, they share approaches and visions, not only about how we can grow food but also about how cultivating food can be a vehicle for social collective activities in public spaces. The process of growing greens can be a metaphor for and at the same time a concrete measure for nurturing and cultivating living things – including plants, animals, humans, and communities.

Many of the urban gardens are run by groups of cultural activists committed to creating a greener and more socially just city through bottom-up initiatives and experimentation with urban form-making. They share visions of how we can grow and harvest our own vegetables and how gardening practices can become meaningful activities in the city. The place-making and social dimensions of urban gardening, along with visions for greening the city and local food production, are driving forces behind many urban gardening projects. Other practical and political agendas are the promotion of regenerative nature management methods and permaculture.

B. Lamm (✉) · A. Tietjen
University of Copenhagen, Copenhagen, Denmark
e-mail: bela@ign.ku.dk

© The Author(s) 2024
B. Sirowy, D. Ruggeri (eds.), *Urban Agriculture in Public Space*, GeoJournal Library 132, https://doi.org/10.1007/978-3-031-41550-0_5

Other urban gardens are created and operated by cities, developers, and organisations to support a variety of strategies, from urban transformation and cultivating new neighbourhoods to public participation and social cohesion. Across Danish cities, urban gardens are used as strategic tool in urban planning and policy (Jensen et al., 2012). Public, private and civic organisations have learned from the knowledge gathered through the activist-driven urban gardening practices: how to design and manage space, cultivate atmosphere, do citizen outreach, and facilitate participation. Urban gardens have proved their worth as a way to achieve political objectives, such as creating citizenship, green and social regeneration of residential areas, citizen volunteering, good neighbourliness, and temporary activation of vacant sites (Jensen et al., 2012).

In 2015, the City of Copenhagen launched a decade long vision for public urban life 'Fællesskab København' (Copenhagen in Common) that aimed to cocreate 'a living city', 'a city with an edge', and a responsible city' (Københavns Kommune, 2015a). That year – and clearly intended as a part of this vision – the city published a handbook for how to start an urban garden on private or public vacant lots, or as a part of existing public spaces (Københavns Kommune, 2015b). The publication marked the culmination of a wave of new common urban gardens in Copenhagen. It also outlined some of the many challenges that public urban gardens can face in the city, from finding and legally renting a plot and organising initiatives to meeting public access requirements and cleaning up pollution.

This book chapter presents the story of four urban gardens in and around Copenhagen, Denmark started between 2011 and 2013. All four urban gardens were community-driven and open to the public but varied widely in their organisation, management, funding, and urban contexts. Two of these urban gardens were bottom-up citizen initiatives, while the two others were part of formal urban development; one was started by a private developer and the other was part of a municipal area renewal project.

The authors were particularly interested in the agendas pursued by the communities who manage the urban gardens, how these agendas relate to the specific site and context, and how the urban garden initiators negotiated demands for public access while creating a lasting urban gardening community. After 4 to 6 years, both of the bottom-up initiatives had ended, so it is relevant to look into what resources were needed to run the urban gardens and what might have led to their closure. The chapter borrows from the authors' direct knowledge of the cases and from various written and online sources.

5.2   Urban Agriculture Cases

Prags Have, PB43, Copenhagen 2011–2015
Byhaven 2200, Nørrebro Park, Copenhagen 2012–2018
Havnehaverne, Opdagelsen, Søndre Havn, Køge 2013 – ongoing
Byhaven, Sundholm, Copenhagen 2013 – ongoing

5.2.1 *Prags Have*

Prags Have (translated Prags Garden) was a temporary urban garden and common space occupying a post-industrial site in the Amager Øst district of Copenhagen that operated between 2011 and 2015. Owned by the Dutch Akzo Nobel, the former Sadolin factory was leased to the cultural entrepreneurs 'Giv rum' that transformed the site into the shared community PB43 hosting creative startups, cultural collaborative activities, as well as the urban garden Prags Have (Andersen & Toft-Jensen, 2012).

The garden was started by a self-organised group of ten committed students and cultural activists, who poured all their creative energy into creating and running the place. None of the initiators had any green competencies but had experience and skills around community building, cultural management, and urban design. Their main agenda was to create an urban practice that could involve local citizens, and they were interested in the shared spatial practices that the garden could become a catalyst for (Andersen & Toft-Jensen, 2012). Though privately owned, Prags Have ran as an open community space with full public access. So that more people would get involved in the day-to-day management, the group formed a citizen association with the aim to be replaced later on by a local citizen association.

Prags Have covered a 230-square-metre triangular site. The 140 planting boxes were built from euro pallets that could be moved around easily to enable the constant reorganisation of the garden and to elevate the planting areas from ground soil. Other amenities included a kitchen, seating areas, shrubs, hedges, a tree house, a chicken coop, and a soil pile. As there was no ownership of the individual planting beds, everyone could participate in growing and harvesting the crops. The produce would either be consumed on-site at community dinners or sold to raise money to support activities in the garden.

Prags Have hosted numerous social events inviting local people and others interested in joining planting days, educational workshops, and community dinners advertised via Facebook events and posters placed around the neighbourhood (Prags Have FB). As the initiators had limited gardening skills, the process of building and cultivating the urban garden became a shared learning experience.

The events attracted some local residents and especially children from neighbouring social housing estates were drawn to the garden and used it as a playground. However, most of the participants in gardening and community dinners were residents of Copenhagen who shared the founders' interest in creative approaches to city-making and urban events, and were attracted by the garden's aesthetics and its successful social gatherings.

With their strong vision for Prags Have, the project initiators managed to create an urban garden that was loved by many and served as a model for how to organise and run community activities. The atmosphere was welcoming, and a large crowd of visitors attended the organised events or hung out informally in the space. Prags Have also hosted activities for the local municipal office, as the garden matched their agenda for increasing spatial and social activities in the neighbourhood. Only the production of vegetables proved to be inconsistent, perhaps because no one had clear responsibility over specific planting boxes. Moreover, projects often started but were not followed upon, and it could prove difficult for newcomers to join and participate in the gardening process.

The urban gardeners wanted to put their energy into community building and gardening but spent most of their time addressing technical and legal challenges around soil conditions or fundraising. The discovery of ground contamination proved challenging to solve. While the Copenhagen municipality supported Prags Have as part of a greater urban strategy, its regulations demanded sudden new and costly measures to address surface coverage, accessibility, and more (Andersen & Toft-Jensen, 2012).

The spatial practices of Prags Have were a tool for collaboration and negotiation both within the urban gardening community and its space and within the external world through fundraising, communication, applications, and the establishing of a dialogue with municipalities, land owners, and neighbours around legal issues and access considerations.

Overwhelmed by administrative challenges and being unsuccessful in establishing a sustainable local group that could take over, the founders eventually ran out of steam. Many looked for more stable jobs, started families, and were unable to help with time- and resource-consuming gardening, facilitation, and management tasks. For the founders, the garden was a stepping stone into positions in the cultural sphere, art world, or urban development. Prags Have also inspired many new community garden projects that had the social and cultural collective as the main driver.

In 2015, 4 years after it started, Prags Have hosted for a few months a school called 'Den Grønne Friskole' (Green Free School), bringing new life into the space. Eventually, the Pelican self-storage company bought the site and tore down all existing structures and gardens to establish a warehouse (Prags Have FB) (Figs. 5.1 and 5.2).

5.2.2   Byhaven 2200

Byhaven 2200 was an urban community garden located in a public park in the dense city district of Nørrebro in Copenhagen. As a bottom-up initiative. 'Byhaven 2200' began in 2012 with the creation of an association that shaped the visions and regulations for a community garden that remained active until 2018 (Urbangardening.dk).

The location of Byhaven 2200 was unusual, as the garden was built in the former dog area within the public green park 'Ny Nørrebroparken'. The materiality, detailing, and processes were a contrast to the surrounding park, yet it fitted, as the park was divided into smaller sections to make room for different programs and community initiatives. Byhaven received permission from the municipality to use the public space in exchange for an assurance that the garden would be publicly accessible and welcome all following the municipal requirements for urban gardens on publicly owned land (Københavns Kommune, 2015b).

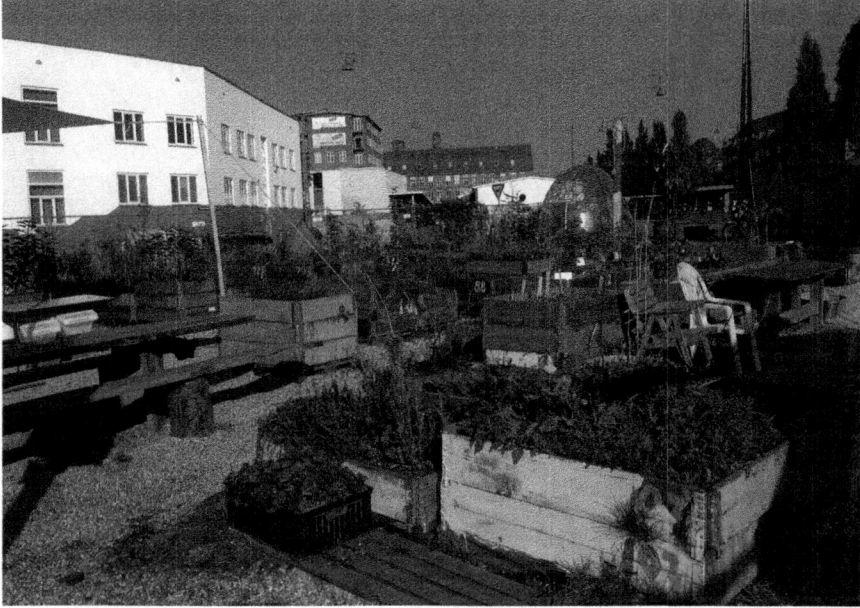

Fig. 5.1 Prags Have sat on a corner site furnished with an eclectic collection of colourful planting beds and a rich variation of seating possibilities. (Photo: Bettina Lamm)

The garden space consisted of 20 DIY (do-it-yourself) raised planting beds built in uneven shapes from half-round barked rafters 'skiers' (Dolleris 2014a). Other features included a pizza oven, a toolshed, water tanks, compost site, various seating arrangements, and many small self-built projects. The garden was a gathering place for urban farming enthusiasts and a source of inspiration for initiatives around permaculture gardening and community building (Urbangardening.dk).

Run by a citizens' association, Byhaven 2200 was based on nine principles informed by permaculture theories and practices that through the cultivation of plants, and ethics of stewardship aim to contribute positively to the local environment and community (Byhaven 2200, Dolleris 2014b).

Every Saturday, Byhaven hosted well-attended gardening workdays open to everyone. Besides gardening, the space served as a hub for social events around pizza making and music. Much effort went into discussing management practices, how to organise the working days, how to communicate and recruit gardeners, and how to distribute maintenance tasks. Educational signs explaining what was in the planting boxes and how they should be cared for were placed across the garden and planting beds. A key concern became the sharing of workload across volunteers, as participants often seemed more interested in socialising than in gardening.

The garden's popularity as a public space and hang-out area proved to be a challenge, with different needs, expectations to be addressed. The agreement with the

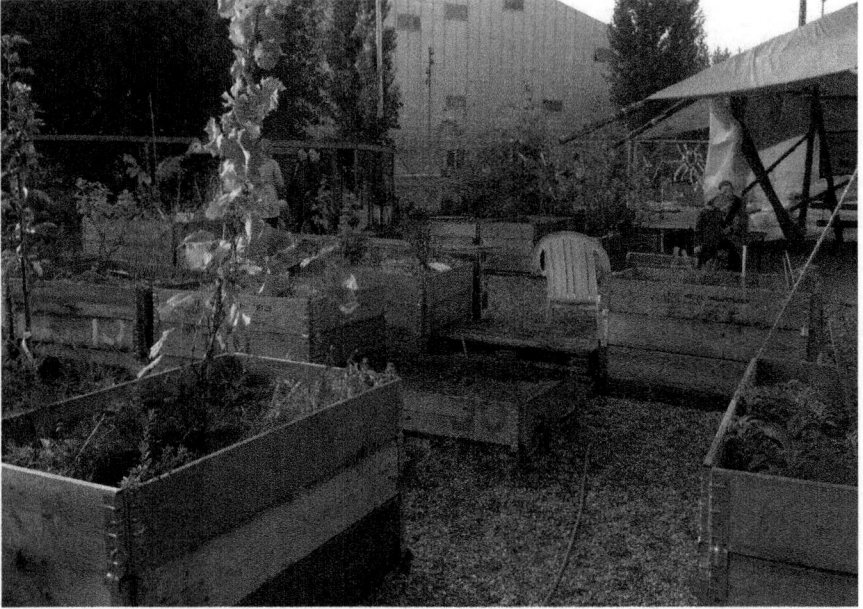

Fig. 5.2 The ground surface of Prags Have had to be covered with a membrane with pebbles on the top to protect against the polluted soil beneath. This required ample time and economic resources. (Photo: Bettina Lamm)

municipality was that the site would be accessible to all and become one of the park's public areas. The publicness goal was consistent with Byhaven's visions of community and inclusivity, and an important question was how to accommodate the more vulnerable groups of citizens minimizing potential conflicts with other user groups. With its material and aesthetic variations of planting beds, colours and vegetation, and cosy corners and seating, the garden became a home base for many individuals who could not find space elsewhere.

The nine permaculture-inspired principles were supplemented by a list of ten more practical 'commandments' to inform people's conduct and behaviour in the garden, including keeping a good tone, disposing of trash, not urinating in the garden, and keeping dogs calm (Poveda 2015). Obviously, there were challenges around how to be in and care for the garden. Pee, dogs, cleaning up, trash, substance abuse, and a sense of unsafety became themes that the garden group had to consider in their gardening visions.

In 2018, due to a lack of resources, Byhaven 2200 finally closed, and its plants and built elements were removed (urbangardening.dk). Without a core group that would commit to the continuous management of the garden, including handling contracts with the city, the site was eventually bulldozed by the municipality of Copenhagen (Tantrumpanda 2019). In a slightly ironic paper, garden activist Tantrumpanda observed that Byhaven 2200 had many 'likes' but not enough local committed participants as many had moved since the garden's inception. He also commented about people's interest in so many other things beyond gardening:

You are in an urban garden, but you really want to have a farm. [...] You are in an urban garden, but you really want to do interviews for your university. [...] You are in an urban garden, but you really want to play guitar. [...] You are in an urban garden, but you really want to make pizza.
    (Tantrumpanda 2019)

As the first urban garden to become nestled in a public urban park, Byhaven 2200 illustrated how spatial practices can connect and create community within the citiy's public spaces. It also showed that managing and tending to an urban garden requires resources that go well beyond what is available in an exclusively volunteer-run project (Figs. 5.3 and 5.4).

5.2.3   Byhaven Sundholm

Sundholm district is an area where several municipal institutions that host different spaces, resources, and activities for some of the city's most vulnerable citizens are located. Amidst this historic district, in 2013 the municipal area regeneration agency, in close collaboration with the adjacent activity centre for vulnerable citizens and municipal social service, established the urban garden Byhaven Sundholm (Konradsen et al., 2013).

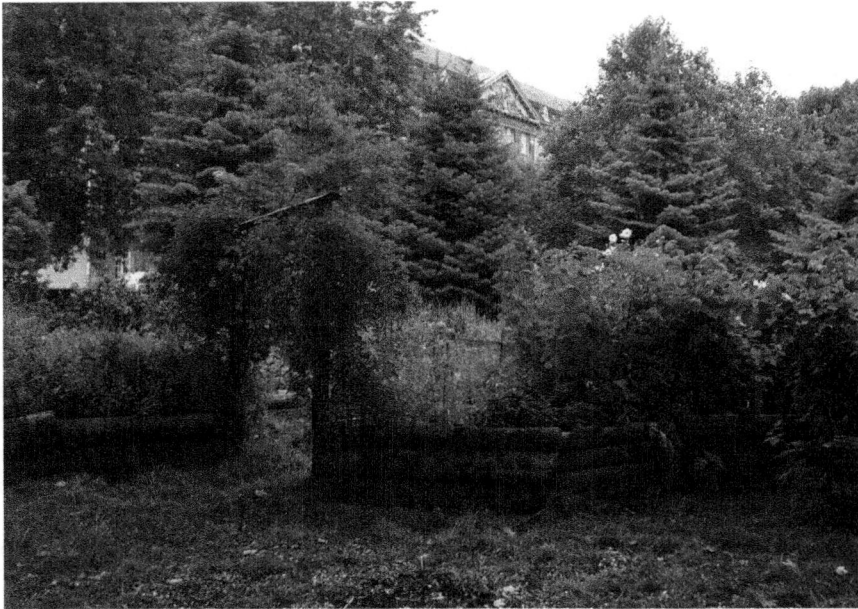

Fig. 5.3 Byhaven 2200 with its edge of vegetation and planting beds towards Ny Nørrebro Park. (Photo: Bettina Lamm)

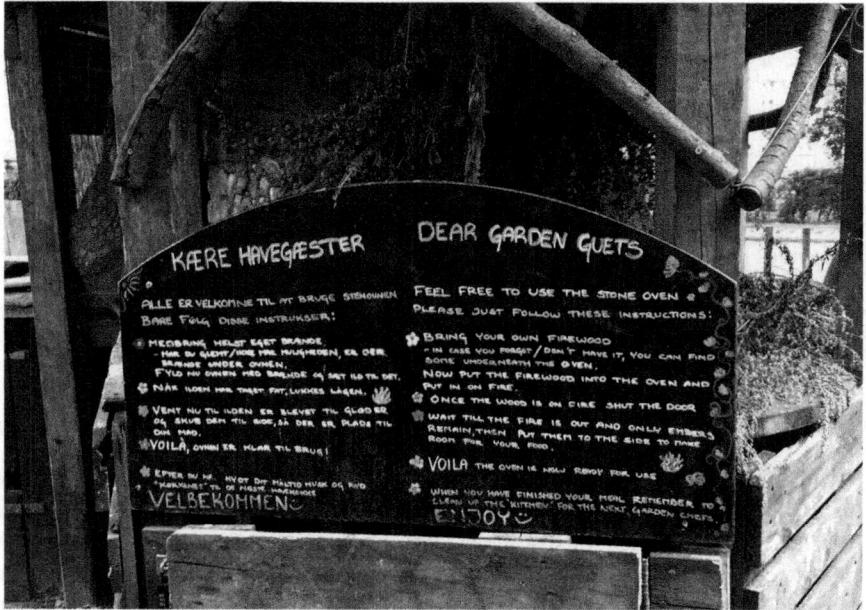

Fig. 5.4 Entering Byhaven 2200 you were welcomed with guidelines for how to use and care for the garden. (Photo: Bettina Lamm)

The urban garden site is open and publicly accessible and flanked by a bicycle path and a social housing estate on one side and a fenced high-security institution on the other. The urban context is complex with many different types of 'neighbours.' Across the street are newer buildings, such as the new Danish television headquarters, banks, offices, and hotels in the new district of Ørestaden.

The garden itself is an intimate oasis-like space with planting beds, lush vegetation, a greenhouse, a chicken coop, rabbits, and a bonfire pit. It is a picturesque and cosy place, which stands in stark contrast to its surroundings. Everyone can come here to garden or recreate. Its public facilities are clearly marked, recycling stations are available, and simple gardening tools are easy to find guided by signage describing how to use the garden and where to find things.

Early in the process, a strategic decision was made to let the activity centre users be part of the startup and establishment of the garden before inviting other local institutions and neighbours to join in (Konradsen et al., 2013). This ensured that vulnerable citizens would be welcome in the garden as the pioneers of the space. Citizens can come and find employment in the activity centre to maintain the garden or feed the chickens (Lygum, 2021).

Partly a social worker, partly a farmer, a staff person manages projects and supports citizens. According to him, even people with substance abuse problems can join as long as they are 'contactable' (Lygum, 2021). The garden project is a bridge-building initiative between vulnerable citizens, dwellers of Sundholm, and the neighbouring community. Besides activity centre workers, residents can get access to individual planting beds, and neighbouring schools and institutions use the garden for educational purposes.

The diversity of users is unique, and most of the social work goes into creating a sense of safety and acceptance for all. This is also where some of the vulnerable citizens can come and seek rest if they have been quarantined from the homeless centre at Sundholm.

At times things do get stolen or burned, and morning clean-ups might require the removal of discarded bottles and containers (Lygum, 2021). The manager stays in constant dialogue with the many different groups to maintain respect for the place and keep it open in a continuous process of cultivation of care. Everyone should feel welcome and everyone should feel responsible. This unique balance of rights and responsibilities makes Byhaven Sundholm a success story for the constant care and attention public landscapes require (Figs. 5.5 and 5.6).

5.2.4 Havnehaverne

Opdagelsen (The Discovery) is an open space in the harbour area of Søndre Havn in Køge, a post-industrial site currently transforming into a new urban district. The developer Køge Kyst initiated a series of temporary urban projects within the open spaces to attract citizens and cultivate new uses and practices amidst the former

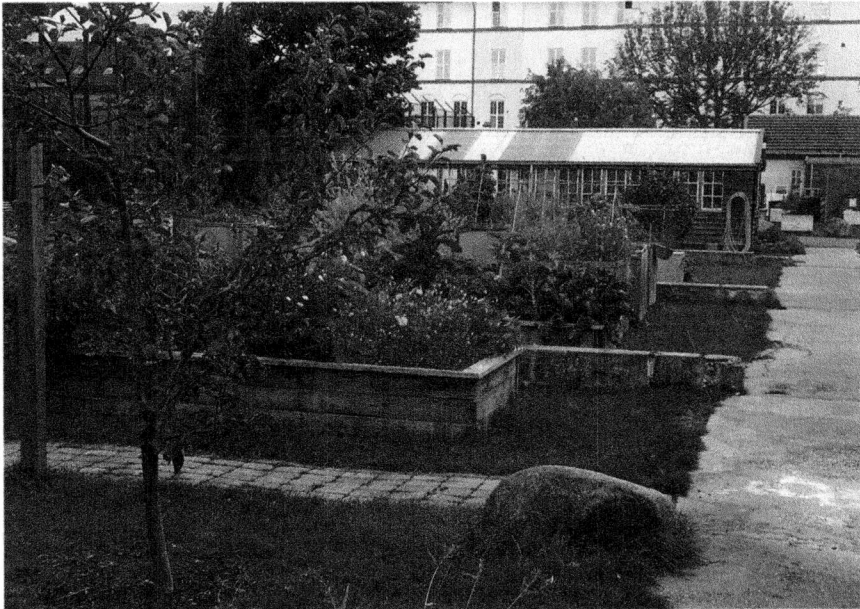

Fig. 5.5 Byhaven Sundholm with planting beds and greenhouse viewed from the public path that crosses through the garden. (Photo: Bettina Lamm)

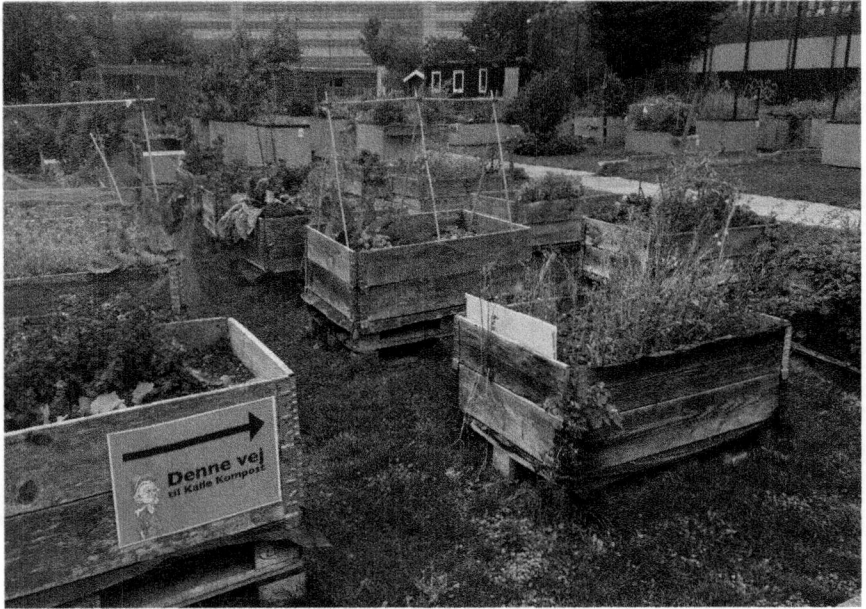

Fig. 5.6 Around Byhaven Sundholm there are educational signs describing where to find and how to use different garden features. Here a sign shows the way to the compost. (Photo: Bettina Lamm)

industrial sites. The 'phase zero' of the planning strategy aimed at cultivating 'The Life before the City' (Køge Kyst, 2011).

One of these projects was the creation of the urban garden 'Havnehaverne'. The project was developed in partnership with Det Grønne Hus (Green projects municipality), that also led the process, BOGL Landscape Architects, and the social carpentry project Køge Bugt Projektcenter. The idea for a community gardening space emerged in 2012 at a local culinary school, as a result of the positive experiences gained with the piloting of a bookable mobile kitchen (Køge Kyst, Opdagelsen). The kitchen was an art piece created in 2012 by Jesper Åbille for the site-specific exhibition Urban Play – another initiative cultivating the former industrial spaces for recreational uses (Lamm & Brandt, 2012).

From the start, the urban garden wanted to not only grow vegetables but also produce and share meals. The garden featured an elaborate outdoor kitchen equipped with four workstations, large grills and access to water, electricity, and bathroom facilities. Citizens in Køge could book the kitchen area for different gatherings from children's birthday celebrations and outdoor dining to cooking school events.

The space holds 85 custom-made raised planting beds prepared by the Køge Bugt Projektcenter workers and assembled on-site with the help of residents. Locals can get their own planting bed if they sign a contract committing to the caretaking of their small lot. Other planting beds are managed by school classes and institutions or used for experimental projects by the Køge Food community (Køge

Fødevarefællesskab). Seven common gardens are shared, and anyone can freely pick herbs and greens, an attempt to compensate for conflicts around access and claimed thefts (Wagner, 2016).

The urban garden Havnehaverne has relied on a consistent flow of resources from the start. The built structures and basic maintenance were funded by the developer Køge Kyst while Det Grønne Hus manage and support the distribution of planting beds, provide know-how and organise gardening and cooking workshops. The individually managed planting beds create a sense of ownership and continuity, as they require frequent visits from local gardeners.

Today, Havnehavene continues to serve as an activator at the former warehouse site in the transforming harbour, while the new city is being constructed around it. Eventually, the site will be absorbed by new city structures, but the plan is that Havnehaverne will relocate to a different space within the neighbourhood, which has so far been impossible. Meanwhile, a new urban gardening project, Køge Fælles Jord, has started in Køge around the experiences Det Grønne Hus, and thanks to the help of some of the citizens engaged in Havnehaverne (Figs. 5.7 and 5.8) (Køge Fælles Jord).

5.3   The Four Urban Gardens: Discussion

Two of the gardens, Prags Have and Byhaven 2200, were created through citizen-driven bottom-up initiatives. The other two, Sundholmen Byhave and Havnehaverne, had public (municipal) or private organisations behind them. While the two citizen-driven urban gardens did not last and only were in existence for a limited number of years, the two urban gardens with public/private organisational support and management are still active. Two of the gardens, Prags Have and Havnehaverne, were conceived as temporary from the start - as they were located on vacant former industrial sites in urban redevelopment areas. Byhaven and Sundholm Byhave were both potentially permanent projects located on municipal land. All four gardens were or are openly accessible to everyone and theoretically open to everyone's participation. The four Danish cases introduced in this chapter are illustrative of the possibilities but also challenges, connected with operating urban gardens in public space. Byhaven 2200 literally *cultivated* public space by creating an urban garden in an existing public park. Being on public land required that the citizens' association managing the space made it publicly accessible and that they actively and strategically worked to allow everyone to participate in it – a task which was not without conflict given the diversity of needs, interests, and resources in the various user groups.

Prags Have, on the other hand, was open to the public even though it was built on private land. Prags Have turned a private plot into a public space by cultivating an urban garden and inviting everybody to participate in the project. Havnehaverne is publicly accessible and explicitly created by the developer to cultivate community

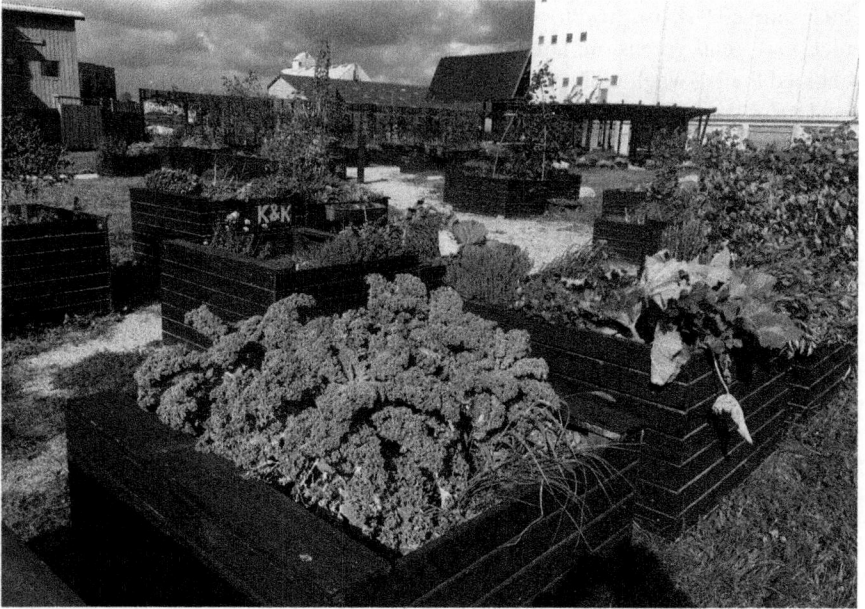

Fig. 5.7 Havnehaverne – the harbour gardens – black planter boxes distributed across the vacant building site in the transforming industrialised Køge harbour. The open kitchen and the seed storage building can be seen in the back. (Photo: Bettina Lamm)

and activate spaces yet to be developed carefully balancing private cultivation and public access.

While also open and accessible, Sundholmen Byhave distinguished itself for a special focus on the inclusion of vulnerable citizens. Here the core idea has been to connect people across social boundaries through the collective practice of gardening in shared, public space.

In both Prags Have and Byhaven 2200, the garden was a tool for community building at the local scale, a goal that became more important than the gardening itself. Both projects exemplify a do-it-yourself (DIY) urbanism of bottom-up initiatives dependent on the voluntary work of local enthusiasts who run and maintain the gardens. Despite being accessible to everyone, the spaces of Prags Have and Byhaven 2200 achieved the character of 'commons' rather than public spaces in the sense that they belonged to and were used by a somewhat stable community of gardeners.

As top-down initiatives by public or private organisations, Havnehaverne and Byhaven Sundholm could rely on sufficient resources to facilitate gardening and community building, yet even here a 'gardening community' emerged which identified with the place and each other, making this public space a commons. But whereas planting beds in Prags Have and Byhaven 2200 were shared, Sundby Byhave and Havnehavern in Køge's growing plots were 'owned' and cared for by individuals or institutions.

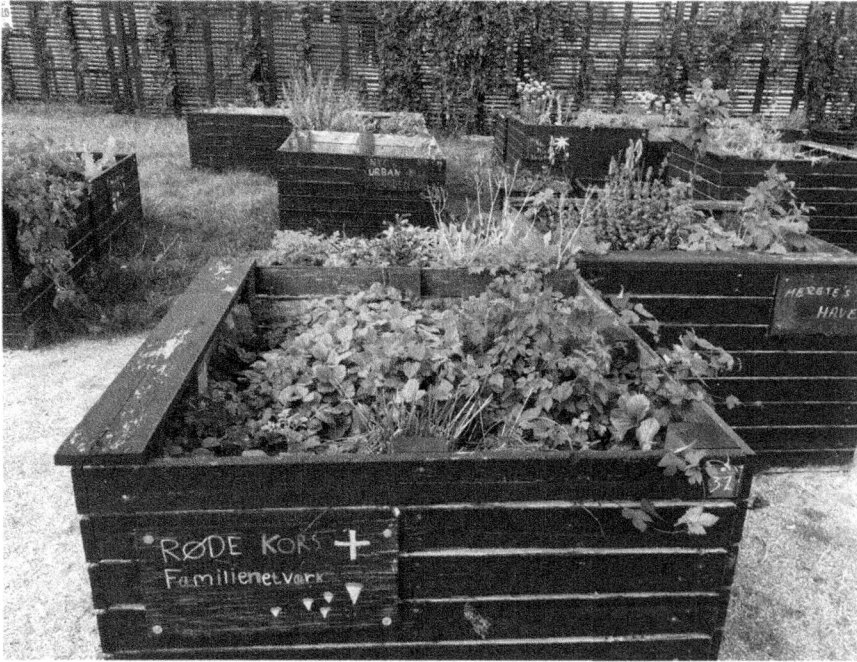

Fig. 5.8 Havnehaverne – the harbour gardens. Individualised planter boxes. (Photo: Bettina Lamm)

Havnehaverne and Byhaven Sundholm did from the start have significant access to resources – something that was not available in Prags Have and Byhaven where all work – both social and gardening as well as fundraising – was carried out by volunteers.

Prags Have and Byhaven 2200 may have failed to improve urban ecologies and nature in the long term, but they did contribute to developing new relationships between people and other living things in the city. They also stimulated community building, supported DiY urbanism initiatives, and encouraged experiments with new ways of public life in public spaces and new ways of taking care of and maintaining public space. While these two urban gardens were temporary, they did support and stimulate a number of capabilities as defined by Nussbaum (2003) during their existence (see also Chap. 2). Beyond bodily health addressed in terms of food production, nutrition and physical activity (C2), the capabilities also included control over one's environment (C10), cultivation of practical reason through opportunities for community engagement and bottom-up initiatives (C6) opportunities for engaging in tactile and creative expressions (C4), sustaining affiliation, inclusion and a sense of belonging (C7), cultivating emotional health (C5) opportunities for interaction with other species (C8).

Both Sundholmen and Havnehaverne took much of their inspiration from Prags Have and Byhaven 2200 as well as other activist-initiated projects. While the explicit aim in Byhaven Sundholmen was the inclusion of vulnerable groups and in Havnehaverne to stimulate community development, both projects used gardening as a tool to advance several human capabilities (Nussbaum, 2003) in a similar manner as Prags Have and Byhaven did. These include the development of physical health (C3), the stimulation of senses and imagination (C4), and the cultivation of relations with other people (C7) as well as other species (C8). The cultivation of capabilities through spatial practices of gardening and caring for a collective green space is perhaps more prominent in the established urban gardens than in the temporary ones, simply because of their longevity and the ability to engage professional staff to facilitate the nourishing of both garden and people. Yet, a top-down management limits some capabilities such as the opportunity to exercise practical reason (C6) and control over one's environment (C10).

In conclusion, creating and cultivating an urban garden – especially when the goal is to establish community and keep public access – requires resources, continuity, and persistent work. The social aspects as well as the tending of plantings require attention and continuous care. One cold hope that in the future public agencies will recognise the widespread community benefits and opportunities for cultivation of capabilities that urban gardens can provide and increase funding and resources in support of community-oriented urban gardening places and practices in public space.

References

Andersen, S., & Toft-Jensen, M. (2012). *Byen bliver til-en urban håndbog*. Forlaget PB43.

Byhaven 2200. *Byhavens grundprincipper*, published at NEXT media production https://nextmedieproduktion.dk/tvaer/uge2013_37/gruppe_7/

Dolleris, C. (2014a). *Film: Copenhagen "Byhaven 2200" Community Garden*. https://youtu.be/iUelW-RogQE

Dolleris, C. (2014b). *What is permaculture*. http://www.geoliv.dk/permaculture

Jensen, L. V., Pedersen, L. R., Hansen, S. S., & Hauxner, K., (2012). *Dyrk din by-fælles byhaver og frivillighed i byfornyelsen*, Hausenberg, Ministeriet for By, Bolig og Landdistrikter. https://byfornyelsesdatabasen.dk/file/335759/dok.pdf

Københavns Kommune. (2015a). Fællesskab København. Vision for 2025. *Københavns Kommune. Teknik-og Miljøforvaltningen* https://kk.sites.itera.dk/apps/kk_pub2/index.asp?mode=detalje&id=1448

Københavns Kommune. (2015b). *Sådan laver du en byhave*. *Københavns Kommune. Teknik-og Miljøforvaltningen*. http://miljopunkt-amager.dk/wp-content/uploads/2018/12/byhaver2015pdf-_1352.pdf

Køge Fælles Jord. http://xn--kgefllesjord-9cb2w.dk/

Køge Fødevarefællesskab. http://www.koeff.dk/1923-2/

Køge Kyst. (2011). *Livet før byen – Byen for Livet, Realdania*. https://realdania.dk/-/media/realdania-by/dokumenter/koege-kyst/k%C3%B8ge-kysts-forslag-til-udviklingsplan.pdf

Køge Kyst, Opdagelsen. https://koegekyst.dk/byen/arkitektur-og-byrum-pa-sondre-havn/opdagelsen/

Konradsen, H.-P., Ishøy, B., & Laursen, D. (2013). *BYHAVEN PÅ SUNDHOLM – Det grønne i det grå*. Roskilde Universitet.

Lamm, B., & Brandt, C. B. (2012). Urban play. *Landskab, 3*, 84–87.

Lygum, V. L. (2021). *Byhaven På Sundholm, Rumsans*. https://www.rumsans.dk/artikler/byhaven-pa-sundholm

Nussbaum, M. (2003). Capabilities as fundamental entitlements: Sen and social justice. *Feminist Economics, 9*(2–3), 33–59. https://doi.org/10.1080/1354570022000077926

Poveda, C. V. (2015). *Byhavens 10 bud.* https://www.facebook.com/legacy/notes/11365413263 73228/

Prags Have Facebook. https://www.facebook.com/PragsHave/

Skytt-Larsen, C. B., Busck, A. G., Lamm, B., & Wagner, A. M. (2022). Temporary urban projects: Proposing a multi-positional framework for critical discussion. *Frontiers in Sustainable Cities, 4*, 722665. https://doi.org/10.3389/frsc.2022.722665

Tantrumpanda. (2019). Death of an urban garden. Write less. https://write.less.dk/index.php/2019/01/13/death-of-an-urban-garden/?fbclid=IwAR1v7Q7yACPVDAUd75uPmU2kyXHuzHw4Vv3YwsMXdPq9OElD-DehwcaCp4g

Urbangardening.dk. http://urbangardening.dk/byhaven-2200/

Wagner, A. M. (2016). *Permitted exceptions: Authorised temporary urban spaces between vision and everyday.* Department of Geosciences and Natural Resource Management, Faculty of Science, University of Copenhagen. https://soeg.kb.dk/permalink/45KBDK_KGL/fbp0ps/alma99122096819505763

Chapter 6
Motivations, Supporting Factors and Challenges for Urban Agriculture in Public Space: Experiences from Oslo

Katinka Horgen Evensen and Vebjørn Egner Stafseng

6.1 Introduction

How do we practice urban agriculture in public space? In this chapter we present case studies from Oslo, in which urban agriculture has been integrated in urban public spaces. We have collected experiences from eight urban agriculture projects of various typologies, scales, and organizational models, from the city farm to small experimental cultivation projects. The projects represent four ways of organizing urban agriculture activities in public space that take aim of being accessible for large and diverse segments of urban populations. In this study we focus on aspects of urban agriculture in public space that can be relevant in the development of socially sustainable compact neighborhoods. We have used Woodcraft and colleagues' (2012) understanding of social sustainability as bearing on "... the infrastructure to support social and cultural life, social amenities, systems for citizen engagement and space for people and places to evolve" (p. 16). The overall objective of this study was to uncover organizational issues of urban agriculture in public space, potential well-being impacts for city dwellers, and publicness aspects for a broader community.

The existing research on urban agriculture and the multifaceted impact on the well-being of those who participate in it has mainly taken a qualitative approach (for a literature review, see Audate et al., 2019). Research has reported benefits of participation in urban agriculture activities that can relate to quality of life in the city, such as aesthetic and social experience (Hale et al., 2011) and social cohesion (Veen et al., 2016). Urban agriculture has also been connected to learning, eco-literacy

K. H. Evensen (✉)
Department of Landscape Architecture, Faculty of Landscape and Society,
Norwegian University of Life Sciences, Ås, Norway
e-mail: katinka.evensen@nmbu.no

V. E. Stafseng
Norwegian University of Life Sciences, Ås, Norway

117

B. Sirowy, D. Ruggeri (eds.), *Urban Agriculture in Public Space*, GeoJournal
Library 132, https://doi.org/10.1007/978-3-031-41550-0_6

(Rogge et al., 2020) and healthy eating (Litt et al., 2015). In a review of quantitative evidence of health impacts of urban agriculture, Tharrey and Darmon (2022) revealed mixed results regarding improved physiological health and physical activity but positive associations between urban agriculture activity and improved mental and social health.

Considering previous research, it seems fruitful to apply a eudemonic understanding of well-being when studying benefits from urban agriculture (see Chap. 1) since many of the benefits reported relate to social interaction, learning, and self-actualization which again relate to the idea of human flourishing. In our research we therefore used the capability approach of Nussbaum (2011) to understand what a good life in the city can entail. Nussbaum draws on the eudemonic traditions for understanding human well-being and opportunity to live a life in dignity. She outlines a set of opportunities, or what she refers to as 'capabilities', that can enable people to live a good life. These capabilities include experiencing safety and bodily integrity, possessing the right to political anticipation, and exerting control over one's own environment. They also encompass feelings of affiliation or belonging, being able to express oneself creatively, engaging with one's senses, as well as maintaining contact with nature and the living world. Employing the capability approach which acknowledges the importance of such wide range of aspects of everyday life, we could explore the potential of urban agriculture as a public space use that contributes to human well-being in the city.

To uncover the potential of urban agriculture to create inclusive, public meeting places, we analyze the cases in terms of publicness, understood as opportunities for interactions in and with physical space that link people (Tornaghi & Knierbein, 2014). We have used the conceptualization of publicness relevant for urban agriculture in public space by Murphy et al. (2023) (see Chap. 4). Using this conceptualization, we could identify how urban agriculture could support publicness in each case through increasing access and animation in urban space, contributing to social services, producing and distributing food, and building communities to spread cultivation knowledge.

6.1.1 Context and Objective

During the last decade, there has been an upsurge of urban agriculture projects in Oslo. Based on the knowledge on the potential benefits of urban agriculture activities, the municipality has developed a strategy for urban agriculture (Oslo Kommune, 2019). The strategy has five goals that focus on the capacity of urban agriculture to green the city, local food production, creating meeting places and learning arenas, and contributing to Oslo becoming a cooperating knowledge city (see Chaps. 11 and 12). The municipality operates with ten typologies of urban agriculture projects, from publicly accessible edible parks to therapeutic gardens for institutions (Oslo Kommune, 2022).

The Cultivating Public Space (CPS) project focuses on how urban agriculture can be systematically integrated in urban public spaces, ensuring its accessibility for large and diverse segments of urban populations (see Chap. 1). In this chapter we explored the range of urban agriculture practices experienced in public space in Oslo through interviews and observations. The objective of this case study was to (1) uncover organizational issues of urban agriculture in public space: identifying typologies of public urban agriculture in Oslo and mapping motives, supporting factors, challenges, and visions for practicing urban agriculture within cases representing these typologies, and (2) identify publicness impacts, addressing the potential of urban agriculture for creating inclusive meeting places for the broader community.

6.2 Methods

6.2.1 Methodological Approach

We analyzed and collected experiences from eight urban agriculture projects in Oslo. Through interviews with project initiators and managers, we mapped experiences of practicing urban agriculture in public space, both in practical terms and in terms of meaning or benefits to the users or local community. We studied the projects over time through field visits and initial and follow-up interviews a year later with initiators and project managers. This research approach allowed us to gain a deeper understanding of the cases that could give insights into how urban agriculture can be systematically integrated in urban public spaces and ensure accessibility to a wider population.

6.2.2 Case Selection and Analysis

Our case selection was a collaborative effort with key public, private, and nongovernmental stakeholders who were gathered in two workshops, organized by the CPS project partners. With additional conversations with urban agriculture project leaders we got a comprehensive overview of the diverse urban agriculture initiatives in public spaces in Oslo, which were active until June 2018. In total, we considered 20 cases, which we categorized using Lohrberg's (2019) typologies of urban agriculture and the primary, secondary, and tertiary users' framework described in Eason (1988) (Appendix 1).

Based on field visits and mapping, we selected cases that were (1) situated in accessible public spaces, (2) within densification areas, and (3) offered collective cultivation/food production. The selection also represented a variety in typologies, scales, and organizational models of public urban agriculture. The cases (Table 6.1, Fig. 6.1) are not an exhaustive overview of all the ways of practicing urban

Table 6.1 Selected cases of urban agriculture projects in Oslo 2018–2019

Typology/ model	City farm	Urban agriculture in central public parks	Neighborhood garden	Innovative urban agriculture-gardens (rooftop/floating)
Urban structure	Development of park in transformation area in central urban area	Existing parks in central urban area	Green space in suburban area	*Publicly accessible rooftop garden in central urban residential area **Floating educational garden on the river/in the Oslo-fjord
Case/ project	Losæter	Schous plass/ Sofienbergparken Snippen	Voksenenga nærmiljøhage Ellingsrud parsellhagelag Dr. Dedichens Drivhus	Sagene takhage (rooftop garden) Grønlands flytende hage (2018) Oslo Fjordhage (2019) (floating garden)

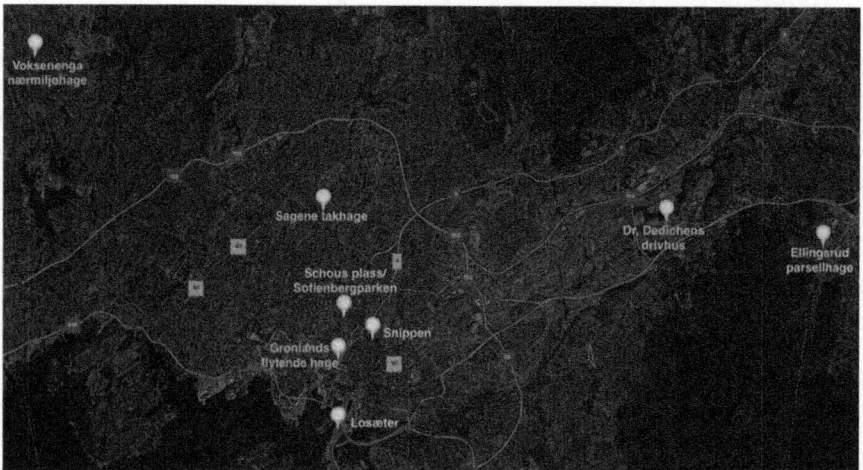

Fig. 6.1 Location of the eight cases in Oslo

agriculture in public space. Rather, they describe typologies and organizational models visible in the Norwegian context. In our study we therefore found it advantageous to differentiate the broad category of collective food production in urban gardening with which Lohrberg (2019) operates, into four typologies/models: the 'City Farm;' Urban agriculture in central public parks the 'Neighborhood Garden;' and Innovative Urban Agriculture-Gardens in Public Spaces.

All the projects was initiated between 2011 and 2018 and received funding from either a foundation or the municipality's urban agriculture funding scheme. Some projects even secured financing through funds in support of public art in urban regeneration areas.

We developed our case descriptions and analyses, applying the conceptualization of publicness relevant to urban agriculture in public space (Murphy et al., 2023; see Chap. 4). Our field visits and interviews detailed the cases in terms of location and connectivity, design and amenities, management, and activities. This approach allowed us to assess how urban agriculture activity could support publicness in each case, by increasing access and animation in public space, contributing to municipal services, producing food, and networking communities to spread cultivation knowledge.

6.2.3   Project Initiators and Managers' Experiences

From March 2018 till February 2020 we conducted 17 semi-structured interviews with project initiators and managers. In the first year, the interviews focused on the background and motivation for the initiative, organizational matters, cooperation with other actors, activities yearly programming and expectations for the coming season. The second year was part evaluation and follow-up and part reflection on the achievements and challenges of the project. Some projects had multiple managers or coordinators whose perspectives could contribute to a deeper understanding of the project. In some projects, new managers took over after the second year, and one project ended after the first year.

We analyzed and transcribed interviews with the project managers, conducting a thematic content analysis on the material (Braun & Clarke, 2006). This helped us identify (1) *motives* for initiating the projects; (2) *supporting factors,* or what made it possible; (3) *challenges* in practicing urban agriculture in public space; and (4) *visions* or potentials for further development. We discussed and decided what characterized each case on these four topics that were especially relevant for understanding urban agriculture in public space. The interviews with project managers were a source of valuable information to describe the cases in addition to the projects' web pages. See Appendix 2 for research ethics.

6.3   Experiences from Oslo

In the following we briefly describe each case and present our findings related to motives, supporting factors, challenges, and visions for practicing urban agriculture in public space based on interviews with initiators or managers' experiences. Then, for each case we present an overall assessment of publicness relevant to urban agriculture activities (Murphy et al., 2023) to draw possible comparisons across the typologies of urban agriculture projects. In the discussion and concluding section, we address aspects relevant to practicing urban agriculture in public spaces and review lessons learnt.

6.3.1   City Farm

Losæter is park of the central Oslo redevelopment area, Bjørvika, and represents the 'city farm' urban agriculture typology. Table 6.2 provides a description of the case. Pictures 6.1 and 6.2 show the site and its surroundings.

Initiating and Managing Urban Agriculture in Public Space

In the following sections, we present our findings derived from interviews with the initiator and the two Losaeter city farmers.

Motives

The project's main objective was described by the initiator of Losæter, to become an *outdoor culture institution* in the city. This can be traced back to its genesis as a public artwork, being a part of the regeneration of the waterfront of Oslo. "They aimed to create a 'cultural institution without walls' with a focus on intangible cultural heritage. A central emphasis of the art project was the importance of tacit knowledge and skills in crafts, such as the baking of traditional bread and the

Table 6.2 Case description Losæter representing the city farm typology

Losæter (est. 2011 as the free allotment garden Herligheten)
Location and connectivity
Public park in high-profile waterfront development area surrounded by major cultural institutions, expensive housing, and corporate headquarters. Transformation area surrounded by construction sites (2018–20). Situated by highway with heavy traffic and noise exposure (65–70 dB) (Miljødirektoratet, 2022). Poorly connected to public transport. Well connected to cycling and walking paths.
Design and amenities
Approx. 7000 m² (total area). Cultivation in fields and hilly terrain. Artfully designed baking house with woodfired ovens and cooking facilities. Outdoor seating. Occasionally sheep/hens in season.
Management
One full-time city farmer was employed to maintain the area and facilitate events, helped by a full-time seasonal worker. In 2019, Agency of Urban Environment, Oslo municipality took over the responsibility from Norges Bondelag (Norwegian Farmers' Union).
Activities
Weekly open workday and dinner. Participants are instructed in the work needed done (weeding, harvesting, compost making, planting, etc.); a meal is prepared, mainly using produce from the garden and bread made on-site. Venue for courses in various cultivation or food-related techniques and crafts, as well as art and cultural happenings. Organized activities for groups from dementia care, vocational training, and internships for gardening students.

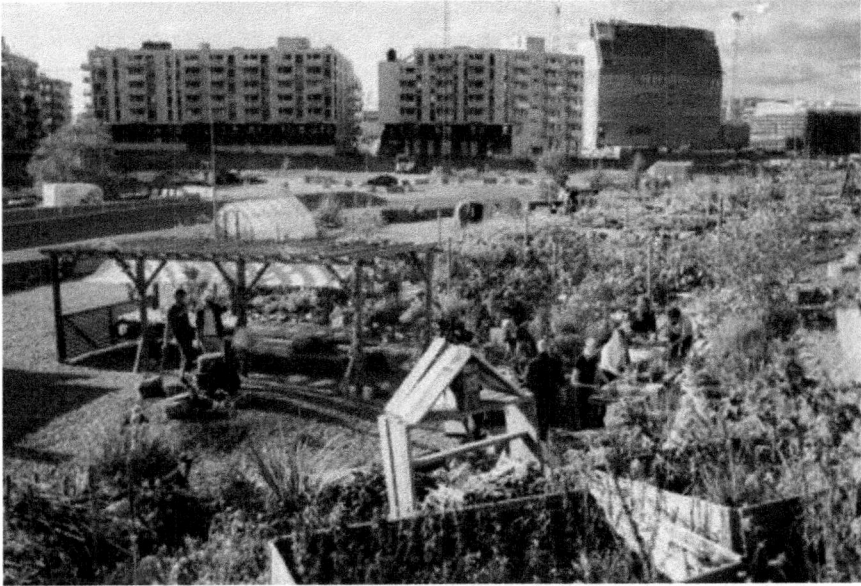

Picture 6.1 The social facilities and vegetable bed at Losæter. (Photo: Brooke Porter)

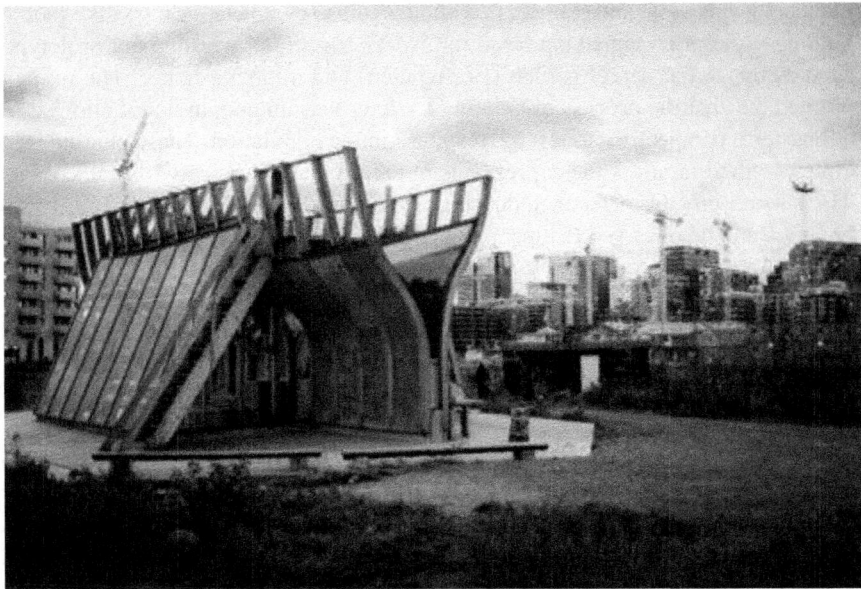

Picture 6.2 The baking house at Losæter. (Photo: Brooke Porter)

handling of wood-fired ovens. Losæter was envisioned as a place where these skills could be practiced, preserved, and passed on. This makes *knowledge dissemination focusing on cultural heritage* another central objective of the project. The activities of cultivating, preparing, and preserving fruits, vegetables, and bread serve as a means to create an arena for arts and creativity. This was also connected to a third objective, *participation and empowerment*. Losæter wanted to provide meaningful experiences to visitors as active contributors to the various activities. According to the initiator, empowering citizens was an important motive for the project, showing people how they "... can act and influence their environment and the city and their own life" and linked this motive directly to public health.

Supporting Factors

In this project some guiding principles of organization were highlighted as supporting factors. The project's success was ascribed to the overarching idea of *organic development* of the place. As the first city farmer described it: "... it's a strength that we do not have a clear strategy plan, because that is exactly what makes room for things to develop organically based on the people who joins, and wants something, or has the knowledge about something." Aesthetically, the project strives to keep it "unfinished" with a rougher surface than elsewhere. This intentional aesthetic choice aims at fostering a sense of inclusivity by making people feel they can join and contribute without extensive knowledge or skills. Another guiding principle was making room for *experimentation* by testing out prototypes such as the initial parcel garden (Herligheten) and a baking house. The initiator pointed out that the process of creating Losæter was unique, in that it allowed for a long-term perspective, to test the response in the population. These guiding principles seemed to affect the expressions of creativity and the activities at Losæter. The second city farmer concluded that less control or rules make people more creative, and he observed that people tend to forget themselves when working in a group and toward a common goal. Although Losæter was open for experimentation and user influence, the cultivation activity was still run by the city farmer securing a high level of *professionality*, which also seemed to characterize the place and its success.

Challenges

Overall, the initiator and the city farmers mentioned a few challenges with the project. Losæter is a designated public park in the waterfront area in central Oslo, but one may question the *perceived publicness* of the place. Combining a welcoming public park with a highly professionalized hub for specialized baking and cultivation may be challenging. Losæter did offer activities for a broad spectrum of user (i.e., pupils, youth in vocational training, people with dementia, local immigrant women). Still, both *social and physical barriers* may exist for entering the park as a visitor and joining the activities. Both the city farmers insisted that the users are diverse and internationally represented. One admitted that it has become a place for engaged young adults that now finally have found their place for cultivation in the city: "I think that also has something to do with the aesthetics out here [...] I think it appeals to that group [...] not those who are stressed by the fact that it is not so damn nice and that we do not have the signs in order and all that." The other city farmer pointed to aesthetics as being a potential social barrier that may be present at Losæter, namely, that some people associate graffiti and pallet collars with alternative, social groups. Examples of physical obstacles were no signs directing people to the place, and the main gate was hidden and situated on a heavily trafficked road. One of the city farmers described this as a key to protecting it from the crowds of the neighboring popular waterfront sites and keeping the atmosphere and contrasting aesthetics of the place.

Visions

At Losæter the above-described organic development strategy kept the management from having too clear a vision for the place instead letting it evolve as freely as possible. However, the first city farmer desired to develop the place as a hub for farmers interested in using regenerative farming[1] as a *unifier of farming movements*, envisioning it as a place where growers from both conventional and organic movements could meet and engage in dialogue. The city farmers also expressed a desire to forge partnerships with local and national arts and culture institutions, such as the Munch Museum and Deichman, Oslo's main public library.

6.3.2 Urban Agriculture in Central Public Parks

The typology *urban agriculture in central urban parks* is exemplified by the case Schous plass/Sofienbergparken described in Table 6.3 and Snippen in Table 6.4. Pictures 6.3, 6.4, and 6.5. show how cultivation areas fit into the two parks.

---

[1] An alternative farming practice focusing on regenerating/building agricultural soil while producing food.

Table 6.3 Case description of Schous plass and Sofienbergparken, representing the typology urban agriculture in central urban parks

Schous plass (est. 2017) /Sofienbergparken (est. 2019) District Grünerløkka
Location and connectivity   Public square (Schous plass) and park (Sofienbergparken) in densely populated central district. Well connected to public transport and walkways.   *Design and amenities*   Schous plass: Public square in front of public library with a combination of cobbles and lawn. Cultivation in existing flower beds on one side of the square with information signs.   Sofienbergparken: Large public park of which about 1500 m² was a newly established garden parcel with greenhouse and shed. Surrounded by low fences (planned removed).   *Management*   The Schous plass project started as a collaboration between the district, the library, and social entrepreneurs working with food, design, and communication. The district green space management has since then integrated urban agriculture in selected parks. Local youth participated in the green space maintenance as part of a vocational training program. The local library was involved through a special focus on cultivation, food systems, and ecology in their dissemination work.   *Activities*   In Schous plass the library hosted community dinner events and an outdoor café in summer in collaboration with the local youth in vocational training, local restaurants, and other food-related organizations. They also wanted to focus on circularity and make and use compost from food waste from local restaurants.   In Sofienbergparken, the district hosted garden activities for local kindergartens and schools (sowing, planting, harvesting, etc.).

Table 6.4 Case description of Snippen representing the typology urban agriculture in central urban parks

Snippen (one season in 2018) District Gamle Oslo - Tøyen
Location and connectivity   Public park next to Oslo's botanical garden in a densely populated central district. Well connected to public transport and walkways.   *Design and amenities*   Cultivation in singular raised oval beds designed for the park which has a theme playground with organic forms. No information signage. The Agency of Urban Environment, Oslo municipality, designated an area of the park to cultivation activities for the local residents.   *Management*   A coordinator from the District Gamle Oslo - Tøyen organized volunteers in cultivation groups of local women and parent groups, kindergartens, and a group of foreign nationals.   *Activities*   Planning, sowing, planting, maintaining, and harvesting. Cultivation courses given to the groups. They had plans for a harvest gathering, but most of the produce was lost for various reasons during the season.

Initiating and Managing Urban Agriculture in Public Space

In the following, we present our findings on practicing urban agriculture in public space based on interviews with the coordinator of park management and the project coordinator in District Gråunerløkka, the head of the District Grünerløkka Library, and the project coordinator for Snippen at District Gamle Oslo.

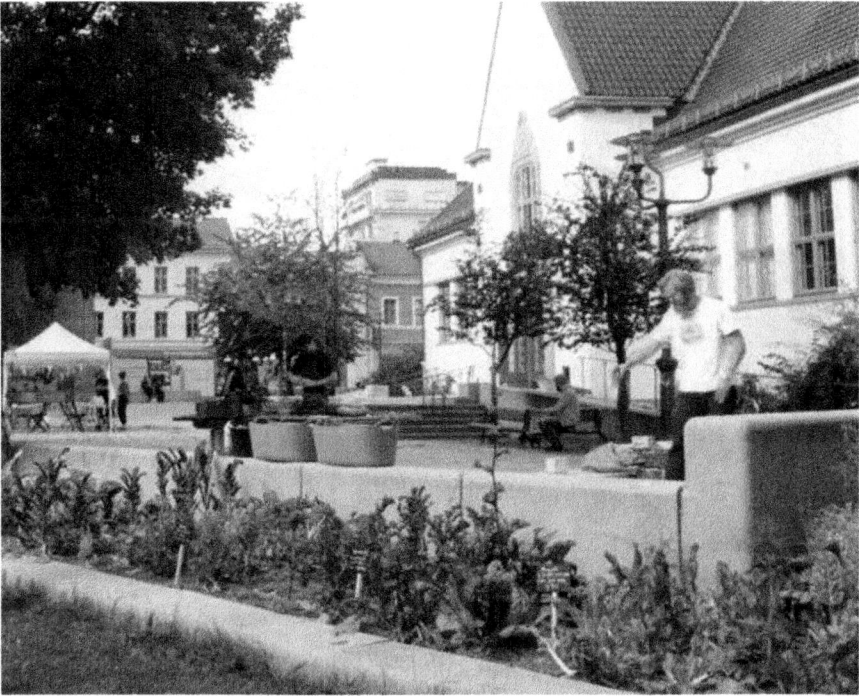

Picture 6.3 Schous plass with cultivation in former flowerbeds around the library. (Photo: Troels Rosenkrantz Fuglsang)

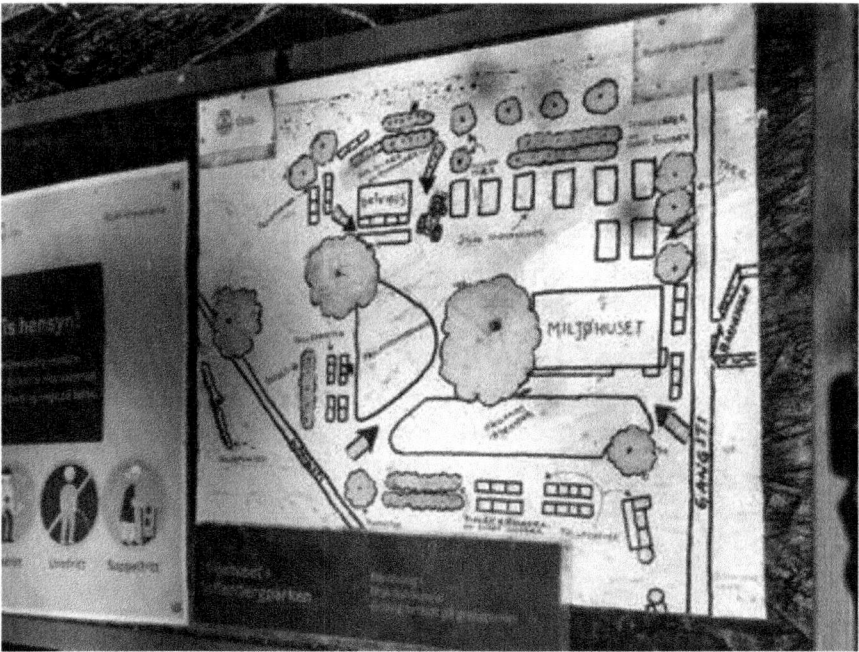

Picture 6.4 Layout of the Sofienbergparken cultivated areas. (Photo: Vebjørn Stafseng)

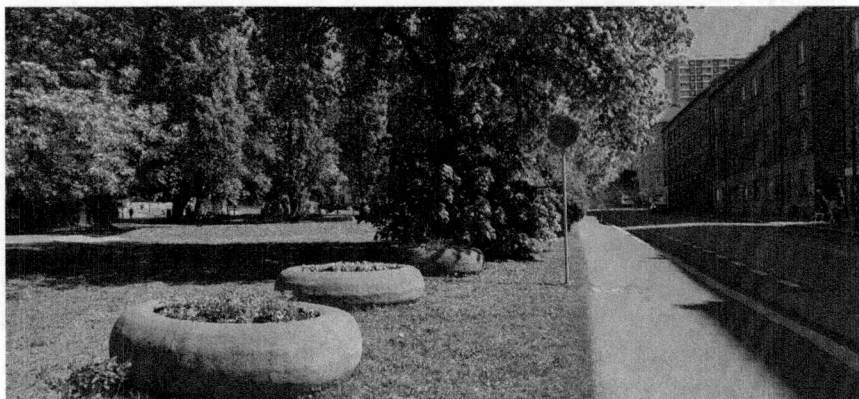

Picture 6.5 Snippen seen from the street. (Photo: Beata Sirowy)

Motives

One primary motivation for introducing urban agriculture into the central public park management of the Grünerløkka District was to *activate the parks,* and thereby enhancing their safety and security. The parks and public squares selected for urban agriculture witnessed significant improvements. Through cultivation, introducing new organized activities, and ensuring the presence of employees, volunteers, and youth employed during the summer. In the Gamle Oslo - Tøyen District, the Snippen Park project wanted urban agriculture to encourage the multicultural community to use public space more actively and in new ways. *Participation and empowerment* were important motivations. In the words of the Snippen Project coordinator: "…instead of saying that a municipal service tries to fix people's problems, you support them, you empower them to make possible what they want. And they want green social meeting places." By engaging local teenagers in green space management, District Grünerløkka also sought to give them essential *vocational training,* as part of a community scheme against child poverty, and improve their sense of belonging. Finally, cooperation between the green space management and the local library was established to *disseminate knowledge on food systems and ecology.* The head of the local library, who had been involved in most of the activities of the Schous project, saw dissemination of knowledge as an essential motivation. He also expressed the wish to change the outdoor space through a programming of activities from Spring to Fall and to create a sense of belonging by facilitating encounters across generations and minorities.

Supporting Factors

The success of the establishment of the projects in District Grünerløkka was ascribed to the *collaboration across sectors and the public-private partnerships* created in the process. Both projects involved a mix of actors from different sectors in the municipality, private enterprises, and volunteers. The head of the local library emphasized the need for careful selection of partners and the reliance on enthusiasts [ildsjeler] or drivers to achieve their goals. The involvement of youth and volunteers in the operation of parks and public spaces underscored the importance of technical expertise, which was instrumental in the projects' success. This is exemplified by the diverse range of competences needed from the various actors involved in the projects, such as in design, horticulture, social work, and pedagog. According to the District Grünerløkka project coordinator, they involved youth vocational training, "but the final touch [is] done by professionals. And I think it has a lot to say in these public spaces, that it [is] proper, it [is] nicely executed." According to the project coordinator, District Grünerløkka professionals affiliated with the project provided special competences and library management offered the requird daily support.

Finally, the willingness to test *innovative practices* seemed to be a key strategy. By innovative practice, we mean new ways of thinking partnerships and collaboration, activating public spaces, and green space maintenance. In the Grünerløkka district, they used existing funding for green space maintenance to cultivate edible instead of ornamentals. At Snippen, they gave volunteers a space to practice vegetable cultivation as well as socialization, while keeping a part of the park lush, publicly accessible and well-kept. These examples all shared a common dimension of multifunctionality in the occupation of public spaces.

Challenges

The projects in Schous plass and Sofienbergparken were described as successful in several ways. Their events were well attended and appreciated, but they would have liked to engage more residents in everyday activities. They describe some instances of *lack of appreciation* of urban agriculture by the general public. The project coordinator in District Grünerløkka was concerned about people's perceptions of urban agriculture as "a gimmick" and that public health benefits from cultivation activities were not given the deserved attention. The projects encountered several design-related challenges, with the Snippen project facing obstacles both practically and in communication. The project manager experienced reactions from the public while working in the park, due to the lack of signage identifying their project. "The reaction we got sometimes was 'you are doing something illegal' 'What are you doing?' 'This is not yours; you cannot do this.'" The practical challenges were a lack of a tool shed and access to water on the site, which made them have to carry all tools and attached hoses to distant water sources. Furthermore, the design of the planter boxes provided by the municipality (Picture 6.6) proved not to be suited for vegetable growing and was too wide for kindergarten children. Finally, both projects had issues relating to their *temporary* mandate for using the space for urban agriculture. Schous plass was planned to be transformed into a paved square, but the project initiators kept developing it in line with the project, and the head of the local library argued that they had transformed the square for less than the official plans. The integration of cultivation within Snippen park remained a pilot project lasting for only one season.

Visions

The project managers saw potential embedding multifunctional cultivation in public green space. The Grünerløkka project coordinator had ideas for smarter and even more useful ways for managing cultivation activity at a district level, like transforming parts of parks into edible gardens that can also function as school garden. They also wished to implement and expand systems for circularity in practice, such as using surplus from local restaurants for compost. The local public library wished to increase the cultivated area in the surrounding public space: "My plan is actually to expand, because I see the whole lawn on this side [of the square], I would like a field there" (head of local library).

6.3.3   Neighborhood Garden

The typology *neighborhood garden* is exemplified by the cases Voksenenga nærmiljøhage, described in Table 6.5, Ellingsrud parsellhage (allotment garden) (Table 6.6) and Dr. Dedichens Drivhus (greenhouse) (Table 6.7). Pictures 6.6, 6.7, and 6.8 show how cultivation areas fit into their public green space.

Initiating and Managing Urban Agriculture in Public Space

In the following we present our findings on practicing urban agriculture in public space based on interviews with two project managers and one board member from one of our chosen *neighborhood gardens*.

Motives

An important objective for all three projects was to become a *social meeting place* for local residents. The manager in Voksenenga nærmiljøhage pointed at a shortage of social meeting places in the neighborhood beyond all the sports arenas. She clarified that the meeting place function was important: "…it probably really trumps the cultivation itself. Cultivation for us is a tool to achieve more social goals." The project manager in Ellingsrud Parsellhage also mentioned using urban

Table 6.5 Description of the case Voksenenga nærmiljøhage, representing the urban agriculture typology neighborhood garden

Voksenenga nærmiljøhage (est. 2017)
Location and connectivity   Public green space characterized by an open field adjacent to cemetery and within urban woodland. Densely populated suburban area with apartment blocks and detached houses. Located on a local walkway and hiking path to the forest and appr. 500 m distance from nearest public transport.
Design and amenities   Fenced area within open field. A common cultivation area (CSA) appr. 2000 m^2 and an allotment garden, 60 lots á 2,5 m^2. Outdoor roofed kitchen with pizza oven and social seating. Greenhouse, hen house, and sheds.
Management   Run by employed coordinator 60–100% 2017–2019, as well as volunteer-based work.
Activities   Open weekly workdays in season, organized groups of various activities, and family club. Cooking classes, school and kindergarten visits, and courses on cultivation all year. Annual open day with cultural activities for the whole neighborhood.

Table 6.6 Description of the case Ellingsrud parsellhage (allotment garden), representing the urban agriculture typology neighborhood garden

Ellingsrud parsellhage (est. 2016)
Location and connectivity   Public green space characterized by lawns, trees, and football fields in suburban area with a mix of apartment blocks and single-unit houses. The allotment garden is located next to a local walkway, about 750 meters, and a steep descent from the nearest metro station.
Design and amenities   Field of 20 x 40 meters with 35 allotments made from eight-pallet collars in an H-formation, some of which are for the community and some for compost. Some benches with tables for seating nearby the allotment area.
Management   Run by a coordinator on a voluntary basis, in addition to volunteer-based work by members. Local youth has also been involved in building and upkeep through a summer-job project run by the district administration.
Activities   Common dugnad/workdays for members. Courses and events related to cultivation all year. Regular school and kindergarten visits in season, events such as "open days," summer, and harvesting parties.

agriculture to cultivate a culture for creating more open and welcoming common outdoor areas. The neighborhood gardens were described as providing a venue for outdoor activities beyond the home. A goal was to create a pleasant and attractive outdoor space for everyone, including those not interested in cultivation, in order to draw people out of their apartments. The cultivation activity in the family club at Voksenenga Nærmiljøhage was at times secondary to providing an outside home arena where especially minority women appreciated getting outside and meeting others. In Ellingsrud Parsellhage, the motive of activating the place and the green space specifically through urban agriculture activity was deemed

Table 6.7 Description of the case Dr. Dedichens' Greenhouse, representing the urban agriculture typology neighborhood garden

Dr. Dedichens Drivhus (est. 2015)
Location and connectivity
Greenhouse surrounded by lawns, a school, two kindergartens, and former barn and farm buildings. The area was part of a psychiatric hospital, later owned by the municipality and listed as a heritage environment. Located in densely populated suburban area with apartment blocks. The greenhouse is around 300 m from the nearest subway station, but not connected to any local paths.
Design and amenities
600 m² greenhouse with one entrance: a regular-sized door and no signs. The door is locked unless there are members working there or during open events. A social area inside for communal meals and cultural events with simple kitchen facilities.
Management
Run by volunteers, loosely organized in a board with head of the board, as well as other responsibilities distributed. No paid employees but some funding for hiring experts for courses, etc.
Activities
Allotment-style vegetable cultivation for members, half of a table per lot. Local schools and kindergartens have some tables and get help from volunteer members. Plant club for school children/after-school activity. Open café with meals and waffles. Annual open plant market with sales of seedlings and food and coffee.

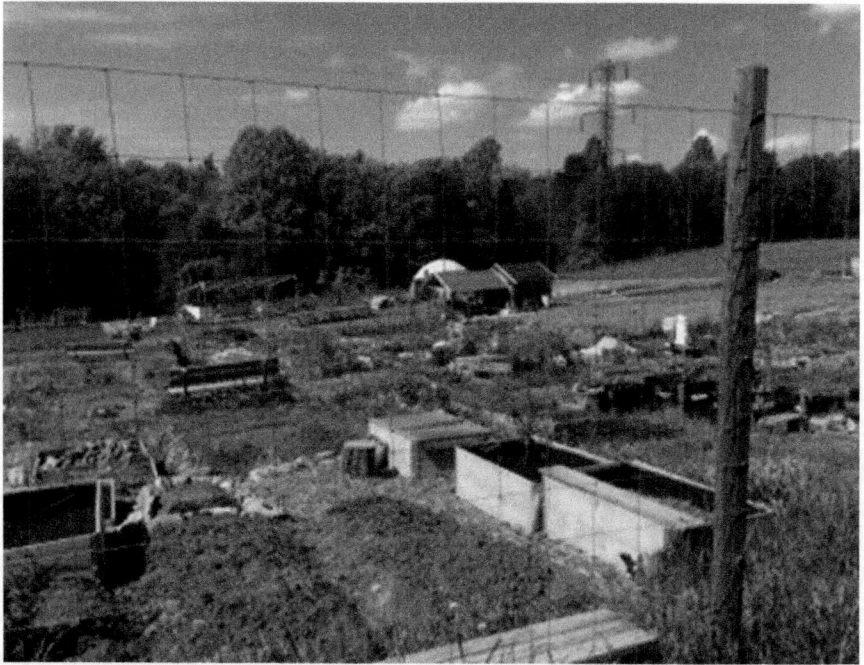

Picture 6.6 Voksenenga nærmiljøhage, its facilities, and the see-through fence surrounding it. (Photo: Katinka Evensen)

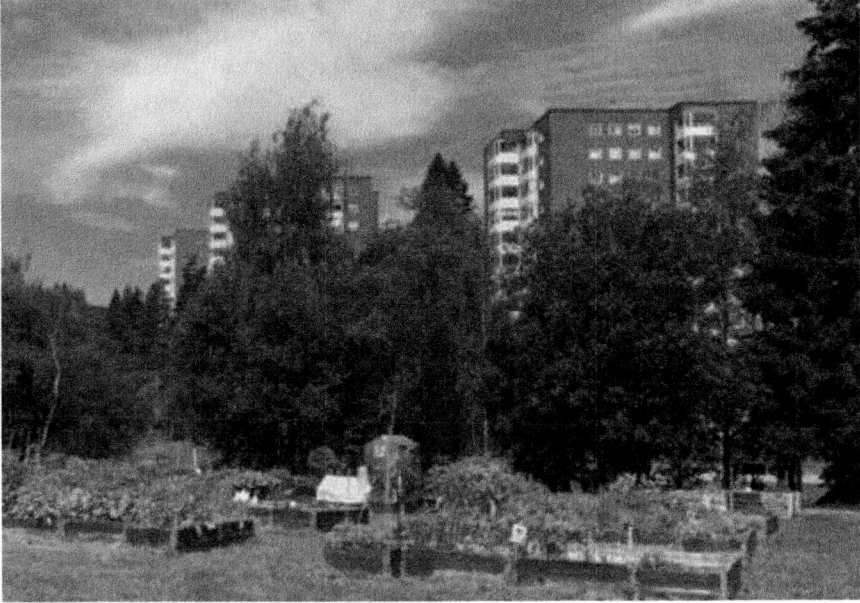

Picture 6.7 The Ellingsrud allotment garden and its surroundings. (Photo: Anne Grete Orlien)

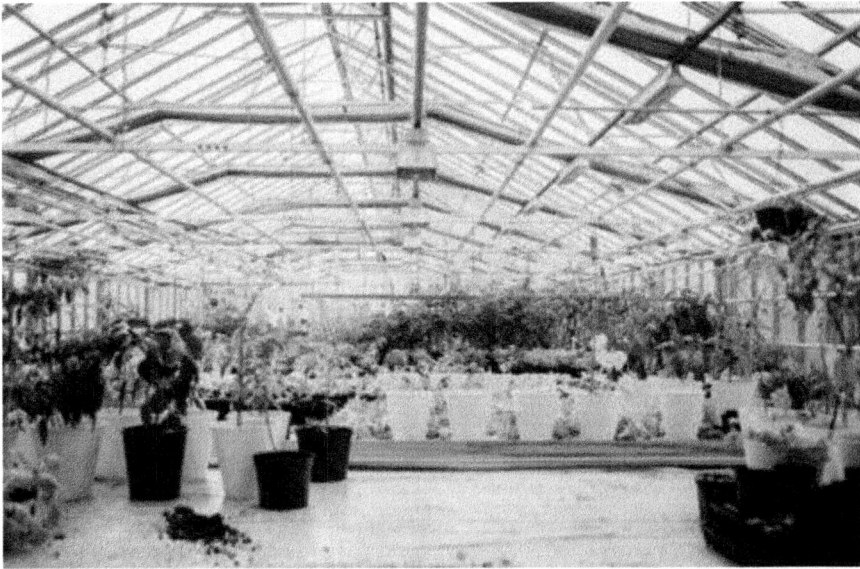

Picture 6.8 Interiors of Dr. Dedichens greenhouse, with activity space and cultivation facilities. (Photo: Brooke Porter)

important, with the aim of improving neighborhood safety. Meanwhile, at Dr. Dedichens Drivhus, the activation of the place was also utilized for the purpose of conserving historical buildings. Lastly, all three projects had the motive of serving as a supplementary educational arena for schools and kindergartens, welcoming groups of children.

Supporting Factors

Having a coordinator to oversee the neighborhood garden was identified as crucial by all the projects. The role of the coordinator was described as being more than just an administrator, like the Voksenenga project manager who emphasized the importance of having time for conversation and recognizing individuals. Networking and collaboration with various local actors, such as the district administration, the local church, farm, and sports clubs, were cited as important in all three projects. The manager of Voksenenga Nærmiljøhage also stated that their project model was a combination of *co-creation/networking* and having a coordinator "There are many collaborations here and it is the model I have seen work elsewhere in Europe, that it is co-creation, but also the fact that it is a project manager in a paid position who holds it." Another supporting factor, particularly described by the managers of Dr. Dedichens Drivhus and Ellingsrud Parsellhage, can be termed as *keeping scale and ambitions low*. The managers described a situation where they allowed volunteers to freely start small projects within their capacity to ensure implementation.

Challenges

Project representatives from all neighborhood gardens saw *organizing volunteers* as a critical challenge, that demanded a lot of time from coordinators. It also demanded caring for the volunteers, making their work pleasurable, and ensuring they did not wear themselves out. They all called for a sound system to organize volunteers. While one of the options would have been to be professionally managed by an external organization, the Voksenenga nærmiljøhage manager argued that it would undermine its role as a meeting place for residents in the local community: "…we wish to be a meeting place for local residents, and if we include organizations that are concerned with ecology, organic agriculture, yes, those values, then I think it may be perceived as excluding to the others." Both Voksenenga Nærmiljøhage and Dr. Dedichens Drivhus worked hard to secure more permanent support for organizing their activities but found a lack of recognition at the district level and felt they were expected to manage on voluntary work. All projects struggled with resources to offer a satisfactory educational program. For instance, Dr. Dedichens Drivhus would have liked to have a pedagogical position to welcome all the schools and kindergartens visiting. In Voksenenga Nærmiljøhage, they cooperated well with the municipality, and they believed that the municipality appreciated their efforts. However, the manager felt that because Voksenenga Nærmiljøhage was a private voluntary organization, neither the Agency for Urban Environment nor the local district administration was willing to assume more financial responsibility. All projects had temporary agreements with the respective landowners, creating uncertainty and difficulties in planning ahead. However, the element of temporality in the projects may have also been one of the reasons for their existence. In Ellingsrud Parsellhage, they had an agreement with the Agency for Urban Environment, and the project manager stated that the collaboration had a degree of reciprocity, in that the municipality had an interest in the place being cared for and maintained.

Visions

The neighborhood gardens we studied all welcomed kindergartens, school classes, and after-school clubs, and in Dr. Dedichens Drivhus and Voksenenga nærmiljøhage, the project managers saw a great potential in receiving even more children if they were not to rely on volunteers only but have a person in a combined pedagogical and administrative position. This also reflects a common wish among the neighborhood gardens: to become publicly funded and be included or part of local public services. Another potential that was expressed was to create a culture for open accessible active outdoor spaces, through cultivation activities. Finally, Dr. Dedichens Drivhus and Ellingsrud parsellhage shared a vision of *preserving local history by activating public space* through cultivation. Dr. Dedichens Drivhus would like to restore the greenhouse and the historical buildings of a psychiatric hospital to become useful for the community (see more in Swensen et al., 2022). In Ellingsrud parsellhage they planned to expand by establishing a community garden on a derelict cotter's farm in the urban forest in collaboration with enthusiasts of local history, making it an activity and hiking destination.

6.3.4 Innovative Urban Agriculture-Gardens in Public Space

Sagenetakhage (rooftop garden) and Grønlands flytende hage (floating garden, the project evolved into Oslo Fjordhage), represent *innovative urban agriculture-gardens in public space* and are described in Tables 6.8 and 6.9. Pictures 6.9, 6.10, and 6.11 show their design and location within the Oslo public realm.

Table 6.8 Description of the case Sagene rooftop garden, representing the urban agriculture typology "Innovative urban agriculture-garden in public space"

Sagene takhage (est. 2018)
Location and connectivity
Publicly accessible rooftop garden on a one-story building belonging to a housing association. Located in the main square of Sagene district, a densely populated area with apartment buildings.
Well connected to public transport and walkways. The garden is not visually accessible from the square or sidewalk but is easily accessed by a staircase from the main entrance to the district's community house. One sign to the garden.
Design and amenities
Garden approx. 300 m^2 with 100 m^2 of cultivation beds. Table(s) and benches.
Management
A community garden initiated and run by volunteers connected to an organization working to promote organic food and agriculture (Økologisk Norge).
Activities
Volunteer workdays in the garden, open lunch/dinner events with produce from the garden, and visits from kindergartens/schools.

Table 6.9 Description of the case Grønlands flytende hage, representing the urban agriculture typology "Innovative urban agriculture-garden in public space"

Grønlands flytende hage (floating garden) (est. 2018)/Oslo Fjordhage (est. 2019)
Location and connectivity
Pilot raft on the bank of the river Akerselva in Grønland, a densely populated area in the city center. Well connected to public transport, but not easily visible, and more accessible for local users than the general public.
Floating greenhouse placed in Sukkerbiten, a central site in the seafront area Bjørvika, visible and easily accessible for the general public on the harbor promenade.
Design and amenities
Pilot raft 3m^2 on the bank of Akerselva made from two wooden logs carved out to rafts with jute coffee bags filled with coir as growing medium attached between.
Floating dome-shaped greenhouse made of wood on top of blue plastic barrels for buoyancy.
Management
One-year pilot project initiated and run by a high school teacher and volunteer pupils. Pilot raft built by teacher and pupils with help from professionals. Floating in the river during the summer of 2018.
Floating greenhouse launched 2019 on the seafront of Oslo, managed by high school teacher and local school.
Activities
Pupils and local youth invited to take part in building and planting the pilot raft. Educational program in natural science for schools offered in the floating greenhouse.

Initiating and Managing Urban Agriculture in Public Space

In the following section, we present our findings on practicing urban agriculture in public space based on interviews with two co-initiators of the rooftop garden and the initiator of the floating garden.

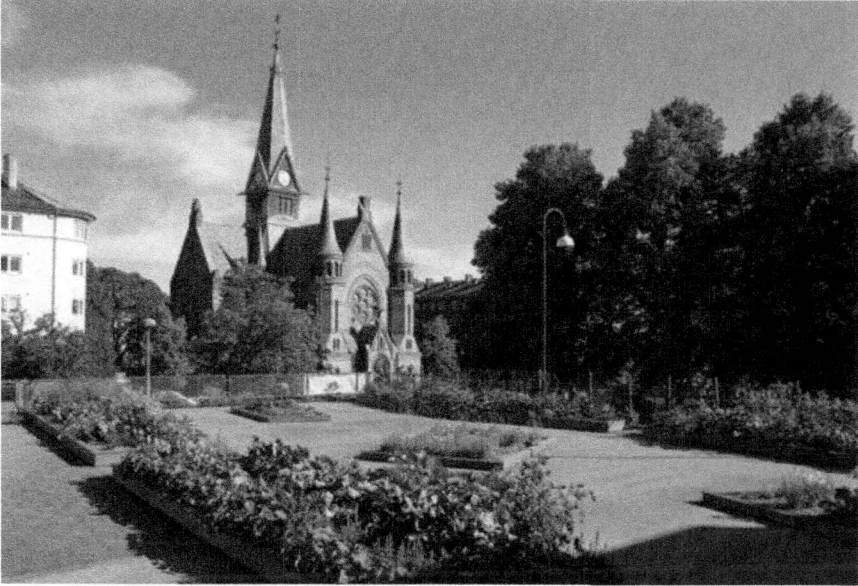

Picture 6.9 Cultivation beds on Sagene rooftop garden. (Photo: Janet Rojas)

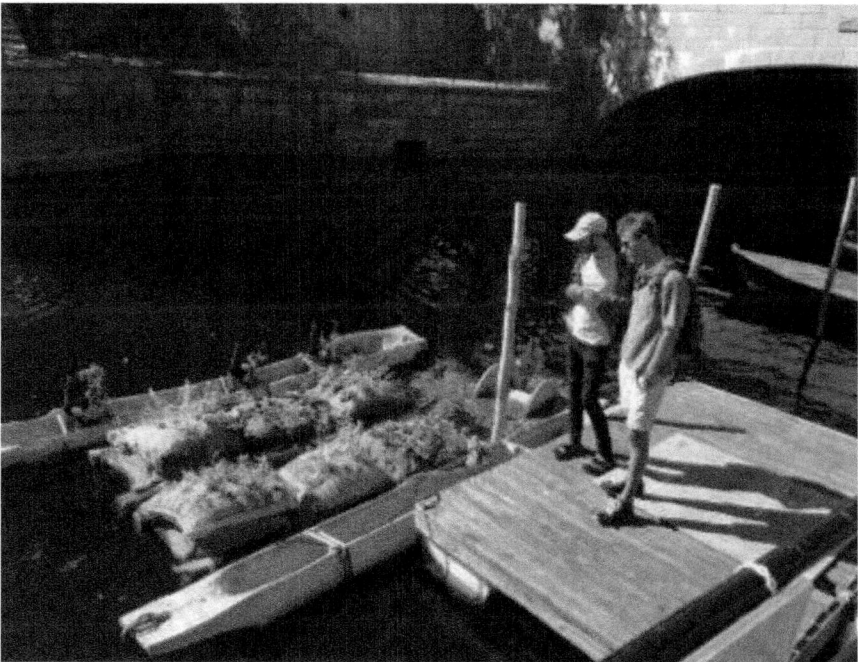

Picture 6.10 The Grønlands floating garden in its initial location along the river Akerselva. (Photo: Jølin Egner Stokke)

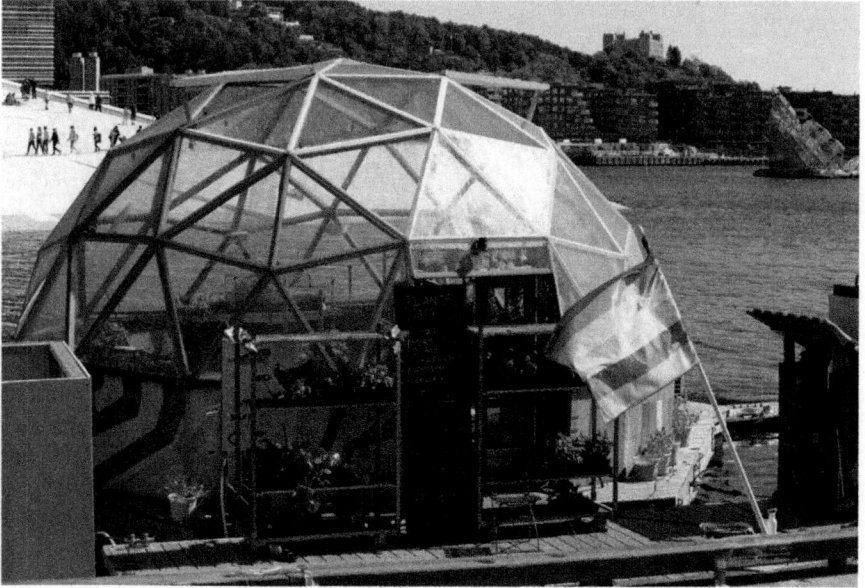

Picture 6.11 The Oslo Fjordhage floating garden on the Oslo waterfront. (Photo: Katinka H. Evensen)

Motives

Albeit different in form and organization, the rooftop and floating garden show some similarities in terms of urban agriculture innovation. Being new and untested in the local context, both projects were motivated by a desire for developing *innovative urban garden typologies*. In Sagene rooftop garden this motive was centered around the issue of unused space in the city when taking rooftops into account. Inspired by European cities like Paris, they wanted to make cultivated rooftop gardens a reality in Oslo and Norway as well. They also aimed to act as agents in local public space development. In the case of Grønland floating garden, one of the main motives was to make a difference in the urban public space especially in areas considered problematic due to drug use: "I want to use it as a showcase, because not only can we make this place nicer [...]. But getting to chat with people, or that there is activity here, can have the ripple effect that makes those who do more shady activities, that they are not chased away, but that they behave properly, that this takes place in civic forms" (Project manager, floating garden). In this way, the goal was to enhance the livability of the area. A transformation process was underway, as part of the waterfront development in Oslo. According to the project leader, this process predominantly benefited major actors and property developers. With this project, they sought to represent non-commercial interests and serve as a productive force in creating a more inclusive space.

The initiator of the floating garden project, a teacher at a local high school, expressed a clear motivation to combine the local urban development impact of the project with his teaching activities. Sagene rooftop garden had no formal connection to schools or kindergartens, but held regular open days. Therefore, developing an *educational arena for schools and kindergarten and showcase for food production in the city* were common motives. For the floating garden, the goal was to get the students out of the classroom and give them more practical experiences. In Sagene rooftop garden, learning was a key motivation, with information signs and organized events for local children as educational moments.

Supporting Factors

The first common supporting factor in these projects was competence. To succeed in these innovative projects, a variety of *competencies* seemed needed. At the rooftop garden, multidisciplinarity was a crucial factor: the whole multidisciplinary group of people, that is part of the success [...] because we are engineers and have no bearing on cultivation, and those who cultivate, they do not like to work with lawyers and contracts (Co-initiator, Sagene rooftop garden). In both the rooftop and floating gardens cultivation of plants on roofs and water required seeking specialized competences on materials. However, the technical expertise would be insufficient in the end they also needed do it in practice, as the initiator of the floating garden expressed it: "I have learned this quite thoroughly; one should not overestimate people with 'papers' in such projects. [...] In the world we operate in, hands-on experience is what truly counts, nothing else."

In the rooftop garden, formal collaborations with prominent actors and entrepreneurs were as crucial as collaboration with local actors. They especially valued their collaboration with the local café and ecological grocery store: "[...] the main reason is to work together in 'dugnad' (community work), so that everyone can have fun." The collaboration with a center for food culture for children nearby was also essential, as it gave them access to the greenhouse. At the floating garden, an important aspect was involving local users of the space, regardless of whether they were considered problematic. By interacting with and involving them, the hope was that they would protect and prevent vandalism of the floating garden and its riverbank neighbor, the wooden boat rental. A third supporting factor is *determination*, which was visible and necessary to all the cases studied in this project. Still, seeing the list of challenges experienced by these innovative projects, it seems reasonable to give it special attention. The floating garden adopted a "just-do-it" mentality exemplified by dealing with municipality regulations. The project manager described lengthy communications with the municipality about bureaucratic requirements. In the end the pilot raft was launched, and they informed the municipality instead of asking.

Challenges

Some primary challenges for the innovative urban agriculture gardens were related to *juridical, technical, and aesthetical issues.* In breaking ground, both gardens experienced overwhelming legal requirements to initiating their projects. For the rooftop garden, most of the juridical and technical issues came from the carrying capacity of the rooftop itself. This kind of calculations required qualified experts' involvement, and formal contracts for insurance issues/reasons. For the floating garden, they found themselves being asked to apply for a building permit, as if they were constructing a permanent structure.

Also connected to issues concerning technical requirements is the aesthetics of an innovative urban agriculture garden. At the rooftop garden, engineers calculated a carrying capacity allowing for certain parts of the rooftop to carry a limited weight. This would allow them to put planter boxes with a lot of space between them spread across the surface. To the project initiator group, this did not meet their esthetical standards, and they had to bring in a landscape architect to draw a design where the weight is spread more evenly. According to them, the fact that the garden is in public space necessitated a certain aesthetics: "I think that Sagene takhage is one of few [rooftop gardens] that are publicly accessible [...] so it's very important that it always looks nice and lush" (Project co-initiator, Sagene rooftop garden).

Another challenge described by both project managers was navigating bureaucracy. Dealing with these technical and legal issues is costly and time-consuming, especially for low-budget, volunteer-based projects. In both projects, they put down hundreds of hours in meetings, inquiries, writing applications, and contract work. A final challenge for both initiatives is *collaboration with landowners.* The initiators of these projects expected that gardens would be considered valuable in the city and that all relevant actors would be collaborative. The floating garden project spent a lot of time getting the right permissions to use the public space. As for the rooftop garden initiators, it came as a surprise to experience that the members of the board of the housing cooperative (the landowner) were skeptical and had concerns about the garden potentially attracting youth and drug-related problems: "[...] for us it was a great surprise that not everyone was jumping for joy to have a rooftop garden" (Co-initiator, Sagene rooftop garden). The project group selected the space as suitable for a rooftop garden. Still, there was no pre-established connection between the project group and the housing cooperative, which may have given the project less grounding.

Visions

The project managers from both innovative urban agriculture gardens we studied seemed to have a vision of developing rooftop garden and floating school garden as typologies for urban public cultivation of the future. They saw potential in exploiting unused and even unexpected public spaces, like the river and fjord, for areas for urban agriculture activity.

6.3.5 Assessments of Urban Agriculture's Contribution to Publicness

Based on Murphy and Grabalov (Chap. 4) we assessed each urban agriculture case's contribution to publicness. The assessments revealed that the location and design of the cultivation area were decisive in whether the place increased accessibility and the space's animation. The Sagene rooftop and Ellingsrud neighborhood garden are examples of urban agriculture projects that succeeded in opening the space to a larger public. However, the same two cases and Snippen, only contributed social services to a smaller public. Being a suitable place to offer social services such as educational, vocational, or therapeutic activities may hence need a degree of enclosure or demarcation provided by fences or signs. Only the city farm Losæter was considered producing food to a smaller public, beyond members due to their regular open common meal served. Finally, all, except Snippen, a project for a small group, were considered to have significantly contributed to building communities to spread cultivation knowledge. The comparison across typologies illustrates their various potential in increasing the publicness of urban space.

Table 6.10 Publicness assessment based on Murphy and Grabalov (Chap. 4 of this book), ● significantly present, reaching a large public, ◐ present, reaching a smaller public, ○ implies not present or not reaching beyond members

Case	Increasing access and animation	Contributing social services	Producing and distributing food	Building communities to spread cultivation knowledge
City farm				
Losæter	◐	●	◐	●
Urban agriculture in central parks				
Schous/Sofeinbergparken	◐	●	○	●
Snippen	◐	◐	○	◐
Neighborhood garden				
Voksenenga	◐	●	○	●
Ellingsrud parsellhage	●	◐	○	●
Dr. Dedichens drivhus	○	●	○	●
Innovative urban agriculture gardens				
Sagene takhage	●	◐	○	●
Grønland flytende hage/Oslo Fjordhage	◐	●	○	●

6.4   Discussion

This chapter presents the main findings from our case studies in Oslo, exploring various ways of integrating urban agriculture into public spaces. In the following, we discuss experiences across the typologies of urban agriculture (see Table 6.11 for overview of main findings). First, we look at organizational aspects of urban agriculture in public space. Then we discuss the potential impact of urban agriculture on well-being urban agriculture city dwellers in public spaces by summarizing the motivations and experiences from the projects. Finally, we address future potentials for urban agriculture in public space to contribute to publicness and increase social sustainability.

6.4.1   Organizational Aspects of Urban Agriculture in Public Space

The experiences from the Oslo cases offer valuable insights into how to succeed with urban agriculture in public space. First, the importance of *co-creation/networking* seemed crucial to making the projects happen and keeping them going. The initiators and project managers highlighted collaborations between local government, community, and private stakeholders. Having a coordinator or *project manager in a paid position*, preferably within the municipality or district, seemed decisive for the longevity of the larger more complex projects like Losæter and Voksenenga nærmiljøhage. Accordingly, another shared experience was that urban agriculture projects need a coordinator of activities, but that they also need to keep room for individual or bottom-up initiatives. The latter was exemplified in Losæter, where their strategy of organic development ensured openness to users' ideas, and in Dr. Dedichens Drivhus where they recognized the importance of letting the users self-initiate manageable small-scale projects. Finding a *balance between professional and local coordinators* also seems important to consider and needs to be adapted to the type and goal of the project, be it a learning hub like Losæter or a local meeting place like a neighborhood garden as the main function.

Furthermore, using urban agriculture to develop more *innovative green space management practices*   seemed to offer many opportunities, the District of Grünerløkka being an interesting case. Furthermore, the *collaboration* between the local library and the green space management in Schous plass, organizing events with free food, and use of play equipment, are examples of reaching a greater audience for disseminating ecological knowledge.

To succeed with practicing urban agriculture in public space seemed to be especially sensitive to *physical design and configuration* of the space itself. First, it seemed important to effectively communicate that cultivation was going on in the space to legitimize the activity, like in Snippen, and second, to make sure the space was perceived as welcoming for passers-by to enjoy, or invite to participate.

Table 6.11 Motivations, supporting factors and challenges for urban agriculture in public space: experiences from Oslo

Typology	City farm	Urban agriculture in central public parks	Neighborhood garden	Innovative urban agriculture gardens in public space (roof/floating)
Motives	Outdoor culture institution Participation – empowerment Knowledge dissemination – cultural heritage	Activation of place Participation – empowerment Vocational training Knowledge dissemination – food and ecology	Social meeting place Arena for outdoor/outside home activity Activation of place Educational arena for schools and kindergartens	Develop roof/floating garden as urban agriculture typology Local urban space development Educational arena for schools and kindergartens Showcase for food production in the city
Supporting factors	Organization: organic development Professionality Room for experimentation	Collaboration across sectors/public-private partnership Horticultural, social, and pedagogical competence Innovative practice	Coordinator Co-creation/networking Keeping scale/ambitions low	Collaboration with local actors Competence Determination
Challenges	Perceived publicness Social barriers Physical barriers	Lack of appreciation/value among local residents Design Temporality	Organizing volunteers Lack of recognition at district level Temporality	Technical, judicial, aesthetical issues Navigating the bureaucracy Collaboration with landowner
Visions	Collaboration with the national art and culture institutions Become a unifier of farming movements	Cultivate entire square(s) Multifunctional urban agriculture gardens Create system for circularity in practice: composting	Become publicly funded and included/part of local public services Creating culture for open accessible active outdoor spaces Preserve local history by activating public space through cultivation	Roof garden/floating school garden as typologies for urban public cultivation

Moreover, when integrating urban agriculture in public space, finding a suitable quantity of space to be taken up by urban agriculture seemed important. In Schous plass urban agriculture was added as "something extra" in the public square, while Losæter offered full-scale urban agriculture, completely leaving behind the neat park design and management. Likewise, considering the aesthetics of the cultivation project seemed important, various aesthetics appealing to some user groups, others not, could influence perceived openness and hence accessibility for a large public. Therefore, it seems relevant to communicate through signage or design that the spaces are open for all people's enjoyment. Furthermore, urban agriculture's typologies in public spaces varied greatly in dimensions of publicness within one typology, like the neighborhood garden. This demonstrates the variety of locations, design, and organizations possible and their respective consequence in perceived accessibility to the public.

6.4.2   Urban Agriculture in Public Space for City Dweller's Well-Being

The motives for initiating the studied urban agriculture projects in Oslo seemed focused on creating green *social meeting places* and *educational arenas* for cultivation and ecology (see Table 6.9). Additionally, the motives of *activation of place* and *empowerment* seemed to have been an underlying motivation for initiating some of the projects. Below we provide our interpretations of these findings.

Previous practice and research focusing on the benefits of urban agriculture have also highlighted urban agriculture's potential role as community builder and capacity for being both social and learning arenas (e.g., Hale et al., 2011; Veen et al., 2016). We found that the project initiators and managers across the typologies of urban agriculture studied shared a nuanced understanding of the potential of urban agriculture in public space as social and learning arenas in the city. Using urban agriculture as a means to create a social meeting place was described as an important goal in itself, especially for the neighborhood gardens, while the other typologies of urban agriculture in public space had wider perspectives on the places' functions as social and learning arenas. Urban agriculture as a learning arena seemed to hold more than learning about cultivation and ecology. The emphasis on cultivation activity in public space as an opportunity for the citizens to have a place to unfold creatively was directly connected to *empowerment*. This function was expressed as important for the city farm in particular, to offer its users and the city dwellers. Having access to an outdoor space where one can actively shape and create the surroundings is related to the capability "senses," described by Nussbaum (2011) as being able to use the senses, develop ideas, and produce works.

Finally, the motive of using urban agriculture in public space as a tool in the local urban space development to activate unused or challenging spaces also seemed to be connected to yet another benefit. The project initiators and managers saw urban agriculture activity as an opportunity for citizens to influence their outdoor space's use and their perceived ownership of it. For example, the city farm and the urban agriculture in central park projects recognize the importance of cultivation activities in facilitating *participation* among city dwellers, which is linked to the capability described by Nussbaum (2011), having "control over one's environment." Hence, we found that the projects seem to recognize benefits related to dimensions of well-being that go beyond using urban agriculture for greening the city, green social meeting places or as arenas for spreading knowledge of ecology.

In summary, we found that the motives or goals for the studied projects correspond with the strategy for urban agriculture in Oslo (Oslo Kommune, 2019). Project initiators and managers saw urban agriculture as a means to create green social meeting places and learning arenas. In contrast, the other goals in the municipality's strategy, greening the city and increasing local food production, were not given much attention. Food production and greening the city as goals were less prominent as motives among the project managers, although mentioned by the innovative urban agriculture projects we studied. This finding may illustrate how urban agriculture is already established as a tool in urban local space development and explored as a catalyst for social services and educational purposes, and not simply being driven by a wish to grow food and make the city greener.

Production of food as a motive is a debated topic in urban agriculture practice and research (Martin et al., 2016). What role does food production have in urban agriculture in public space? What our findings suggest is that the activity of producing food was mostly the tool for achieving the benefits mentioned above. This can also be explained by the types of gardening we have studied. Having crops in public space, like in the studied cases, is liable to "theft" and sabotage, which could be a challenging. In the sociopolitical context of Oslo, the need to produce food to alleviate food scarcity has not been a priority. However, the recent events like pandemic and war may have caused instability in the food supply chain that can alter this notion.[2]

6.4.3 Methodological Considerations and Future Studies

In this study, we followed the development of a selection of urban agriculture projects in public space. The project initiators and managers shared their experiences, their reflections on challenges, and critical issues in organizing urban agriculture in public space. Similarly, the analysis of dimensions of publicness of the projects was

---

[2] It's been reported that garden centers experience increased interest in gardening supplies for growing vegetables. See, e.g., https://www.nrk.no/innlandet/enorm-interesse-for-a-dyrke-gronsaker-pa-grunn-av-pandemi-og-krig.-espen-nordbekk-er-i-gang.-1.15919578.

conducted by the research team and could have benefitted from being more systematically studied from the perspective of the neighbors and visitors to get a broader picture of these urban agriculture projects' perceived publicness and accessibility.

6.5 Conclusions

This case study in Oslo (2018–2020) exemplified several ways of organizing urban agriculture in public space and their accessibility to the urban population. Experiences from eight urban agriculture projects of various typologies, scales, and organizational models, from the city farm to small experimental cultivation projects, were collected. The urban agriculture projects' motivations emphasized creating social meeting places and learning arenas for cultivation and ecological knowledge. They also utilized urban agriculture as a tool in local urban space development and to improve city dwellers' well-being by using urban agriculture in public spaces to activate and make unused space safer. They also integrated cultivation in green space management in new and innovative ways. Significant supporting factors for the success of urban agriculture in public space were related to co-creation or wide networks of collaborators, preferably with coordinators employed by the municipality or city district. However, finding the right balance between professional organization and room for users' initiatives seemed important for social sustainability. The main challenges described by the project managers concerned issues of recognizing urban agriculture as spaces offering social and public services and navigating bureaucracy with innovative uses of public spaces. To ensure accessibility for large and diverse segments of urban populations, we found that perceived publicness of spaces could improve through purposeful design.

6.5.1 Visions and Potentials for Urban Agriculture in Public Space

The projects initiators and managers had ideas for further development of their projects and saw potential for urban agriculture in public space. Most of the potentials envisioned were related to how to organize urban agriculture in public space. The most prominent potential described by the project managers was to better utilize urban agriculture as part of the local municipal services. They function as both educational arenas and social meeting places and, as such, hold an important function for local environments' social sustainability. However, for urban agriculture in public spaces to succeed with such functions, it seemed to demand stable leadership and competencies in both social work and cultivation.

The further potential was to expand in size or develop new typologies of urban agriculture in public space and to make urban agriculture a more integrated part of the green space structure as multifunctional gardens. Another idea was to create a system for circularity in practice through collaboration with local restaurants and using their compost. Further, some see the potential of urban agriculture in public space to be a unifying meeting place for various farmer movements from conventional and organic agriculture. On the cultural side, developing a closer collaboration with art and culture institutions was mentioned, as well as using urban agriculture in public space as a means to preserve local cultural heritage buildings. The visions and potentials found among the coordinators interviewed for this study correlate well with the findings of Chap. 8. In that study, some of the same initiatives partook in student-facilitated processes to develop a shared, tangible vision for their initiatives. Additionally, they worked with action plans for how to reach this vision.

The projects included in this study received their funding either from a foundation or the municipality's budgets and were established, while the Oslo municipal and central government of Norway were developing a strategy for urban agriculture (The Norwegian Ministries, 2021), the impact of which may have resulted in positively influencing the initiatives. The role of the municipal policy in successfully integrating urban agriculture in public space is the focus of Chaps. 11 and 12.

Appendix

Appendix 1 (Table 6.12)

Table 6.12 Categorization scheme of cases

Variety/differences in:
Types of users: primary (active members/users), secondary (neighbors or local people belonging to the place), and tertiary (passers-by, visitors, users of the public space, not living in the neighborhood).
Objectives/motives
Functions/activities
Opportunities for engagement
Stage and organization
Well-established/newly started/planned
Top-down (planning, governance, maintenance, etc.)/bottom-up initiative
Short-term/long-term funding
Volunteer-based (social entrepreneurship)/employment-based
Degree of publicness and accessibility
Ownership status of public space (privately owned and regulated as public space vs. publicly owned and regulated as public space)
Urban structure

Appendix 2

The interviews with the project managers lasted between 45 and 110 minutes and were recorded with the informants' written consent. They were given the opportunity to read and comment on citations used for this publication. The study was registered and approved by the Norwegian Centre for Research Data (NSD) (Reference number 251173).

References

Audate, P. P., Fernandez, M. A., Cloutier, G., & Lebel, A. (2019). Scoping review of the impacts of urban agriculture on the determinants of health. *BMC Public Health, 19*, 672. https://doi.org/10.1186/s12889-019-6885-z

Braun, V., & Clarke, V. (2006). Using thematic analysis in psychology. *Qualitative Research in Psychology, 3*(2), 77–101. https://doi.org/10.1191/1478088706qp063oa

Eason, K. D. (1988). *Information technology and Organisational change* (1st ed.). CRC Press. https://doi.org/10.1201/9781482275469

Hale, J., Knapp, C., Bardwell, L., Buchenau, M., Marshall, J., Sancar, F., & Litt, J. S. (2011). Connecting food environments and health through the relational nature of aesthetics: Gaining insight through the community gardening experience. *Social Science & Medicine, 72*(11), 1853–1863.

Litt, J. S., Schmiege, S. J., Hale, J. W., Buchenau, M., & Sancar, F. (2015). Exploring ecological, emotional and social levers of self-rated health for urban gardeners and non-gardeners: A path analysis. *Social Science & Medicine, 144*, 1–8. https://doi.org/10.1016/j.socscimed.2015.09.004

Lohrberg, F. (2019). Urban agriculture forms in Europe. In E. Gottero (Ed.), *Agrourbanism: Tools for governance and planning of agrarian landscape* (pp. 133–147). Springer International Publishing. https://doi.org/10.1007/978-3-319-95576-6_9

Martin, G., Clift, R., & Christie, I. (2016). Urban cultivation and its contributions to sustainability: Nibbles of food but oodles of social capital. *Sustainability, 8*(5), 18, Article 409. https://doi.org/10.3390/su8050409

Miljødirektoratet. (2022). *Miljøstatus – Støy*. Retrieved 06/03/2023 from https://miljostatus.miljodirektoratet.no/tema/forurensning/stoy/

Murphy, M. A., Parker, P., & Hermus, M. (2023). Cultivating inclusive public space with urban gardens. *Local Environment, 28*(1), 99–116. https://doi.org/10.1080/13549839.2022.2120461

Nussbaum, M. C. (2011). *Creating capabilities: The human development approach*. Harvard University Press.

Oslo Kommune. (2019). *Sprouting Oslo – Room for everyone in the city's green spaces. A strategy for urban agriculture 2019–2030*. Oslo Kommune. Retrieved 06/03/2023 from https://www.oslo.kommune.no/getfile.php/13398183-1614956203/Tjenester%20og%20tilbud/Natur%2C%20kultur%20og%20fritid/Urbant%20landbruk/BYM_SpirendeOslo_engelsk_A4_digital.pdf

Oslo Kommune. (2022). *Ulike typer urbant landbruk*. Retrieved 06/03/2023 from https://www.oslo.kommune.no/natur-kultur-og-fritid/urbant-landbruk/ulike-typer-urbant-landbruk/0

Rogge, N., Theesfeld, I., & Strassner, C. (2020). The potential of social learning in community gardens and the impact of community heterogeneity. *Learning Culture and Social Interaction, 24*, 100351. https://doi.org/10.1016/j.lcsi.2019.100351

Swensen, G., Stafseng, V. E., & Nielsen, V. K. S. (2022). Visionscapes: Combining heritage and urban gardening to enhance areas requiring regeneration. *International Journal of Heritage Studies, 28*(4), 511–537. https://doi.org/10.1080/13527258.2021.2020879

Tharrey, M., & Darmon, N. (2022). Urban collective garden participation and health: A systematic literature review of potential benefits for free-living adults. *Nutrition Reviews, 80*(1), 6–21. https://doi.org/10.1093/nutrit/nuaa147

The Norwegian Ministries. (2021). *Dyrk byer og tettsteder. Nasjonal strategi for urbant landbruk.* Landbruks og matdepartementet, Kommunal og moderniseringsdepartementet, Helse og omsorgsdepartementet, Klima og miljødepartementet, Arbeids og sosialdepartementet og Kunnskapsdepartementet. Retrieved 06/03/2023 from https://www.regjeringen.no/conte ntassets/4be68221de654236b85b76bd77535571/207980-strategi-for-urbant-landbruk-web. cleaned-1.pdf

Tornaghi, C., & Knierbein, S. (Eds.). (2014). *Public space and relational perspectives.* Routledge.

Veen, E. J., Bock, B. B., Van den Berg, W., Visser, A. J., & Wiskerke, J. S. C. (2016). Community gardening and social cohesion: Different designs, different motivations. *Local Environment, 21*(10), 1271–1287. https://doi.org/10.1080/13549839.2015.1101433

Woodcraft, S., Bacon, N., Hackett, T., Caistor-Arendar, L., & Hall, F. (2012). *Design for Social Sustainability: A framework for creating thriving new communities.* Retrieved 06/03/2023 from https://planning.ri.gov/sites/g/files/xkgbur826/files/documents/comp/Design_for_Social_ Sustainability.pdf

Chapter 7
The Importance of Social Programming in Urban Agriculture: A Practitioner's Experiences from Norway

Helene Gallis, Kimberly Weger, and Adam Curtis

7.1   Sowing the Seeds of Change

Founded in 2013, the Norwegian social enterprise Nabolagshager literally means "community gardens" or "neighborhood gardens." Urban agriculture, as such, has always been at the heart of the organization's work. The organization dates back to 2011, inspired by a deep motivation to work on the transition to sustainability by engaging communities in hands-on action. Sowing a seed, watching it grow, caring for the plant, and enjoying the harvest at the end of the season seemed to me like the best pedagogical tool to begin a conversation on sustainability and the state of our urban landscapes. Nabolagshager closed it's operations in 2023, but the projects described in this text are continuing, and building on the insights from this essay.

From these early experiences, over a decade Nabolagshager grew into a renowned organization in the field of urban agriculture in Norway. Combining hands-on experiences with a focus on developing knowledge, sharing tools and best practices in entrepreneurship, placemaking, social inclusion, and circular economics, the Nabolagshager team was a significant contributor to the popularity and mainstreaming of urban agriculture.

Nabolagshager staff worked with prestigious universities, think-tanks, cities, and municipalities in Oslo, Europe, and worldwide. Our mission embodied the "think global, act local" motto. We played an active role in facilitating the development of urban agriculture by developing and sharing knowledge, providing a networking forum, and seeking visibility in media and social media for agriculture in the city. Some of our key experiences included running a rooftop farm, an indoor aquaponic facility, and an incubator program for urban agriculture startups and entrepreneurs. Additionally, we coordinated a variety of large and small urban gardens with private or public sector partners. More than 2000 people attended our courses and training

H. Gallis (✉) · K. Weger · A. Curtis
Nabolagshager, Oslo, Norway

© The Author(s) 2024   151
B. Sirowy, D. Ruggeri (eds.), *Urban Agriculture in Public Space*, GeoJournal
Library 132, https://doi.org/10.1007/978-3-031-41550-0_7

sessions, and the organization offered hundreds of young people their first job experience, often in community gardens around Oslo.

Today, we think of ourselves as social designers who utilized sustainability and urban agriculture as tools to build better cities. The significant experiences we gained around urban agriculture – both practically and theoretically and locally and internationally – have given us an understanding of urban gardens as projects that produce public life and social meeting places, rather than food alone. In this essay I share some stories of Nabolagshager's and my journey and vision for the urban agriculture of the future.

7.2   An Emerging Field Where Practitioners Need to Learn from Each Other

When asked to list the key elements for a thriving and resilient urban garden in public space, most people would list seeds, plants, and soil, nurtured by sun, water, and compost. However, from an experienced practitioner's perspective, I have observed that a project's success rarely depends on these basic elements but on the active cultivation of social connections and a project team skilled at facilitating community dialogue and nurturing local pride and ownership.

At their best, community gardens are multifunctional spaces where we cultivate zero-km organic food, improve urban biodiversity, engage in physical activity while nurturing urbanites' biophilia, and contribute to writing a captivating story that illustrates what a transition to a sustainable and resilient urban future can look, feel, and taste like. However, there is a flipside to this coin (Fig. 7.1).

Having seen many projects come and go and having had over the years many informal conversations with urban farmers to find out what worked and what went wrong, I am aware of a few common experiences and answers. Most often, failure of urban agriculture sites is due to an overestimation of the capacity and interest from the local community, or the fluctuating availability and willingness to commit and contribute, even among interested people. Very often the initiators suffer "burnout" after trying to carry out the project responsibilities – including gardening, fundraising, community outreach, and coordination with the municipality and local civil society, alongside day-to-day chores, watering, and weeding. We all need a better understanding of the complexities of an urban agriculture community, along with communication strategies to connect stakeholders.

Urban agriculture continues to be an emerging field. Across the world, practitioners are still exploring, piloting, and adjusting strategies to ensure the maximum positive impact of a systemic and integrated urban agriculture on our communities. This essay digs deeper into some of the challenges I have observed over the years and shares key lessons and tools for addressing and overcoming current and future challenges.

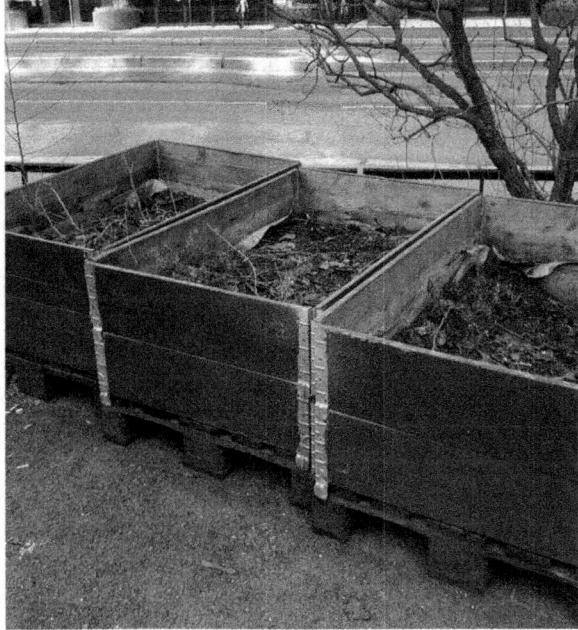

Fig. 7.1 Abandoned pallet garden boxes in a public space, Nabolagshager

As practitioners ourselves, we are continuously evolving, learning, and becoming better at connecting people and creating community. We understand our agency and impact as going well beyond a few bunches of leafy greens and a handful of cherry tomatoes. At the Stensparken Community Garden, one of Nabolagshager's current projects in Oslo, we have applied the lessons we learned over the past decades, gained insights from other "urban farmers," and explored placemaking strategies to help our projects excel, be impactful, and be sustainable. I share these findings in the sections below as proof-in-point of the power of urban agriculture to transform us and the landscapes we live in.

7.2.1 Beer and Hotdogs in the Garden (Fig. 7.2)

"We have found beer and hotdogs to be the secret to a successful urban garden," said Mads Boserup Lauritzen. I met the Danish architect and founder of TagTomat in Copenhagen, Denmark, in 2014, when I was researching my first book, *Dyrk Byen!* (Grow the city), a compilation of experiences from urban agriculture projects in Copenhagen, Stockholm, and Oslo.

Mads soon became a mentor for me, and in many ways we were each other's only colleagues as we both tried to establish ourselves as professional urban gardeners in two Scandinavian capitals. Mads had developed a design for self-watering raised beds made of upcycled materials that became quickly popular both in public

Fig. 7.2 Beer and
hotdogs, Nabolagshager

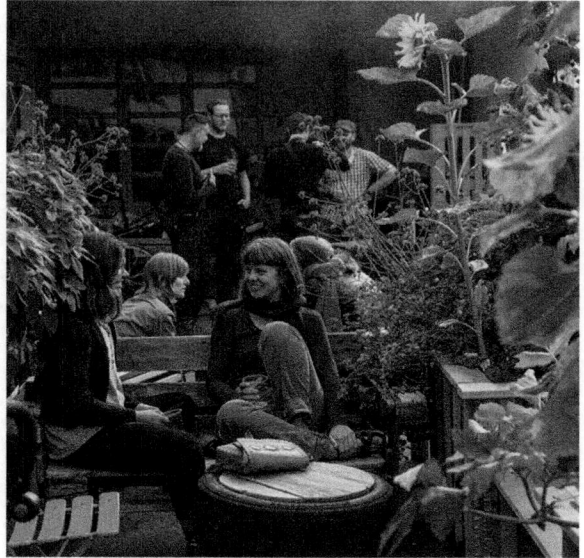

Fig. 7.2 Beer and hotdogs, Nabolagshager

spaces commissioned by city administrators and in private housing associations. The moveable raised beds allowed for an almost instant makeover of any urban space into an edible garden.

"It is extremely important to instantly ignite the social sparks that convert a new garden project into a social meeting place, where people are given a pretext to strike up a conversation and where connections between neighbors are made," explained the architect. By tapping into the favorite Danish past times of socializing with a beer in one hand and a hotdog in the other, he demonstrated a solid understanding of the social dimensions of urban gardening. Every time he and his colleagues built a new garden with neighbors, they ensured that the sharing of food and drinks was an integral part of the process. Sharing a meal helped define the new garden as a place for social encounters and conversations with neighbors and strangers.

Mads' experience resonated strongly with my own experiences of urban agriculture in Oslo, as a project manager and volunteer composter. I understood that building garden beds, planting seeds, and watering plants is the easy part of creating an edible garden. Engaging a wider community in the process, ensuring their ownership of the process and their vested interest in the crops that are cultivated, proves to be more complex. Where garden skills fluctuate over the seasons, community building requires persistence and can take years for results to materialize. Often, people with skills or an interest in vegetable gardening will have little or no skills in community building, co-creation, and social inclusion. I came to these conclusions early on, but I did not yet have appropriate tools to address them.

7.2.2 Urtehagen: Early Experiences with Social Programming

Back in 2012, "Urtehagen" was the first public urban agriculture project I started in Oslo. Before that I had helped out at various other private gardens in the city. I was inspired by the global surge in local initiatives to bring ecologically produced seasonal vegetables to communities that were in one way or another broken (Fig. 7.3).

Urtehagen was one of Oslo's first "new wave" urban agriculture projects of the 2010s to happen in public space. As a pilot project, it illustrated that to be successful, a public urban gardening project needs to play a "social connector" function. The project consisted of over 30 simple raised beds in the sunny corner of Urtehagen, a public plaza.

I lived in the area, had worked as a substitute teacher at the local primary school, and had firsthand knowledge of the local social networks, needs, and challenges. Spending more time in Urtehagen led to in-depth conversations with neighbors, including the alcoholics, drug dealers, and "troublemakers" that were at the time the most frequent users of the space. I made it very clear to them that I was neither a social worker nor the police. I had no intention to interfere nor judge their buying or using drugs or engaging in daytime drinking.

Through a mutually respectful dialogue, we came to a shared understanding that the space would be a public resource prioritizing local kids, at least during the daytime. By day, when children were around, so-called troublemakers would use a different space. I could appeal to universal values such as kindness and helpfulness – most people inherently want to be seen as useful to others. Many of

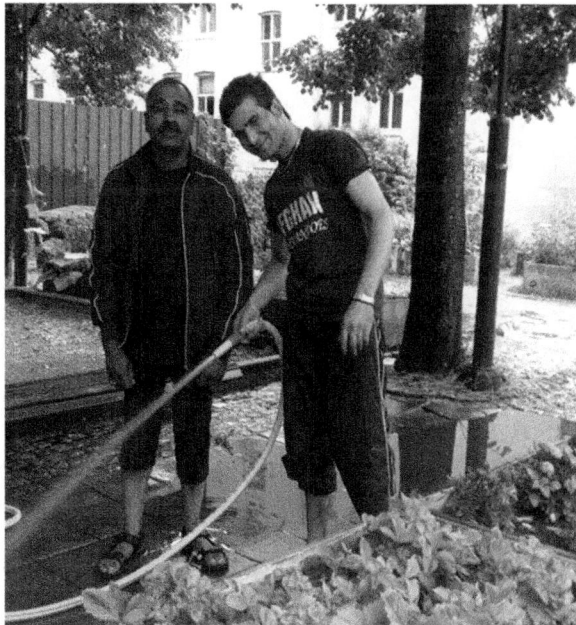

Fig. 7.3 Neighbors, Nabolagshager

the current users had younger siblings or family members, could remember their childhood in public space, and could empathize with local children needing a place to play and feel safe and the children's joy of exploring the urban garden. After all, in addition to being a drug dealer or alcoholic, these were people just like you and me. This dialogue process leveraged the negative elements of the plaza into becoming key players in its success.

The garden witnessed no significant vandalism, and neighbors happily volunteered to water and weed, and many harvested the herbs and vegetables that grew in the garden. Fresh cilantro became a particularly popular crop.

"I have lived here for almost twenty years" said Cecilia, one of the neighbors, "and it's the first time I sit down on this bench," explaining how she had never felt safe in the area. Haroon, a young male refugee from Afghanistan, told us about how this garden helped him feel connected to his family back home. "In Afghanistan, my family always had a garden, and we would grow tomatoes there too. When I am here, tending to the plants, I know that my family, far, far away, are doing the exact same thing" he said, "It's a way of being together, even when we are apart," he explained.

As the project became more established, we realized that there was no funding to support the social programming and gardening activities or simply to support an active presence in it. A very high turnover of inhabitants in the neighborhood made it challenging to have continuity in the activities, as networks had to be continuously updated and re-established. Gradually the project degraded, vandalism damaged plants and planter boxes, and waste accumulated. We had to retract from the project, formally handling it over to the district administration, who would try to make it part of other publicly run social programs. After a successful season, with children as the joyful users of the space, the area was reclaimed by drug dealers and substance abusers.

7.2.3   Sjakkplassen: Empowering and Giving Community Members Responsibility (Fig. 7.4)

In 2015, Nabolagshager took on another challenging public space project. Vaterlandsparken, a small downtown public park, with a reputation for being "Oslo's most dangerous place" was transformed into "Sjakkplassen." This pilot project by the City of Oslo took place between 2015 and 2016 and explored new design processes to integrate urban agriculture in public space. For years, the city had struggled with insecurity in the space, where a combination of homeless Roma migrants, drug users, and drug dealers occupied the area. The project team again had to emphasize our role as being neither social workers nor policemen and explain this to the city administrators. We did not want to alienate or remove certain groups from the public space, rather to empower and give them responsibilities, while also proactively inviting other groups to join the process.

Fig. 7.4 Sjakkplassen, Nabolagshager

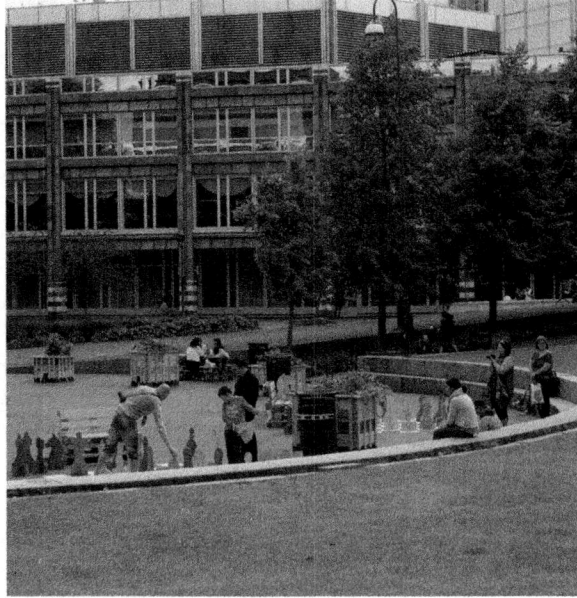

Early in the process we reached out to many community groups in Grønland but aimed especially at the people lacking access to well-functioning public spaces. We also considered their vulnerability as a factor for whether they would be able to act as "pioneers" in the renewed space alongside current users. This meant limiting the involvement of kids or families with small children (Fig. 7.5).

A key target group was Pakistani male seniors that congregated daily in a nearby crowded public space due to its proximity to one of the city's main mosques. By involving them we hoped that they would have a calming effect and instill a sense of mutual respect on the sometimes rough clientele frequenting Sjakkplassen. These seniors would then become responsible for keeping "eyes on the street (Jacobs, 1961)," acting as a sort of community conscience. By incorporating street chess and adapting some of the designs of the benches – including back support and relatively high seating – we worked to create an attractive future space for a relaxed, peaceful, and mature audience.

The rigging of the garden, done in collaboration with Mads from TagTomat (my first so-called colleague in urban agriculture as mentioned earlier in this chapter), happened over a 2-day intensive weekend event. The core team was instructed to treat each person with the same kindness and respect and to talk to and engage everyone – regardless of their social and economic status. We were consciously talking *with* people, not *at* or *to* them. We broke bread with them and served copious amounts of warm food, coffee, lemonade, and fruit over the weekend.

"By offering tasty food, served in an esthetically pleasing place, in a respectful and enthusiastic manner, and not at all expecting anything in return, we created a unique social dimension to the project," explains Tatiana, one of the organizers.

Fig. 7.5 Seniors,
Nabolagshager

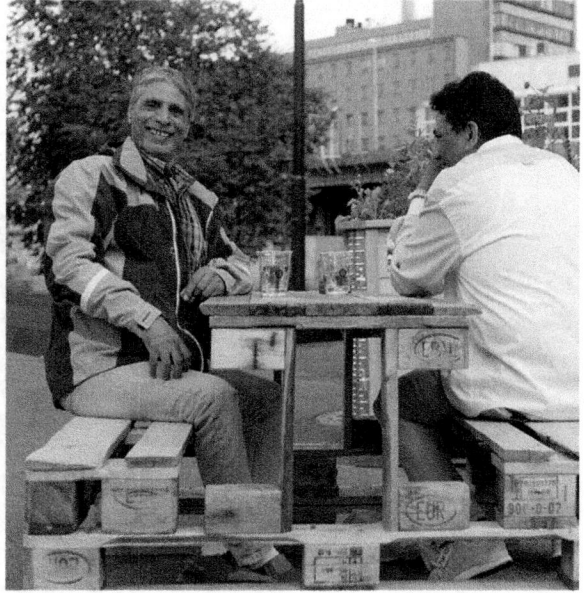

There were no strings attached to the food, and people were free to continue on with their day, after having a bite to eat with us. However; "it baffles people," she says, "gestures of receiving something really nice, for free, in a public space is not something we are used to. When there are no expectations to pay, or do something in return, it can trigger kindness in the most unexpected of places."

By proactively engaging a wide range of current and potential future users, neighbors, and passers-by and engaging them in volunteering for the project, carrying soil bags, planting herbs, or distributing food, participants were empowered and inspired to individual and collective ownership of the project.

"It was a great day, it felt so good to be invited in, being included, and being able to give a hand and feel useful for once," said one of the local contributors when I ran into him a few weeks later. As an immigrant with a longtime struggle with alcoholism, being included in a community activity meant experiencing something new. "I'm clean now," said another one of the locals, referring to his history of substance abuse, "but I know everybody who comes here. I will keep an eye on the place to make sure that people respect what we've all built" (Fig. 7.6).

Throughout the summer of 2015, the community garden at Sjakkplassen transformed into a well-functioning, peaceful, and inclusive social space. Families felt more comfortable bringing their kids to play or socialize in the space. Guests of the nearby Oslo Plaza Radisson Hotel were no longer directed to avoid the plaza when heading to the Munch Museum, and employees in nearby offices could be seen bringing their lunches to this sunny space at midday.

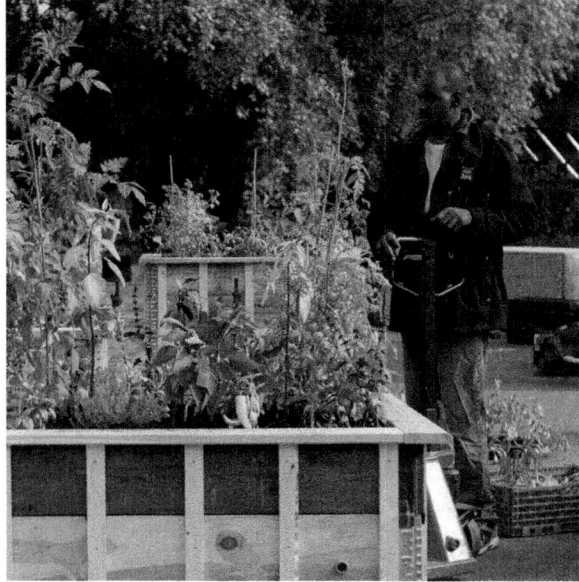

Fig. 7.6 Stakeholders, Nabolagshager

Our observations also matched those of the welfare services outreach team and the police forces. In interviews with anthropologist Katja Bratseth for our project reporting (Brantseth, 2015), local police confirmed that the vibe of the space had changed when more people started using it. They noted that the integration of urban agriculture had a soft, but noticeable regulatory, calming effect on the vulnerable groups they work with. Members of the City Administration told us that during the lifetime of the project on their daily walk-throughs, they did not observe any evidence of violence, vandalism, fighting, drug use, or drug selling, with only one account of littering.

By late October 2015, the city removed the planter boxes and furniture and put everything into storage. In spite of the success, this project was discontinued. It seemed that administrators were not yet ready to fully embrace socially inclusive urban agriculture in the public spaces of the city. Perhaps as a side effect of our strong focus on building community, we had failed to build a stronger rapport with the municipal bureaucracy and thus failed to instill a sense of ownership in them.

A few years later, the district's government tried to revive the project but never managed to actively involve the wider community and ensure their pride and ownership in the project. At the time of writing this chapter, the site has returned to being an asphalt jungle, and there are currently no plans for edible gardens or well-functioning, inclusive social spaces at Sjakkplassen.

7.2.4   The Search for Better Solutions for Lasting Community Impact

Our urban agriculture examples show that ensuring that plants thrive is not sufficient to successfully cultivate a public space. Design and planning practitioners need to continue to experiment with novel approaches to urban agriculture integration in public space and new practices of community engagement. Similarly, they should look beyond their existing networks to become more inclusive of a diversity of traditions of gardening and new practices for cultivating food, as well as community.

The global placemaking community is a practitioner-led source of practical knowledge and solutions to expand the impact of urban agriculture on our cities. This streetwise, practical knowledge can prove easier for practitioners to respond to than the more formal advice of academics and public institutions. Evidence of successful placemaking is widely available, and stories of human impact are easily found on social media, on TED talks, and other web-based platforms and can be a source of inspiration. I will introduce the placemaking community further in the following section.

7.3   Discovering the Global Placemaking Movement

Around the middle of the 2010s, the term "placemaking" was gaining popularity, appearing in all sorts of discussions, and it intrigued me. It described community gardens, bottom-up affordable housing initiatives, temporary projects converting parking lots into public parks, and also large-scale urban developments with sustainability ambitions. I could see that the people involved were just like me – they believed in the community *superpowers* of igniting conversations, giving people an excuse to discuss and untangle local challenges. They were optimists who believed that change was possible and that community could play a key role.

There is no universally accepted definition of the term "placemaking," but the term commonly refers to human interactions that are key to addressing local and global challenges. Dr. Cara Courage, a renowned expert in placemaking and the arts, explained the term in her 2017 *TEDxIndianapolis* talk: "Placemaking is a set of tools and it's an approach to put the community right at the front and center of changes where they live." She continues "it's about bringing people together, in their place, and about getting them talking to each other. When people tell stories of themselves and their places, they begin to understand their places better, and they begin to understand they can have an impact in changing these places for the better (Courage, 2017)."

"Placemaking is a form of community organizing, facilitating, bringing together people and challenging communities to get involved" explains Ethan Kent, the Executive Director of Placemaking X, a global network of leaders that work to accelerate placemaking as a way to create healthy, beloved and inclusive communities. "Placemaking is all about how we all help create our public realm, the world beyond our front door, we challenge each other to be participants in shaping that space," Kent continues "We see it as a new environmental movement that focus on place as a way to bring together many different issues and causes in a city, involving many different departments and disciplines to create value" (Kent, 2018).

In a 2022 article in *The Guardian*, Charlot Schans, the director of the Placemaking Europe network, explains that "We need people-centered cities and public spaces that work towards public life," adding "placemaking is the idea that we own and create these spaces together (Yeung, 2022)." As of today, Placemaking Europe network, whose development Nabolagshager has been a partner in, has members in more than 30 countries, ranging from city administrations and architectural and design firms to community initiatives.

7.3.1   Becoming a Part of a Global Movement That Was Not About Urban Farming

In 2017, I traveled to Amsterdam, Netherlands, to join the Placemaking Week conference. I went there as an urban farmer and left the conference a placemaker. In the keynote presentation by Fred Kent, Project for Public Spaces (PPS) founder, I learned that across the world a huge wave of *changemakers* are transforming urban spaces like streets, parks, and plazas as stages for community building. Many projects involved some aspect of urban agriculture, seen as a means to bring the community together and get a conversation started, not as the end goal itself.

This way of looking at green urban interventions resonated strongly with me. I had increasingly become uneasy with the term "urban agriculture," as I felt that it cultivated human relationships rather than just edible crops. These human connections made a significant difference in people's lives, while edible crops were often negligible in volume and rarely make a significant impact on the local food system. Often, we even hesitated to harvest and eat what was grown in a public space, worried it would be polluted or "dirty" from growing near traffic and litter. The human connections, however, felt like the sparks of something much greater, initiating conversations about making our communities and cities friendlier, more creative, and sustainable.

In his keynote, Fred Kent also observed that public space had become the convergence of many social movements and that this would hold the key to tackling many of our communities' challenges, including equity, sustainability, and public health. Placemaking would help facilitate community champions, alongside lighthouse thinkers in architecture and design, governance, mobility, arts, innovation, and entrepreneurship to come together in our streets to shape visions of a better tomorrow and take the first steps toward a bottom-up urbanism. Placemaking theory proposes that the most important changemaker can be a local grandmother just as well as an important politician or a famous architect. This democratic aspect is to me its most appealing principle that one does not need to be an expert to have a voice that matters.

7.4   Three Key Principles of Placemaking and How They Can Benefit Urban Farmers

Based on decades of work analyzing public spaces and designs that help or hinder human connections, Kathy Madden and Fred Kent, founders of PPS, have developed 11 placemaking principles. These have been shared widely within the placemaking movement as open-source tools, guide PPSs' design work, and inspire other placemakers globally. Many of these principles can be effectively adopted by urban farmers and used in the context of community gardens. Some examples of these principles, as well as their updated applications related to the cultivation of public spaces, are outlined below.

7.4.1   PPS Placemaking Principle #1: The Community Is the Expert

> The important starting point in developing a concept for any public space is to identify the talents and assets within the community. In any community there are people who can provide historical perspective, valuable insights into how the area functions, and an understanding of critical issues. Tapping into this information at the beginning of the process will help to create a sense of community ownership in the project that can be of great benefit to both the project sponsor and community. (PPS, 2013)

Conventional definitions of community tend to be abstract, encompassing anything from a unified body of individuals to society at large. Placemakers also interpret community broadly, but they always set it in a geographical context. In placemaking, community is defined as "anyone who has an interest or stake in a particular place. It is made up of the people who live near the place (whether they use it or not), own businesses or work in the area, or attend institutions like schools or churches there. It also includes elected officials who represent the area and groups that advocate or organize activities there, such as a social justice group, a gardening club, a bicycle coalition, or a merchants' association (Madden, 2018, p. 45)."

The principle of letting the community be the expert is important, because they are the ones who know – through personal experience and local knowledge – what are the strengths and weaknesses of a place. They are the ones who will benefit, or suffer, from any changes happening. Some community members may have already identified potentials for improvement, while others may be more aware of the underlying threats. Most importantly, some community members may function as gatekeepers to others and encourage or hinder participation.

Involving a larger number of people at the early stages of a project means more people will have ownership of the process and outcomes in the long run. The ideas and suggestions generated by a larger and more representative pool of participants are likely to also communicate the perspectives of vulnerable or underrepresented groups and individuals. This is particularly true compared to conventional, top-down public consultations, often dominated by *NIMBY* (not-in-my-backyard) attitudes and also not fully representing the average citizen in income or education levels.

"The Community is the Expert": Experiences from Stensparken Community Garden

At Stensparken Community Garden, a small public space within a larger neighborhood park, Nabolagshager has been creating and running an edible public garden. The community garden is run in close collaboration with the municipal district administration. Getting solid input and triggering community ideas and visions for the future has been a process of mutual learning and inspiration.

We spent the first months of the project performing qualitative and quantitative community mapping and research. We employed a team of young researchers living in the district to help us in this process as part-time collaborators. In order to map ideas and visions from neighbors, we also hosted pilot events to ensure that many demographic groups would be represented. Our collaboration with the district administration was also helpful for sending out digital invitations to residents within a 500-meter radius of the project site.

We began by mapping community ideas, interests, and visions through a quick and effective impact diagnosis. We used the Place Game originally developed by PPS (PPS, 2016) a well-known tool for placemakers worldwide. The youth researchers began by filling out the Place Game questionnaires themselves, before extending the questionnaires to other users of the space.

The Place Game questionnaire evaluates the current status and the potential of a space. The Place Game allows for a group of citizens to dive deep into four categories: sociability, uses and activities, comfort and image, and accesses and linkages. Impressions of the current state of a place are scored in a table, and ideas for short-term and long-term improvements are jotted down and shared (Fig. 7.7).

A low total score showed us where we most urgently needed to take action. The Place Game has been repeated with each group of youth in the Stensparken project, and it has been central to our outreach. In addition to the initial mapping, we have used it over the project life to monitor improvements and prioritize tasks.

Some of the other mapping and monitoring activities at Stensparken included:

- Interviewing seniors at a local senior center about their current but also historical uses of parks
- Sensory exercises to get a better understanding of how the space is experienced if one has some sensory limitations such as being visually impaired
- Quantitative monitoring of different uses and users at different times during the week and during the day
- Interactive and creative sticker voting to rank potential future activities

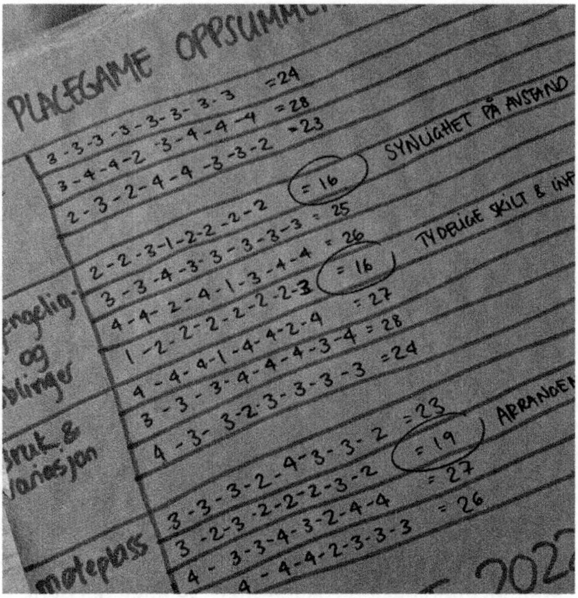

Fig. 7.7 Alternative Place
Game, Nabolagshager

7.4.2   PPS Placemaking Principle #8: Triangulate

> Triangulation is the process by which some external stimulus provides a linkage between
> people and prompts strangers to talk to other strangers as if they knew each other. In a pub-
> lic space, the choice and arrangement of different elements in relation to each other can put
> the triangulation process in motion (or not). For example, if a bench, a waste basket and a
> telephone are placed with no connection to each other, each may receive a very limited use,
> but when they are arranged together along with other amenities such as a coffee cart, they
> will naturally bring people together (or triangulate!). On a broader level, if a children's
> reading room in a new library is located so that it is next to a children's playground in a park
> and a food kiosk is added, more activity will occur than if these facilities were located sepa-
> rately. (PPS, 2013)

Many urban gardens in public space fail to attract community members beyond the avid gardeners and struggle to keep up motivation throughout the growing season, particularly since the harvest is often limited. Indeed, most community gardens are simply uninteresting to the majority of the community members – especially if the only perceived activity there is to watch plants grow. Inherently, the seasons also affect community gardens, and activity levels drop dramatically during the long Norwegian winter. Every spring, many community gardens find themselves starting practically from scratch, needing to mobilize new volunteers and participants.

Most projects would therefore benefit strongly by thinking of complementary ways to attract other demographics. Applying the triangulation thinking typical of placemaking means adding extra elements, functions, or activities to the urban gar-den to appeal to a wider audience. This can ensure that more people visit the place, stay longer, and strike up a conversation once they are there – leading to a more vibrant and friendly place overall. The human scale is also important: activities or elements must happen within a short distance, close to people, so that they can easily interact and participate.

Triangulation Experiences from Stensparken Community Garden in Oslo

In Stensparken Community garden, we are working on developing the community garden into an attractive destination for many demographic groups in the neighborhood. A triangulation element that emerged early in the participatory mappings was that several neighbors expressed an interest in getting a pizza oven in the space to use for community events (Fig. 7.8).

To build the pizza oven, we contracted a natural building materials expert who built it with the help of youth with summer jobs in the community garden. Other community members added designs and decorations to the oven during one of our open community events. Over the course of a month, the local youth had built a pizza oven in the shape of a frog, an instant hit on social media. Involving the community in its design of the oven ensured a sense of ownership and lots of excitement about the process in the neighborhood.

Other triangulation elements in the community garden included beehives, which were run as a job training program for young adults with learning disabilities and the refurbishment of existing seating and placement of new benches. Simple infrastructural improvements included an outdoor water fountain for dogs and the installation of a recycling station by the gate to invite regular park users to stop by. A

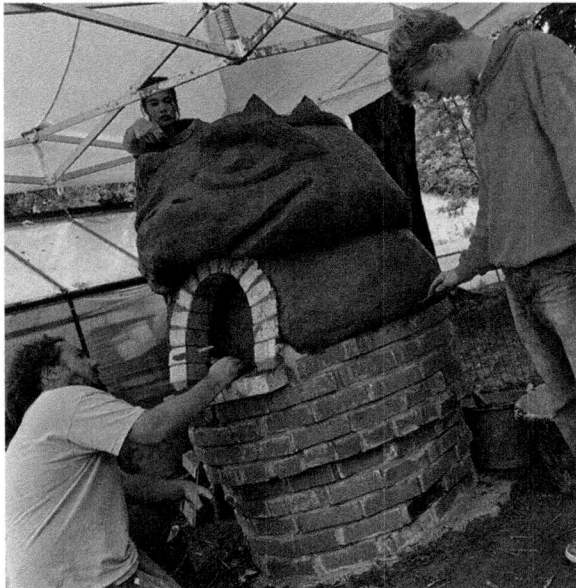

Fig. 7.8 Triangulation in the community Stensparken, Nabolagshager

small covered patio provided shelter when it rains, and the community garden became a stop on a very popular local "map quest" game called "Stolpejakten."

A range of events have been crucial to spreading word-of-mouth through community members about the new venue, and local kindergartens and playgrounds have been key targets in our communications. The events did not focus on gardening – creating instead a rewarding social space for the local community. We especially wanted to engage families with small children, a demographic group who has access to few local facilities beyond outdoor playgrounds. The events were scheduled throughout the year, including successful Halloween and winter festivals.

Triangulations Experiences from Sjakkplassen

Triangulation was also key to the success of Sjakkplassen. In addition to the raised beds, there were various seating areas so that people could enjoy the space alone or in small groups. By dividing the plaza into smaller subspaces and appealing to a more human scale, we found that people were more likely to sit and spend time there (Fig. 7.9).

A signature element of this space was the large-sized street chess set. Before the project started, we had been unsure whether chess would be suitable for the space. However, it proved to be a magnet for many user groups. For instance, it turned out that some of the homeless Roma people were keen to engage other community members in friendly chess matches. As chess games follow internationally understood rules, I observed people of very diverse backgrounds interacting as

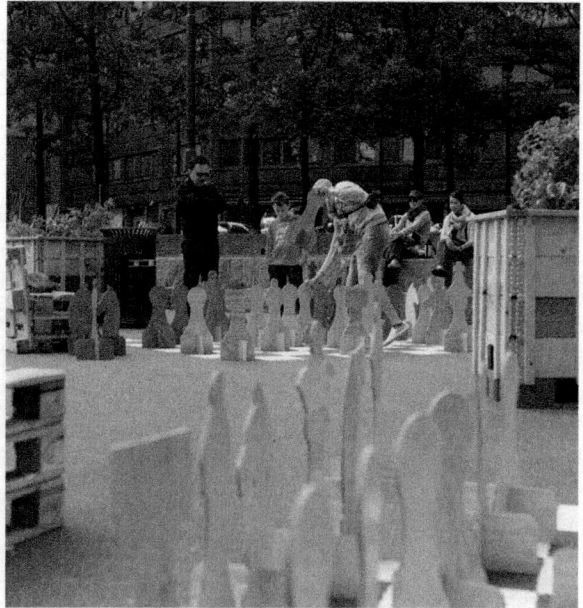

Fig. 7.9 Triangulation Sjakkplassen, Nabolagshager

players–sometimes communicating through body language and nonverbal chess jokes. Adding the outdoor street chess set was a key factor in creating a positive, 24-hour ambience in the urban garden which in itself contributed to Sjakkplassen becoming a well-functioning public space.

Had the project at Sjakkplassen continued, it would have been a logical next step to add other functions to build off the early successes. Within placemaking this is often referred to as "the power of ten (PPS, 2009)" – a principle of providing at least ten complementary activities for each site, ranging from people watching or newspapers reading (requiring comfortable seating) to playing games or engaging in site-specific activities.

Triangulation Experiences from Sandaker Center and Linderud Manor

Oftentimes, an urban garden can serve as a triangulation element within a larger vision. At Sandaker Byhage in Oslo, Nabolagshager runs a small urban garden for the neighborhood shopping center, and at Linderud Community Garden, we are a part of developing an urban gardening space as a part of the museum and heritage site of Linderud Manor in one of Oslo's suburban districts.

Sandaker Senter is a small shopping center in inner Oslo dating back to the 1970s. Part of the building complex is made up of public housing apartments often housing inhabitants who struggle with substance abuse or mental health issues. The complex also houses a municipal library and a community center frequented by many elderly people. As a part of an ongoing dialogue with OBOS, the owner and largest housing developer in Norway, we were commissioned to develop and run an urban public garden around a plaza and terrace on the sunny southern tip of the center. This was a part of a larger upgrade and overhaul of the shopping center, coinciding with the expansion and upgrade of the library, indoor renovations, and an upgrade of the municipal park on the back of the complex.

By investing in a public community garden, the shopping center received a visual makeover and also managed to attract a more balanced clientele to the terrace with a positive ripple effect on other nearby businesses. Community members told us that they appreciated walking past the garden and being able to take in nature's beauty on a day-to-day basis, rather than worrying about hearing cuss words or aggressive outbursts from the heavy drinkers that used to dominate the terrace.

An important part of the success of this triangulation element was our approach in dealing with the locals, who were quite negative to begin with, seeing this as just another gentrification effort. Time and again, we repeated and emphasized that the lush garden would not make beer more expensive or force them to leave their favorite hangout, even as it was becoming more popular and the clientele changed. Over the 5 years we have managed this garden; we gradually built a good relationship with many of the bar guests, who became fond of the beautiful surroundings, were inspired by the seasonal change, and felt a part of a community of caretakers.

This urban garden, which we manage on behalf of the shopping center owners, has also been an important experiment in developing a low-maintenance pollinator-friendly garden that is more visually appealing than edible, although there are several berry bushes, herbs, and edible plants included in the garden design from which one could eat.

At Linderud Manor our role has been more as a facilitator helping to kick-start some of the social aspects of the Museum's vision. The Manor's management has over the last few years radically changed the museum from being an introverted, closed-off, "storage of historical artifacts," to becoming a busy hub of many activities that cater both to the local community as well as maintaining the interest of those with an interest in local history. In addition to their historical baroque gardens, the Museum has set aside a large field as a multifaceted urban farm. This field has now become a large and bustling community garden managed in collaboration with local community groups and startup businesses. There is land allocated for startups related to urban agriculture, such as cultivation of flowers for sale for weddings and events, and a Community Supported Agriculture garden (CSA) providing abundant organic vegetables to their members.

Throughout the year, Linderud Manor hosts market days and workshops and invites local kindergarten and primary school students to garden. Local teenagers are employed as garden helpers during the summer, and once a week there are guided tours, with an eco-philosophical twist. All these triangulation elements help develop a site with a multitude of attractions, ample possibilities for connecting with other people, and multiple partners from the local community.

The Power of 10

The power of triangulation is so effective that, among placemakers, it is easy to think "the more the better." The most well-functioning public spaces are where a wide range of people can find attractive reasons to hang out, and it's argued that at least ten such attractions should exist in every place. At a larger level, each city should have at least ten such well-functioning and attractive places.

In the context of urban gardens, few manage to have as many as ten attractions. Prinzessinnengärten in Berlin, Germany, illustrates a successful application of very varied and inclusive triangulation experiments. The site hosts a popular café, beekeeping, plants, seeds, and seedlings for sale for those interested in gardening themselves. The garden organizes solidarity events, features educational gardens for local school children, and hosts a wide range of events catering to all interests, including beer brewing, flower arrangements, upcycling workshops, concerts, lectures, and food-related workshops such as making sauerkraut and spice mixes. Crops from the garden are sold at the café, and excess produce is sold to visitors.

Prinzessinnengärten is a multifaceted attractive destination for local foodies, environmentalists, urbanists, and social entrepreneurs, as well as people simply looking for a green and peaceful corner to spend time with friends or read a book. Children of all ages find great pleasure in exploring the site, roam free, and connect with urban nature. As a space for self-organized initiatives, it is popular among people wanting to share a skill with the community. Activities such as pop-up bike repair workshops or DIY building of insect hotels or garden beds from upcycled materials take place throughout the year. The garden attracts a significant number of national and international tourists interested in sustainable urban development and edible city solutions. Prinzessinnengärten has successfully developed into a multi-faceted destination, partly due to the longevity of the project, as it has been an active site since 2009.

The Power of 10 principle also advocates working on the city scale – that every city should have at least ten such hotspots within its city limits. In 2010, the town of Andernach in Southern Germany, with a population of 20,000, launched its initiative to become an "edible city." All over the city, there are large and small edible gardens, ranging from a public fruit garden along the wall of the medieval castle in the city center to a mobile school garden in a trailer parked in one of the downtown pedestrian streets. At a local archeological site, a historical garden showcases varieties commonly grown during Roman and Medieval times, which has been developed in consultation with local historians. People can harvest freely from any edible garden located within a public space. Schools are heavily involved, as are the social welfare services that use the gardening and maintenance of the various urban garden plots as part of the city job training programs.

When Triangulation Fails

Triangulation in itself does not work if it does not integrate the input from current and future users of the public space and build their capabilities to be involved – the first of all placemaking principles. At Sjakkplassen, for example, after the initial project ended, later top-down attempts to reinstate the urban garden involved adding new chess pieces, a slackline, a community swap shed, and a pop-up art gallery. These initiatives failed however, as they never sought to build the ownership and capacities of the existing user groups and encourage them to see themselves as valuable guardians of an important community asset.

7.4.3 PPS Placemaking Principle #9: Experiment – Lighter, Quicker, Cheaper

The complexity of public spaces is such that you cannot expect to do everything right initially. The best spaces experiment with short-term improvements that can be tested and refined over many years! Elements such as seating, outdoor cafés, public art, striping of crosswalks and pedestrian havens, community gardens and murals are examples of improvements that can be accomplished in a short time. (PPS, 2013)

This principle emphasizes how top-down projects led by public sector or private investors can alienate genuine participation, while also being costly and taking a long time from ideation to realization. After they have been a part of a community hearing or participatory meeting with the city administration, a community wants to witness tangible change, especially given that the project completion may be years away.

Experimenting with lighter, quicker, cheaper installations is a great way to experiment with these changes within a timeline that is more acceptable to the community, as well as a way to work with a community in prototyping and co-designing the changes that are going to happen and even gently breaking down resistance from potential negative voices.

Lighter, Quicker, Cheaper at Stensparken Community Garden

Although the district administration's ambitions for the community garden are high, at Stensparken community garden, we have been careful to be experimental and iterative in our design of the public space, testing out formats and adding functions as we have gone along. Throughout the process, we strive to ensure the largest possible buy-in from the local community toward a shared vision. The gradual implementations of changes have helped tame the critical voices from the few, but vocal, neighbors who were initially opposed to any changes or upgrades to the space.

One of the ideas that originated during early discussions was having a greenhouse so that we could extend the garden season. With the limited funding of the first session, we decided to reallocate the funds that we had saved to build a small outdoor tool shed and rather settle for a cheaper, small but multifunctional 5-square meter greenhouse that could work as a shed during the winter months. As the ambition level of the project increased, we are currently looking to hire an architect to design a greenhouse that can provide better storage opportunities and help us activate the community year-round.

Recently, a comment that came up from various of the youth participants as they were doing the Place Game was wanting to add more colors and flowers. We took the youth up on their placemaking idea, went to a garden center and picked out perennial flowers, and built a flower bed. In addition to the instant gratification of making a tangible improvement to the space, it also helped define the place identity. By having two colorful flower beds at the entrance, we hoped to signal to the public that this was a place where they were welcome.

Building on our experience from Sjakkplassen, we have been careful to document these processes and gathered data on the increasing popularity of the community garden and the successful events as we have gone along, building a strong relationship with the local authorities and making it easier for them to formally and informally support this placemaking initiative.

Lighter, Quicker, Cheaper at Linderud Manor

As another local example of experimenting with lighter, quicker, cheaper installations, Nabolagshager has worked with partners in the much larger community garden space at Linderud Manor to do extensive testing over two seasons to find the most functional spots for seating arrangements. Together with youth hired from the local high school, we used hay bales as temporary seating arrangements, and along the way, a wide range of community members gave us their input as they tested different seating configurations.

The temporary hay bales gave us people's time and attention, soliciting input and building local buy-in for the space. By the time the hay bales were replaced by semipermanent and sturdy wooden furniture made of recycled wood, the community had been active in the space for over a year, and the early critics (some of whom initially wanted the whole area to be cultivated) had been convinced about the need for a more permanent social area.

7.5 Key Takeaway: Seek Complimentary Skills and Knowledge from Placemakers to Ensure Resilience, Longevity, and Impact

Having followed the evolution of urban agriculture in Oslo since its renaissance about a decade ago, it has been exciting to see how it has morphed, pivoted, and taken different forms according to the people who are involved. The public sector, especially in larger cities such as Oslo, Bergen and Trondheim, has made significant strides toward including urban agriculture in their other policies and sectoral plans, including urban planning, public health, education, and many other fields.

At the same time, the project lifecycle of an urban agriculture project is remarkably short. Very few projects live longer than a couple of years, and very often the person who initiated the project ends up abandoning the ship, either because they take on all the work and responsibilities or because of challenges in mobilizing the wider community.

By looking to placemaking practitioners, networking with them, and learning from their toolboxes, practices, and examples, urban farmers can help generate projects that are more resilient, last longer, and have stronger community impacts than if the urban farmer had only looked to their green-thumbed peers for inspiration.

References

Brantseth, K. (2015, December 3). Erfaringer fra Sjakkplassen 2015. *Issuuu.com*. Retrieved february 24, 2023 from Erfaringer fra Sjakkplassen 2015 by Stedsantropolog Katja Bratseth – Issuu.

Courage, C. (2017, Jun 2). TEDxIndianapolis: Placemaking and community (Video). *Youtube*. Retrieved on February 24, 2023 from https://www.youtube.com/watch?v=Sfk1ZW9NRDY

Jacobs, J. (1961). *The death and life of great American cities*. Random House.

Kent, F., & as seen on Shophouse & Co. (2018, July 3). Making places, episode 1 – What is placemaking? (Video). *Youtube*. Retrieved February 24, 2023 from https://www.youtube.com/watch?v=fvCCzLOOHe0

Madden, K. (2018). *How to turn a place around: A placemaking handbook.* Project for Public Spaces, Inc.

Project for Public Spaces. (2009, January 2). The Place Game, how we make the community the expert. *PPS.org.* Retrieved february 24, 2023 from The Power of 10+ (pps.org)

Project for Public Spaces. (2013). Eleven Principles for Creating Great Community Places. *PPS. org.* Retrieved february 24, 2023 from https://www.pps.org/article/11steps

Project for Public Spaces. (2016, June 14). *The Place Game, how we make the community the expert. PPS.org.* Retrieved february 24, 2023 from https://www.pps.org/article/place-game-community

Yeung, P., (2022, July 14). It's a beautiful thing: How one Paris district rediscovered conviviality. *The Guardian online.* Retrieved february 24, 2023 from https://www.theguardian.com/world/2022/jul/14/its-a-beautiful-thing-how-one-paris-district-rediscovered-conviviality

Part III
When Education Gets in the Urban Agriculture Mix

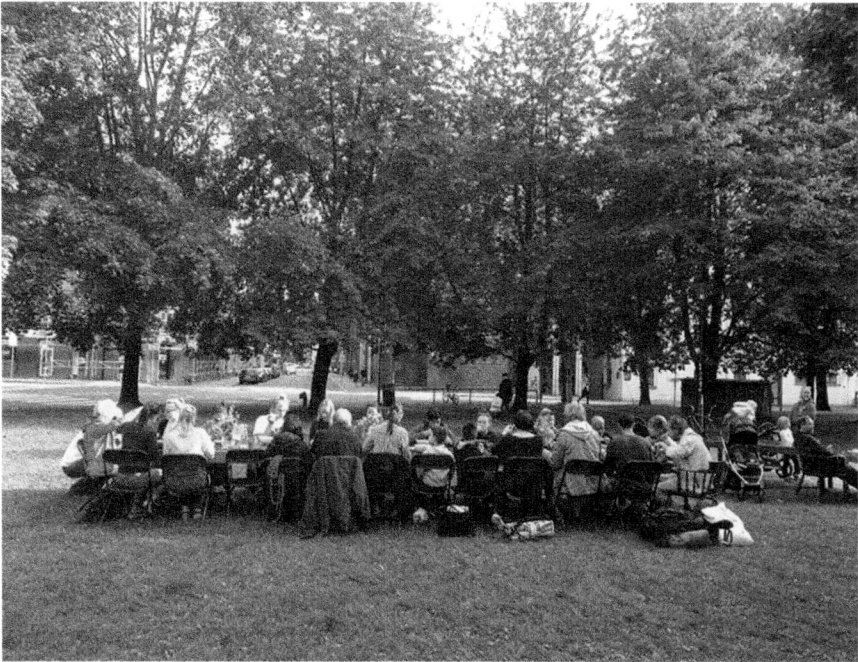

Chapter 8
Key Characteristics of Co-produced Urban Agriculture Visions in Oslo

Vebjørn Egner Stafseng, Anna Marie Nicolaysen, and Geir Lieblein

8.1   Introduction

Urban agriculture – defined here as "all the food production initiatives in and around urban areas" (Prove et al., 2018 p. 17) – plays an indisputable role in sustainable urban development and urban food systems (Halloran & Magid, 2013). However, due to widely accepted strategies of building compact cities, urban public space has become increasingly scarce and contested. Well-functioning processes are needed to decide what urban space should include and how to manage it. One such process is visioning, where the activity of creating a shared vision, "a desirable state in the future" (Wiek & Iwaniec, 2014), is essential to directing of concrete action steps. In this chapter we present results from an integrated research-education effort with students from an MSc Agroecology programme on urban agriculture initiatives. The context was Oslo, Norway, where the interest in urban agriculture is relatively new but growing. The focus was on co-production of visions and action plans in partnership with stakeholders.

Co-creation and public participation are necessary for a successful implementation of urban agriculture. Van der Jagt et al. (2017) conclude that for communal urban gardens "to achieve community buy-in and flourishing, ultimately we need an approach that enables local people to discover, nourish, adapt and co-create their own culture" (p. 273). In the case of requalification of vacant areas in Bologna, Italy, authors Gasperi et al. found that "the integration of the different stakeholders related to urban horticulture (e.g., citizens, agronomists, environmentalists, ecologists, sociologists and urban planners) would ensure a successful process for valuing vacant areas towards the regeneration of cities" (2016, p. 17).

V. E. Stafseng (✉)
Department of Plant Sciences, Norwegian University of Life Sciences, Ås, Norway
e-mail: vebjorn.egner.stafseng@nmbu.no

A. M. Nicolaysen · G. Lieblein
Norwegian University of Life Sciences, Ås, Norway

© The Author(s) 2024
B. Sirowy, D. Ruggeri (eds.), *Urban Agriculture in Public Space*, GeoJournal Library 132, https://doi.org/10.1007/978-3-031-41550-0_8

Public participation in this context can be defined as "the practice of consulting and involving members of the public in the agenda-setting, decision-making, and policy-forming activities of organizations or institutions responsible for policy development" (Rowe & Frewer, 2004, p. 512). The participatory processes we dealt with here were mostly focused on members of the public, more specifically participants and relevant stakeholders in the urban agriculture initiatives. In this study, we chose to make the connection between public participation and action education. The students worked with real-life urban agriculture cases and facilitated participatory change processes. We define action learning as "learning through action and for action" (Lieblein et al., 2004). The Agroecology course and our research for this chapter were inspired by Lewin's (1946) definition of action research as "research which will help the practitioner" (Lewin, 1946, p. 34), and his three-step model of change and force field theory (Burnes, 2020).

Urban agriculture can be practiced and defined in a variety of ways. As in the other chapters of this volume, we focus on the publicly accessible forms of food production that take place in public space. Following the typology from Chap. 6, we explored case studies of urban agriculture in the categories: (1) urban farm, (2) urban agriculture in central parks and (3) neighbourhood gardens.

The student action learning strategy had three major aims: (1) to facilitate student learning, (2) to facilitate positive change in the initiatives and (3) to generate new knowledge about urban agriculture initiatives for research purposes, or practical theory building, to use a framework coined by Peters and Wals (2013). The focus in this chapter is on (3) the product of the student work and the way it can be utilized in research. Our overall question is: *What is the desired future state of urban agriculture in public spaces, and how can we get there?* To help answer this, we ask the following sub-questions: *What are the key characteristics of student and stakeholder co-produced visions for urban agriculture in Oslo? What are the supporting and hindering forces for reaching these visions? What action steps can be taken to reach the visions?*

8.2 Context and Methods: Action Learning and Food System Education for Change

In this chapter we present the action learning, project-based work of master students in the MSc Agroecology programme at the Norwegian University of Life Sciences (NMBU). The work was conducted as part of the semester-long-course "Agroecology: Action Learning in Farming and Food Systems" and was focused on urban agriculture cases in Oslo. In the Agroecology program, we focus on action learning to enable students to overcome the 'knowing-doing' gap (Pfeffer, 1998), through cultivation of their competences to work with complex situations and take informed, responsible action (Francis et al., 2013; Wiek & Kay, 2015). In agreement with

UNESCO (2017), we believe these competences are needed to understand and work with sustainability challenges.

The students worked in groups of four or five and partnered with selected urban agriculture cases, where the aim was to take part in change-oriented activities. The project work design is inspired by Kolb (2014), who presents learning as a cyclical process. The students were asked to (1) describe the *present situation*, (2) identify *themes and key issues*, (3) explore the *desired future* and (4) generate *action plans* for how to improve the situation towards the desired future. For the first two tasks, we encouraged the students to use interviews, participant observation and data-structuring tools like rich pictures (from Soft Systems Methodology; see Checkland (2000, p. 22) and Picture 8.1) to get a rich overview of the present situation. For the third and fourth tasks, students organized an open meeting or a workshop with relevant stakeholders, where they facilitated the creation of a shared vision. Each student group adapted the workshop design to their context, but the basic structure was a three to four-hour workshop, inspired by Lieblein et al. (2001) and the work of Pool and Parker (2017), that contained (1) information about the student project, (2) a guided imagery (that includes a relaxation exercise), (3) individual time to write or visualize the vision, (4) each member share their vision with the group to develop a group vision, (5) each group share their vision in plenary, (6) all agree on a shared vision, (7) all look at hindering and supporting forces and (8) all decide on initial action steps for reaching the vision.

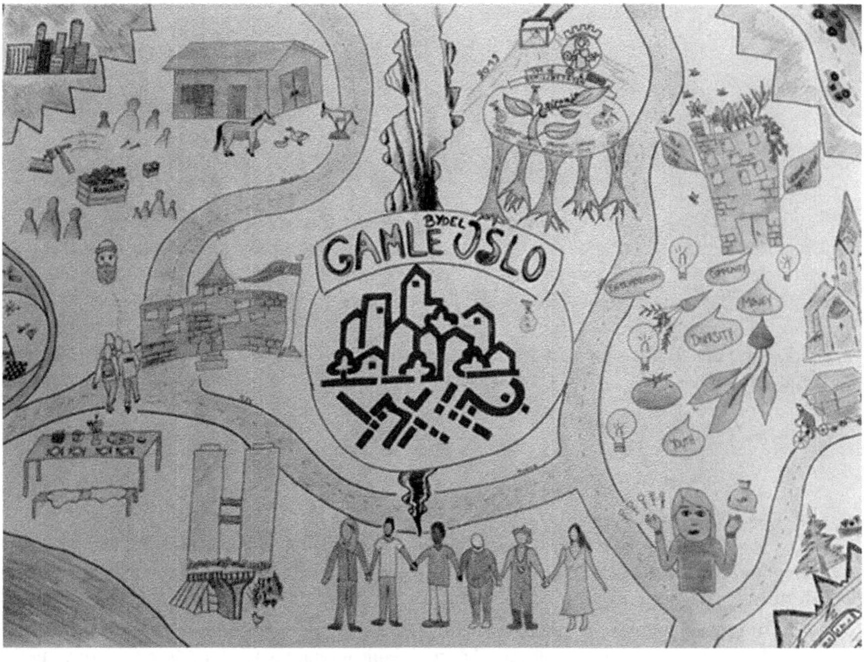

Picture 8.1 Example of a rich picture from the case study of Bydel Gamle Oslo

After the workshop, the student groups refined the action steps and prepared a report addressed to key stakeholders.[1] In the report, they described the critical elements of the current situation, the shared vision, the most relevant hindering and supporting forces and their proposed plan of action. Each year, the interdisciplinary Agroecology programme at NMBU admits around 20 students, of which about 75% are international. Students come from a variety of educational and professional backgrounds, which in 2018 and 2019 included, amongst other, development studies, plant science, agriculture, biology, business and management. When we formed the groups for the project work, the aim was to have diversity in terms of background, age, and gender.

In September 2018 and 2019, the teaching team[2] introduced the project work to the students. We established a collaboration with relevant urban agriculture initiatives, and signed agreements with key stakeholders. We selected the project sites based on availability and relevance to the student work. In 2019, we collaborated with the central municipal unit responsible for urban agriculture in Oslo, the Agency of Urban Environment, to identify District administrations actively involved in urban agriculture, and selected two of them as our partners. The students conducted their first case visit with a focus on the current situation of their case area (see Fig. 8.1 for a complete timeline). During their second visit in November, they organized workshops to develop a shared vision and documented it in their reports to the stakeholders. The workshops were held predominantly in English as groups included many international students. Our team conducted a total of seven workshops with a range in objectives and engagement modalities. In Table 8.1, we compiled essential information about these workshops.

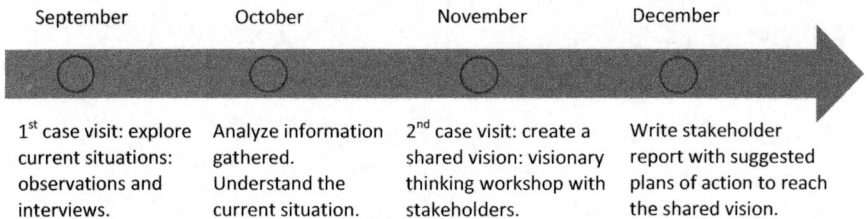

September	October	November	December
1st case visit: explore current situations: observations and interviews.	Analyze information gathered. Understand the current situation.	2nd case visit: create a shared vision: visionary thinking workshop with stakeholders.	Write stakeholder report with suggested plans of action to reach the shared vision.

Fig. 8.1 Timeline for the student work with the case studies. The process was the same both years, with different case studies. 2018: Case studies 1-5; 2019: Case studies 6 and 7.

---

[1]The key stakeholder is the contact person for the students in the collaborating organization. This person helps the students get the information they need and the one who will have to take the process further.

[2]The teaching team is three full-time teachers, and two to three part time teachers involved each fall in PAE302. We are all agroecologists but with educational background in agronomy, applied botany, horticulture, cultural studies, medical anthropology and soil biology.

Table 8.1 Overview of the case studies and their workshops

Case Study	Year	Participants	Report name (as cited in findings section)
(1) Dr. Dedichens Drivhus and Trosterud Parsellhage	2018	30 participants: members from both cases, 1 city official from the planning department and 2 of the authors of this chapter	Dr. Dedichens report 2018
(2) Ellingsrud Parsellhage	2018	Members of the allotment garden and some external people who were interested	Ellingsrud report 2018
(3) Losæter	2018	Main stakeholders: two project leaders, one city farmer and two volunteers leading each their group	Losæter report 2018
(4) Voksenenga Nærmiljøhage	2018	12 members of the garden, including coordinator	Voksenenga report 2018
(5) På Schous	2018	Six participants (employees at the library) for visioning workshop + public meeting/ idea workshop ten participants	På Shous report 2018
(6) Bydel Gamle Oslo	2019	Five participants: one consultant, three municipal officials, one researcher (first author)	Gamle Oslo report 2019
(7) Bydel Grünerløkka	2019	Six participants: two library employees, one municipal official, two entrepreneurs, one researcher (first author)	Grünerløkka report 2019

8.3 Case Locations

The following is a description of each of the urban agriculture communities we partnered with (see Fig. 8.2 for overview of their locations).

8.3.1 Case Study 1: Dr. Dedichens Drivhus and Trosterud Parsellhage

In 2015, a group of local enthusiasts reclaimed a large greenhouse (*Drivhus*) built by the municipality for vocational training in the former Dr. Dedichen's Asylum. They formed an association, got a deal with Oslo municipality, the owner of the building and obtained funding for renting it from the District. The aim was to revitalize the greenhouse and create a place where people of all ages and cultures could meet, exchange knowledge, and promote integration of immigrants. Today, the greenhouse is run by volunteers with some financial support for events and equipment from different funding sources (for more in-depth information about this case, see Swensen et al., 2022). Its structure is similar to an allotment garden: members pay a small annual fee to have a table in the greenhouse at their disposal for cultivation in containers (see Picture 8.2). The association (Dr. Dedichens' Green Square)

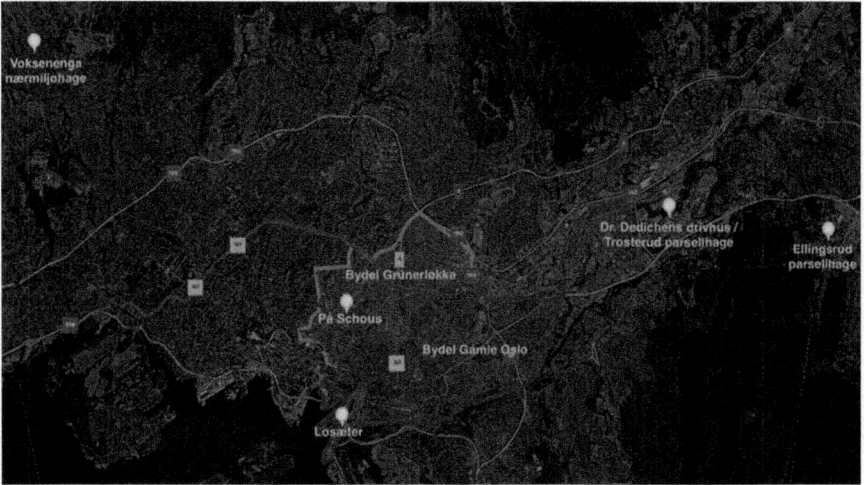

Fig. 8.2 Map of Oslo with the location of the cases. The individual cases from 2018 are marked with yellow pins; the district cases from 2019 are marked in blue and yellow borders. The red line marks the road Ring 2; the second of three ring roads in Oslo. Source: Google Earth

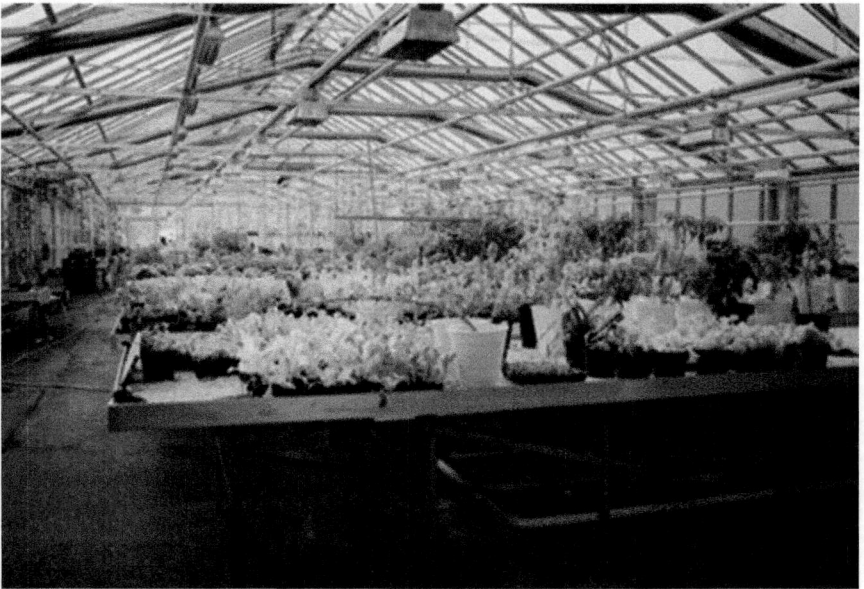

Picture 8.2 Inside Dr. Dedichens' greenhouse. Photo: Brooke Porter

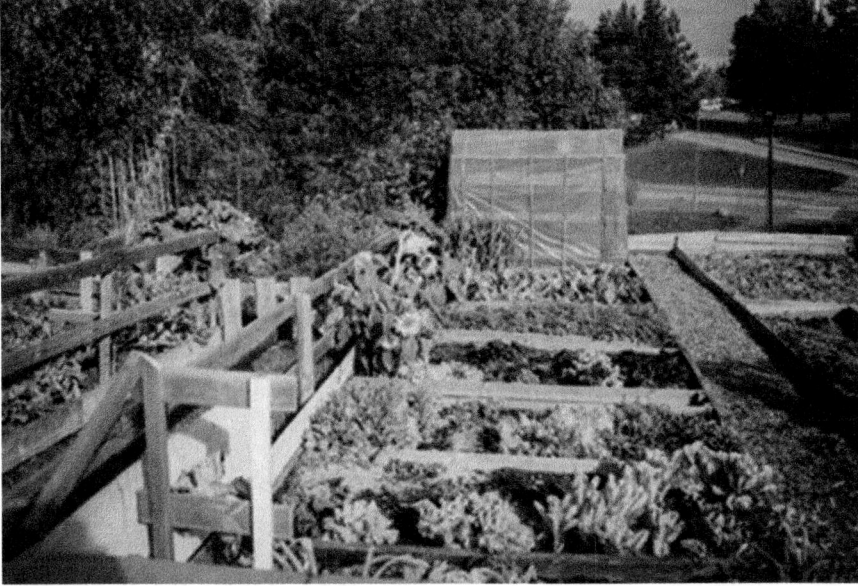

Picture 8.3 Trosterud Parsellhage. Photo: Brooke Porter

collaborates with the neighbouring Trosterud allotment garden (*Parsellhage* in Norwegian; see Picture 8.3), which with new development plans would be relocated next to the greenhouse, making it an urban gardening park. This process was slow and frustrating for the people involved, and was a major area of focus for the student work.

8.3.2   Case Study 2: Ellingsrud Parsellhage

In 2016 a retired woman who wanted to do something for the neighbourhood in memory of her two deceased sons started an allotment garden. The garden, characterized by the lack of a fence, was created on a disused football field to the East of Oslo. At present, the place has grown to include 50 allotments, organized by a board led by the founder. The gardeners each have their "house" of eight pallet collars laid out in a H-shaped configuration (see Picture 8.4). The members include local residents, kindergartens, and primary schools in the area. These groups regularly host events, such as courses, barbecue dinner events, and festivals for special occasions.

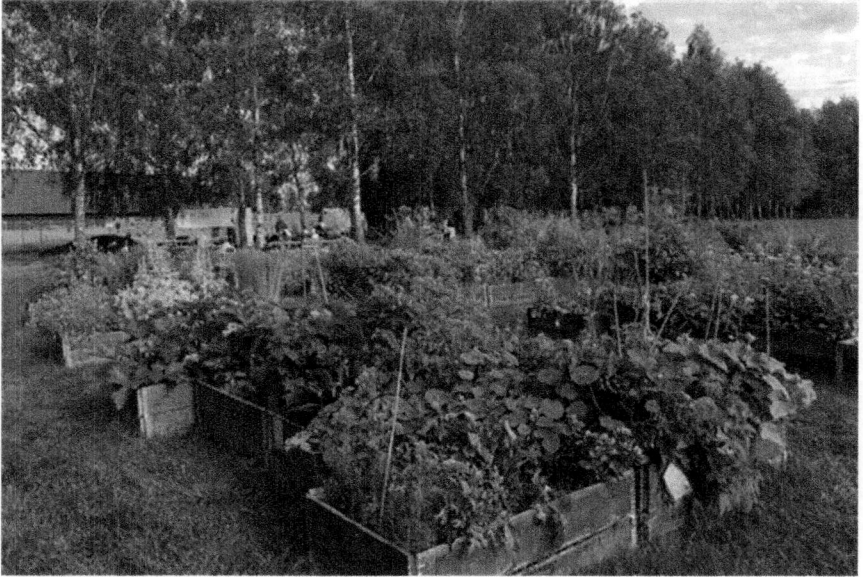

Picture 8.4 The Ellingsrud allotment garden with its H-shaped lots during a fall event. Photo: Vebjørn Stafseng

8.3.3 Case Study 3: Losæter

Losæter was initiated by Bjørvika Utvikling on behalf of the landowners in the redevelopment district of Bjørvika, on the newly developed Oslo waterfront (see Picture 8.5). The name refers to the Norwegian term *Sæter*, a mountainous pasture where animals can graze in the summer season. It started as public art installation space, and was initiated by an artists' collective. The initial 100 allotments that formed its structure in 2012 have since developed to include a grain field, and later a public community garden employing a full-time professional farmer. In 2016, the artists themselves designed a boat-shaped bakehouse at the barycentre of the site. Today, the community garden is managed by *Bybonden*, a full-time urban farmer hired by the municipality. The *Bybonden's* tasks include giving courses, organizing volunteers and hosting a variety of visitors, from foreign journalists to local kindergarten children. Amongst the volunteers are organizations who work on topics of interest to the place, passers-by and other neighbours.

8.3.4 Case Study 4: Voksenenga Nærmiljøhage

Voksenenga Nærmiljøhage (community garden) was ideated in 2016 by a landscape architect living in the area, the northwest end of Oslo. In partnership with the local district administration and church, the initiator received funding from a private

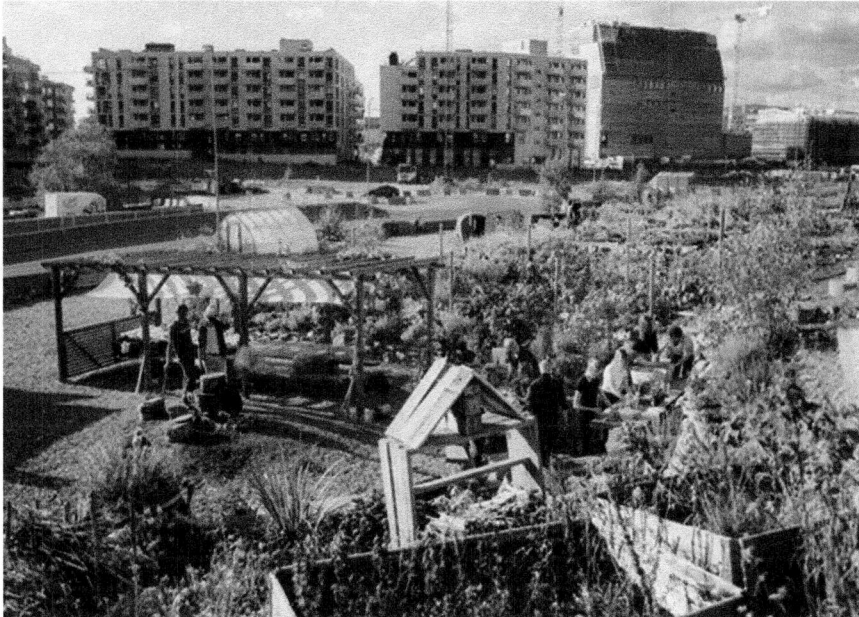

Picture 8.5 The social area of Losæter surrounded by vegetable fields, apartment blocks, with the Munch museum in the background. Photo: Brooke Porter

foundation to start the project but has had no steady income to cover expenses (such as a full-time project manager). The garden comprises of an area with allotments, an area for community gardening, an outdoor kitchen, a tool shed, a chicken coop and social areas with tables and benches (see Picture 8.6). Over the growing season, the garden organizes many activities for residents, participants in the community garden, and allotment holders. They employ youth and have a garden club summer camp for children. Funding for these activities comes from district, municipal and national sources.

8.3.5   Case Study 5: På Schous

The På Schous urban agriculture opened in 2018 thanks to a collaboration between the Grünerløkka District in and the local library. The project encompassed the cultivation of vegetables in beds on the square outside the library (see Picture 8.7) and vocational training for local youth that involved food cultivation, park maintenance and café work. An essential activity was the hosting of dinners where the employed youth, in collaboration with professional chefs cooked dinner for district residents. They used surplus food from stores, bakeries and restaurants in the area and vegetables from the garden to prepare the meals. The project employed hundreds of youths

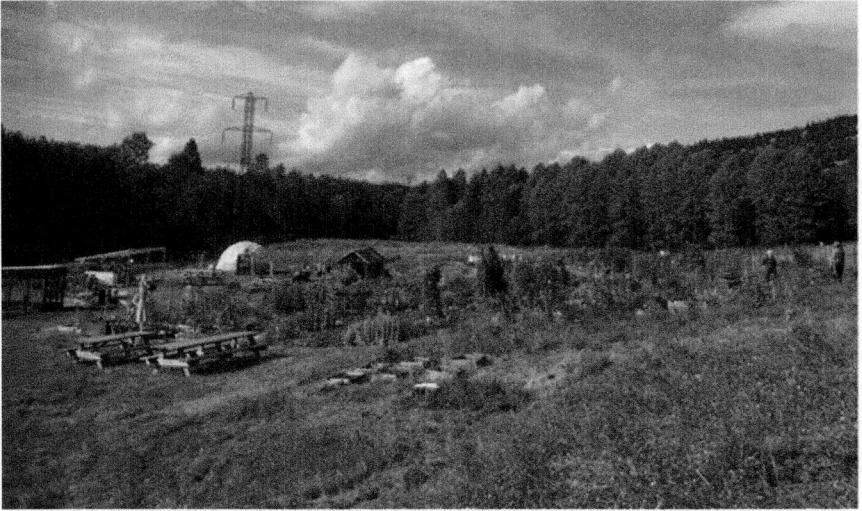

Picture 8.6 Voksenenga with its garden, outdoor kitchen and geodome greenhouse in the summer. Photo: Katinka Evensen

in the summer, and retained some of them for year-round positions. The work included tending to vegetable plants in the various beds around the district and maintaining parks and public spaces managed by the district.

8.3.6 Case Studies 6 and 7: The Districts of Gamle Oslo and Grünerløkka

In 2019 our research focus became the municipality's role in urban agriculture development in Oslo (see also the discussion in Chaps. 11 and 12). The Agency for Urban Environment is the office in Oslo municipality responsible for urban development and planning, but much of the local decision-making is the purview of 15 municipal districts. Our team collaborated with the districts of *Gamle Oslo* (Old Oslo) and *Grünerløkka* both located by the city centre. In recent years, these districts have taken an active role in the development of urban agriculture, supporting projects by local actors and neighbourhood groups.

The findings used in this chapter originate from seven reports written by first-year graduate students in the Agroecology programme at NMBU to synthesize the activities that took place between 2018 and 2019.[3] As course instructors, the authors were involved in the planning and execution of the field work; some also participated in the workshops conducted by the students. Thus, our impressions and

---

[3] The reports are not available to the public due to GDPR and are treated here as data sources. A list of the reports can be found in Appendix 1

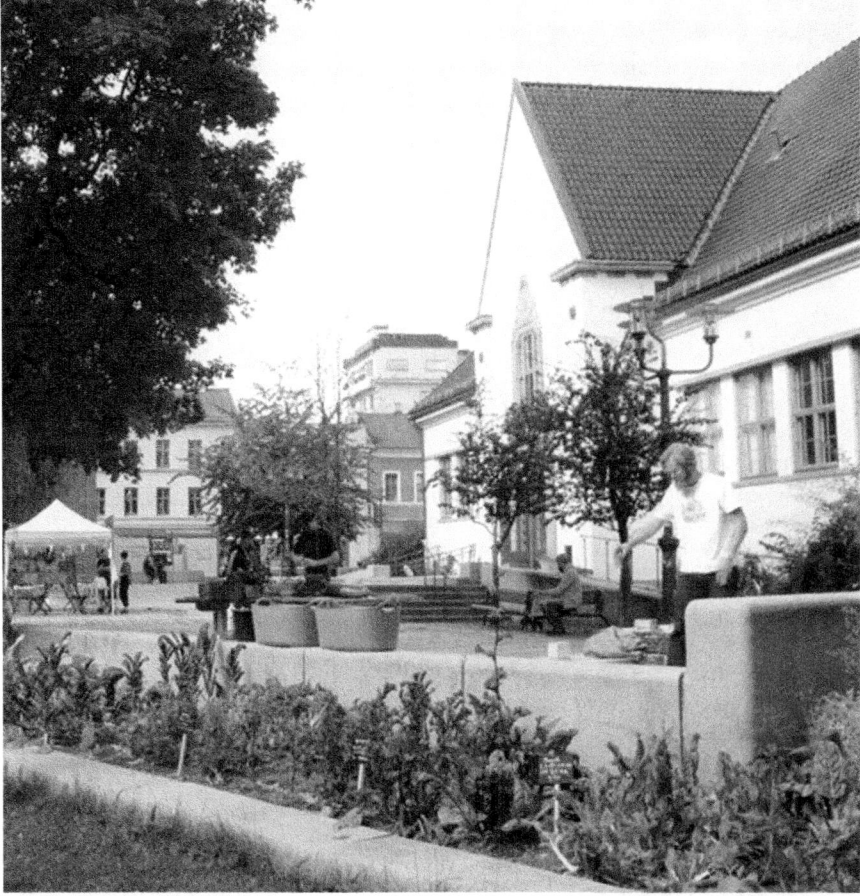

Picture 8.7 Schous square in front of the library, with cultivated beds in the foreground. Photo: Troels Rosenkrantz Fuglsang

experiences from the process also play a role in the interpretation of the results. We used NVivo software to analyze the reports by coding them for the overall categories: *visions, supporting and hindering forces* and *action plans*. We finally grouped the codes in common categories and themes.

8.4   Findings: Visions of Resource Cycling and Empowerment

Figure 8.3, illustrates that the visions of urban agriculture in public space involve elements of nature, the social and governance. To reach them urban gardeners must overcome   common   hindering   forces,   most   importantly,   nonfunctioning

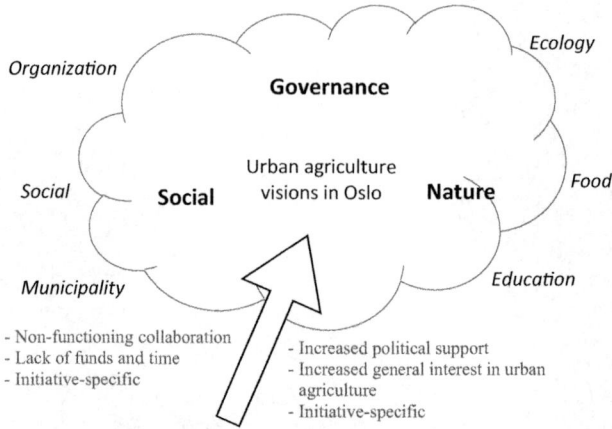

Fig. 8.3 Key characteristics of urban agriculture visions in Oslo (in bold), challenges for improvement (in red), supporting forces for improvement (in green) and areas of suggested action (in italics)

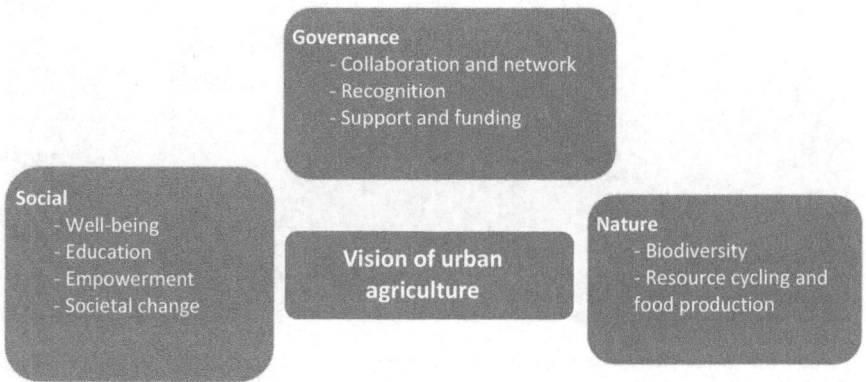

Fig. 8.4 Three categories of a vision of urban agriculture in Oslo

collaboration and limited financial and time resources. Support from higher political bodies and increased general interest in urban agriculture are forces that can support their efforts. Action steps that can help propel their vision relate to the municipality, food, organization, ecology, social improvements and education. In the following sections, we dive deeper into these categories.

Our analysis of the student reports found three main categories that capture the essence of the visions developed in the seven case studies. These are (1) **nature** and (2) societal and individual goods of various forms, a category we have termed **the social**. Further, an overarching vision is related to (3) **governance** of the initiatives, to ensure their development and resilience (see Fig. 8.4). Below we elaborate on these categories and illustrate with examples from the visions.

8.4.1 Social

Visions that relate to the social can be both individual and collective. Well-being is primarily individual-oriented, societal changes are mostly collective and education and empowerment have elements of both.

At Ellingsrud, part of the vision is to promote *well-being*, health and access to nature. In Grünerløkka, well-being is prominent in how urban agriculture can create healthy, aesthetically pleasing, safe and green spaces to elevate the health and interactions of the local community. To be active and in harmony with nature amongst a diversity of trees and plants can put the mind and body at ease and improve one's physical and mental state. In addition, creating a safe, well-designed public space through urban agriculture promotes social interaction between generations and between people with different ethnic and economic backgrounds (Grünerløkka report 2019). Overall, increased social interaction can contribute to a neighborhood's collective well-being. In a district challenged for many years by petty crime and substance abuse in public space, introducing urban agriculture elements could be particularly valuable in ongoing efforts to improve the situation. Year-round activities could help fight degradation and consistently sustain people's well-being.

In Trosterud and Ellingsrud, there is a desire to design social, open and inclusive areas and to involve the community in the process. The proposal includes the establishment of an outdoor kitchen and the organization of various volunteer activities. These initiatives aim to transform public spaces into hubs for urban food production and multifunctional activities. The envisioned community kitchens and meeting places will serve as arenas for social interaction and learning, fostering a sense of inclusivity by bringing together people from diverse backgrounds.

Education, both formal and informal, is another theme that recur in the visions and include the educational effects on the general population, kindergarteners, and pupils from schools of all levels. For the Gamle Oslo district, a part of the vision is a better connection to food; it includes a deep understanding of the importance of nutrition and genuine care for community resilience, personal health and education. Ellingsrud's vision targets education and sustainable development knowledge-sharing across generations. Finally, in the Grünerløkka, the focus is on food production education, and the re-envisioning of school- and kindergarten environments to include gardening lessons and practice.

As an effect of education and a prerequisite for societal change, the visions of urban agriculture include *empowerment* of participants. This can be seen both as a collective and an individual theme. As a collective theme, the focus is on how people can unite, self-organize, and host various events. From an individual point of view, empowerment means to provide space for personal development, and a place to teach, learn and evolve.

The theme of *societal change* encompasses all the elements of the visions where the initiative contributes to change society. This can include making participants of the initiative aware of problematic situations and providing them with tools to contribute to changing them. The Gamle Oslo district vision consists of using urban agriculture as a platform for an alternative sharing-economy. The ultimate goal is to work so that "human connections and sustainability will be valued over accumulation of physical possessions and the striving for socio-economic status" (Gamle Oslo report 2019). Similarly, the larger context of the vision for På Schous is that the project will contribute to environmental consciousness and foster noncommercial networks (På Schous report 2018).

8.4.2 Nature

Another essential part of the vision for urban agriculture is its contribution to urban ecology. The first subcategory under *Nature* is *biodiversity*, and there are various elements that contribute to it. For Trosterud, student visions suggested the introduction of beehives, ponds, ecological pathways, and apple trees. In the Ellingsrud, the vision promoted biodiversity and natural cycles. For Grünerløkka, the vision included buildings with hanging gardens with climbing plants, green rooftops, fruit trees, insects, pollinators and greenhouses with edible and non-edible plants to increase biodiversity in public space, making it more aesthetically rich and attractive to the community.

The visions include resource cycling to make the most of the urban resources and fulfill the role of urban agriculture in this context. This consists of the improvement of water systems to make better use of this scarce resource, and bringing nutrients back to the soil in a closed-loop system using compost, as in the case of Losæter and Bydel Grünerløkka: "There are closed loop systems for food production. People are selling and buying local food. Soils and nutrients from the waste are brought back to the ecosystem and there is composting in every food production site" (Grünerløkka report 2019).

8.4.3 Governance: Initiative Sustainability

Governance is an overarching theme for the visions and a prerequisite for the existence and healthy functioning of the initiatives. We define governance as "an analytical framework to identify different governance structures and governance practices within these structures with regard to the socio-political and spatial regulation of urban gardening" (Fox-Kamper et al., 2018, p. 60). This includes both internal governance in the initiatives and the structures given by the municipality or the state.

The central theme of *collaboration and network* covers how initiatives will connect to other initiatives, the municipality, the district, the private sector, and other relevant actors. In Gamle Oslo they seek tight collaboration between the public and private sectors, NGOs, academic institutions and citizen/volunteer groups. This implies a high level of communication as well as participatory, inclusive planning and decision-making processes.

Another subtheme is *recognition from government and population*. One example of this is Gamle Oslo, a district whose vision includes urban agriculture as a civic priority: "a fundamental element is that all levels of society, including the various public institutions, genuinely consider urban agriculture as an essential component of city dwellers well-being" (Gamle Oslo report 2019). The final subtheme we identified is *support and funding* that initiatives in the visions are supported and have sufficient funding: "There are funds for the urban agriculture initiatives and circular economy activities. The urban agriculture initiatives have employed experts from the Oslo municipality and district who are helping to manage the public parks' projects" (Grünerløkka report 2019).

In this section, we identify forces that could either hinder or propel the visions. One reccurring force for reaching the visions is the *support coming from the higher political bodies*. This includes the municipal, district, and state government levels. This support comes from funding schemes, goodwill in managing the bureaucracy and promoting new initiatives. In their report for Losæter the students share this perception of the municipality: "Having spoken to Oslo Kommune it is clear that there is municipal interest in the proposed changes as they are in line with the city's desire for a transition to a more sustainable future" (Losæter report 2018).

Interest in urban agriculture, is a growing trend attracting also media attention. The students report a sense of urgency, especially amongst the younger members of the population. In addition, it has become ever more popular in new housing developments to include and advertise access to rooftop gardens or gardening spaces as amenities for potential buyers. With greater political support, unused urban spaces in the neighbourhoods could also become gardening projects.

Finally, some of the identified supporting forces are specific to certain initiatives. Densely populated neighbourhoods have "an advantage as there are more people who may be interested in urban agriculture projects and there is the potential for a large pool of capable volunteers and project initiators" (Gamle Oslo report 2019). In the case of both Voksenenga and Losæter, students found evidence of a high number of members and their networks and considered these to be strengths for the implementation of their future visions. At På Schous, the partnership between the involved organizers could be instrumental to support future urban agriculture development.

In the students' reports, *collaboration* appears as a hindering force operating in two ways. One way the collaboration between initiatives and the municipal government can be an obstacle is visible in the *uncertain timeframe of initiatives* and in the *zoning and regulation* and *fragmented bureaucracy*. *Fragmented bureaucracy* may occur when several agencies are responsible for various parts of an urban agriculture initiative. *Zoning and regulation* are hindering forces to the Losæter vision, as it will be challenging to irrigate with grey water and cultivate the walls of a concrete ventilation tower. In addition, the vision of the På Schous is not aligned with the current zoning plans for the square, and this needs to be dealt with to achieve the vision. A second way in which collaboration may be hindering involves the private sector. The Gamle Oslo report puts it clearly: "the private sector is not always willing to actively contribute without having an immediate perceived benefit" (2019).

Two elements seem to hinder the visions when they are either in shortage or absent: *funding for expenses* and *time for involvement* amongst the various participants of an initiative. Expenses can include materials for building new structures and labor for short-term and long-term project coordination and maintenance. This time-related challenge is visible in community gardens like Voksenenga, where the vision entails involvement from the members who "have busy lives and other responsibilities" (Voksenenga report 2018). In Gamle Oslo, the demographic with an above-average low-income population is key to participation in urban gardening as "availability of time is a luxury and participating in urban food initiatives may not be a priority" (Gamle Oslo report 2019). When the vision is to have diverse participants, gentrification and population turnover are real challenges. They can lead to more homogenous and less socially stable community identities. As for the supporting or hindering forces, these may be specific to certain initiatives but likely to apply to several others. This is the case of aesthetics, mentioned in the Losæter report. Some improvements, like a new irrigation system, could help to make the sites more manageable, but would not fit in with the place's aesthetics. When the vision is to create a community, individualism is a challenge: "people often lack the personal relationships necessary to be a part of a greater community" (Gamle Oslo report 2019).

These supporting and hindering forces contribute to the action steps suggested to further the visions. In the following section, we have identified six categories of action steps that benefit the development of urban agriculture initiatives in public spaces.

8.4.4 Ecological

Urban agriculture should integrate closed-loop systems involving compost, composting toilets and food forest initiatives to promote *nutrient cycling*. Related to this, designers and planners can achieve *increased biodiversity* through the establishment of ecological corridors, to increase both the number of habitats afforded and the presence of edible landscapes. At both Dr. Dedichens' greenhouse and Schous, an action step is to establish a seed library "by obtaining, organizing and storing seed, in order to encourage resource sharing and increase biodiversity" (Dr. Dedichens' report 2018). Finally, we also suggest introducing *systems for irrigation,* including instalment of rainwater catchment systems, and diversionary swales in Dr. Dedichens' greenhouse and Losæter.

8.4.5   Education

Related to educational dimension of urban agriculture, the students suggest *establishing a mini book-swap box* in Trosterud's garden. This also has the potential effect to open the gardens to people who are less interested in the gardening but like reading. Additionally, students present ideas for *facilitating education around urban agriculture* and propose to *integrate urban agriculture in the educational system.* This could be achieved through contributions to a new curriculum in local schools and includes cultivation in collaboration with the Ellingsrud garden members. To this end, parents should be involved in the process to gain support for the initiative (Ellingsrud report 2018). The idea of integrating urban agriculture into the educational system is also elaborated in the Grünerløkka report. This report focuses on the concept of "garden-based learning" (from Desmond et al., 2004) and aims to have urban gardens available for all schools in Oslo.

8.4.6   Food

Under the food category, we locate two subcategories of actions: *grow more food* and *strengthen local (food) consumption.* The first is based on the insight that for most urban agriculture initiatives, food production is not the primary motivation, and thus, that there is growth potential (Schous report). To achieve the latter, students suggested revitalizing food preservation techniques through workshops and involve people knowledgeable in the subject (Grünerløkka report) and, setting up alternative distribution systems for local food (Gamle Oslo report).

8.4.7   Organization

Actions to improve and better organize initiatives include *building partnerships* through workshops and food (or other) events as "opportunity for people to learn, spend time together and share their knowledge and experiences. In addition, these social and educational events could increase people's interest in joining the garden" (Ellingsrud report 2018). In the Voksenenga report, the students argue that more workshops "would accomplish one of the garden's higher goals of 'empowering members and the community through education and skill building'"

(Voksenenga report 2018). This group also suggests adopting a care farm model inspired by the Green Care concept for the provision of welfare services on farms[4]: "This practice could be an opportunity to build and promote the recognition of the garden, and ultimately strengthen its relationship with the community". The Schous report focuses on how this initiative can *become an urban agriculture hub* by developing a website and organizing a festival. These actions "would position PÅ Schous as a hub for urban agriculture in Oslo. In addition, an urban agriculture festival can promote and boost urban agriculture and develop a strong network of actors in Oslo" (På Schous report 2018).

An action point that reoccurs in the reports is *establishing work groups* to organize the members and volunteers. This includes obtaining an overview of volunteers' skills, improving functionality of task and responsibility distribution, and fostering member empowerment. A hope is that this will help both with how the garden functions and to sustain volunteer and member motivation. *Communication* is also an essential action point. Some of the reports suggest having a stronger social media presence, creating or improving websites, and promoting the garden in other ways. These action points refer mainly to external communication. In contrast, the Ellingsrud report also stresses the need to enhance communication within groups to counteract existing weaknesses like 'Low sense of ownership' and 'Low motivation for a bigger cause' through the creation of a garden manual.

8.4.8   Social

Based on the insight that positive social outcomes rely in part on a garden's physical design and structures, a suggested action step is to *create social spaces*. In the Losæter report, the students suggest ways to improve visitors' experience through clear entrances to the garden, wayfinding and signage. At Trosterud, the student group focused on creating a social space, including a barbeque and outdoor kitchen area to include the larger community.

8.4.9   Municipality

The final category is the municipality, and what they can do to help urban agriculture initiatives succeed. Some of the suggested action points relate to *citizen engagement*. An important thing the municipality can do is to engage citizens in

---

[4]See more at https://www.regjeringen.no/globalassets/upload/lmd/vedlegg/brosjyrer_veiledere_rapporter/m-0734_green_care_national_strategy.pdf.

policy-making related to urban agriculture and food issues, for instance, by creating a non-governmental Urban Agriculture Food Policy Council (Gamle Oslo report 2019). Such a council could include "gardeners and farmers, project leaders, organizational representatives, city officials, citizens and other players" (Gamle Oslo report 2019), foster collaboration between the various actors, and make policy more grounded. Municipalities should encourage platforms to valuate time as an exchangeable resource[5] and that urban agriculture activities are included.

Lastly, the two groups who worked with municipalities suggested *expanding municipal support*. This could be in the form of added and longer-term funding opportunities for initiatives, or an improved extension/advising service for urban agriculture (inspired by the extension service in traditional agriculture). Additionally, we suggest expanding and improving websites and apps with information about urban agriculture and maps of urban agriculture initiatives in the city. Another suggested action point is that the municipality should think more about their resources in terms of buildings and areas and that they can facilitate multipurpose use of these resources. One example is the "Oslonøkkelen"[6] [translated 'The key to Oslo'] *to* "offer access to public facilities outside of office-hours" (Gamle Oslo report 2019).

8.5 Discussion: What Are the Key Characteristics of Urban Agriculture Visions in Oslo?

Through an action-oriented inquiry into urban agriculture initiatives in Oslo, our team of students and faculty gained valuable insights into what urban agriculture is, and what it means to the stakeholders we involved. Through co-creation, we generated three types of visions catering to the social, nature and governance. The social has elements of both collective and individual focus. In the visions, the urban individual can flourish, develop, feel a sense of belonging and access places that encourage interaction with fellow citizens. The collective aspects of the visions involve changes in education and making citizens aware of issues and their unique social and nature-related character at both a local and global scale. The visions also offer tools to tackle such problems and improve the situation.

---

[5] See, for instance, TimeKred https://www.timekred.no.

[6] Oslonøkkelen is an app provided by Oslo Municipality that gives organizations, etc. access to public buildings to host meetings and events. See more at https://www.oslo.kommune.no/natur-kultur-og-fritid/lokaler-og-uteomrader-til-lan-og-leie/.

8.5.1 Visions vs. Motivations

These findings align with the interviews with project leaders and coordinators in Chap. 6, which revealed that their main motivations are to create social meeting places and educational arenas, to activate public spaces and to empower the citizens (Chap. 6). Our findings expand on these categories, both in terms of method (through the inclusion of urban agriculture participants as well as other stakeholders) and in the detail and description of the elements of these categories. In the workshops, participants were encouraged to be very concrete about the future they desired, and give a detailed picture of what they envisioned. Their motivations, and visions tell us something about what desires individuals have for urban agriculture in the future and what positive benefits could come from such initiatives.

Under the social category, we find the themes of *well-being, empowerment, education* and *societal change*. These can be seen in relation to the other findings of Chap. 6. When we analysed the findings through the lens of the capability approach (see Chap. 2, Chap. 6 and Nussbaum, 2011, p. 33–34). We witnessed how participation in urban agriculture can improve the capability affiliation. Participants reported seeing the gardens as a place to meet new people and feeling a sense of community belonging. In our case, we can say that the vision of well-being, including, for instance, a promotion of interaction between generations and all-year-round activities, relates to the capability of affiliation. Similarly, well-being also includes being in harmony with nature for improved mental and physical heath, which corresponds to the capabilities of *other species, bodily health* and *emotions, senses* and *thought*. Education and empowerment relate to the capabilities *control over one's environment* and *practical reason*.

The distinction between the individual and the collective might be misleading when seen in relation to capabilities. According to Nussbaum, "capabilities belong first and foremost to individual persons, and only derivatively to groups" (2011, p. 35). As such, the approach seems to be most relevant in the context of *individual* well-being. However, when we look more closely, the *collective* and the *individual* are not opposites but complement each other. When individuals come together around an issue and have a desire to bring about change in their surroundings they align with the capabilities of *control over one's environment* in a *political* sense and *practical reason*. According to Nussbaum, this is about "being able to participate effectively in political choices that govern one's life" (Nussbaum, 2011, p. 34). Thus, the focus is on the individual, yet the effects will be visible on a community scale when several individuals unite and participate in a shared political act.

The subcategory of *governance* represents a twofold concept. One way to see this is through internal organization of each urban agriculture initiative. We found collaboration and networking to prevail in the visions. Initiatives collaborate fruitfully with each other and involve volunteers, the public and the private sector. All the initiatives inescapably must relate to municipal governance. How a municipality facilitates urban agriculture, be it through active strategies and funding opportunities or as through their authority to approve zoning of urban agriculture, will impact the development of the initiatives. This relates to findings in Chap. 12, where Oslo municipality serves as a case study of institutionalization of urban agriculture and its impact on policy. Oslo has come far in the institutionalization of urban agriculture, having incorporated it in the municipal plan and in strategic documents (see Chap. 12). Unlike Bergen and Trondheim, Oslo has a strong political involvement in urban agriculture, which makes it a top-down effort. The visions do not specifically address which type of municipal governance is needed, but call for recognition and support, in addition to networking and collaboration. In accordance with Chap. 12, it becomes apparent that the visions embody a blend of the "Oslo model" (with its emphasis on recognition and support) and the "Trondheim model" (with focus on networks and collaboration). This raises an intriguing question: to what extent these models harmoniously coexist and complement each other?

8.5.2 Reflections on Our Method

This paper used and analyzed data from students' written reports and observations as a source of urban agriculture knowledge. This adds one degree of separation from the field, and possibly limits the scope of our research. For this reason, we chose a focus on co-production between students and stakeholders and an analysis of the products of these interactions. Integrating the perspective of students and stakeholders gave us access to new and visionary thoughts and ideas, which are necessary and indeed needed in urban agriculture research.

According to Wiek and Iwaniec (2014), visionary thinking is a good tool for working with change processes. Yet, our team has experienced people's reluctance to participate in the visioning process. In one of the case studies, the students encountered the coordinators' resistance to developing a clear vision, and a preference to keep the future open and "organically" adapt and evolve. In their minds, a clear vision could prevent the unexpected and unplanned. We argue that this open-endedness is also a vision, and that they could still benefit from a visioning workshop, both as an educational experience and as a forum for an open dialogue on the future.

In a visionary thinking exercise, participants think creatively about the future. In contrast to semi-structured interviews and participant observation, visioning is an active, action-oriented, and participatory process. The participants are encouraged to contribute with their ideas and visions for the future, rather than just share experiences and facts. Egmose et al. (2020) argue that this relates to democracy: "it is by democratizing the ways by which new insights emerge that research can make substantial contributions to broader societal democratizations" (p. 234). In this study, we did not collect scientific data on participants's perceptions of the visioning workshops, except for informal conversations with project coordinators. Future research should gather these perceptions through interviews, focus groups or surveys preceding the workshops. Such activities would provide insights into the second aim of student action learning: positive change in the initiatives. From a pedagogical point of view, further research should also provide more knowledge of student learning as a result of their participation in these kinds of project.

8.6   Conclusions: Competing Visions of Urban Agriculture in Public Space?

To imagine means to transcend existing thought and, as a result, cultivate the capacity to seek completely new solutions. We propose that in the development from a known past to an unknown future, where sustainability is at stake, this visionary thinking competences will be vital. This action research endeavour involved students and urban agriculture stakeholders to *help achieve integration of urban agriculture* in public spaces. The students planned and organized the visioning workshops and summarized their outcomes in the reports. We analyzed these documents to find the key characteristics of the cocreated visions, the supporting forces and challenges and the suggested action steps. Our findings predominantly align with prior research done on motivations for urban agriculture and the quality of participants' experiences. One category that stands out more in the visions than in the findings of motivations in Chap. 6 is the greater focus on ecological benefits of urban agriculture, including food production. Our study's visionary aspect is that it revealed what people would really like urban agriculture to be. It is about advancing social and economic benefits and food production, but these goals are challenging to achieve. Another explanation could be the added perspectives in our study, where a diverse group of stakeholders have been involved in making the visions. Might there be a difference in the motivations and desires of project leaders vs. those of the residents and community participants? More research is needed to fully answer these questions.

Appendix 1: List of Unpublished Student Reports

Bhérer-Breton, P., Buckley, R., Liegmann, L., & Nair, M. (2018). *Urban agriculture in Oslo – The study case of Voksenenga Naermiljøhage* [Unpublished student report]. Norwegian University of Life Sciences.

Blindheim, M., Conrotte, M., Durand, A., Hnatiuk, S., & Neault, A. (2019). *A vision of urban agriculture in Gamle Oslo – A case study as part of the course PAE302 action learning in farming and food systems* [Unpublished student report]. Norwegian University of Life Sciences.

Brennsæter, J., Lang, K., Chopin, L., D'orazio, M., & Giraud, N. (2018). *Ellingsrud Parsellhage stakeholder document* [Unpublished student report]. Norwegian University of Life Sciences.

Genneper, R., Attard, P., Demavivas, C., Karuga, J., & Brumer, A. (2019). *The future of urban agriculture in Oslo – A case study on Grünerløkka district* [Report, unpublished]. Norwegian University of Life Sciences.

Kapalla, D., Fausko, M., Brannan, T., & Vernier, T. (2018). *PÅ Schous – Growing the community through food* [Unpublished student report]. Norwegian University of Life Sciences.

Lunder, O. E., Porter, B., Asieduwaa, G. A., & Homulle, Z. (2018). *PAE302 Food Case Document: The cross pollination of Dr. Dedichens Drivhus and Trosterud Parsellhage* [Unpublished student report]. Norwegian University of Life Sciences.

Western, B., Schillinger, M., Reid, E., Faury, A., & Colbert, E. (2018). *Roots of urban change: Climate and community adaptation in water and social systems* (Losæter report) [Unpublished student report]. Norwegian University of Life Sciences.

References

Burnes, B. (2020). The origins of Lewin's three-step model of change. *The Journal of Applied Behavioral Science, 56*(1), 32–59. https://doi.org/10.1177/0021886319892685

Checkland, P. (2000). Soft systems methodology: A thirty year retrospective. *Systems Research, 17*, S11–S58. https://doi.org/10.1002/1099-1743(200011)17:1+<::AID-SRES374>3.0.CO;2-O

Desmond, D., Grieshop, J., & Subramaniam, A. (2004). Revisiting garden-based learning in basic education. *Education for rural people*. UNESCO-IIEP.

Egmose, J., Gleerup, J., & Nielsen, B. S. (2020). Critical utopian action research: Methodological inspiration for democratization? *International Review of Qualitative Research, 13*(2), 233–246. https://doi.org/10.1177/1940844720933236

Fox-Kamper, R., Wesener, A., Munderlein, D., Sondermann, M., McWilliam, W., & Kirk, N. (2018). Urban community gardens: An evaluation of governance approaches and related enablers and barriers at different development stages. *Landscape and Urban Planning, 170*, 59–68. https://doi.org/10.1016/j.landurbplan.2017.06.023

Francis, C., Breland, T. A., Østergaard, E., Lieblein, G., & Morse, S. (2013). Phenomenon-based learning in agroecology: A prerequisite for transdisciplinarity and responsible action. *Agroecology and Sustainable Food Systems, 37*, 60–75. https://doi.org/10.1080/1044004 6.2012.717905

Gasperi, D., Pennisi, G., Rizzati, N., Magrefi, F., Bazzocchi, G., Mezzacapo, U., Stefani, M. C., Sanye-Mengual, E., Orsini, F., & Gianquinto, G. (2016). Towards regenerated and productive vacant areas through urban horticulture: Lessons from Bologna, Italy. *Sustainability, 8*(12), 1347. https://doi.org/10.3390/su8121347

Halloran, A., & Magid, J. (2013). The role of local government in promoting sustainable urban agriculture in Dar Es Salaam and Copenhagen. *Geografisk Tidsskrift-Danish Journal of Geography, 113*(2), 121–132. https://doi.org/10.1080/00167223.2013.848612

Kolb, D. A. (2014). *Experiential learning: Experience as the source of learning and development* (2nd ed.). Pearson Education.

Lewin, K. (1946). Action research and minority problems. *Journal of Social Issues, 2*(4), 34–46. https://doi.org/10.1111/j.1540-4560.1946.tb02295.x

Lieblein, G., Francis, C. A. & Torjusen, H. (2001). Future interconnections among ecological farmers, processors, marketers, and consumers in Hedmark County, Norway: Creating shared vision. *Human Ecology Review, 8*(1), 60–71.

Lieblein, G., Østergaard, E., & Francis, C. (2004). Becoming an agroecologist through action education. *International Journal of Agricultural Sustainability, 2*(3), 147–153. https://doi.org/1 0.1080/14735903.2004.9684574

Nussbaum, M. C. (2011). *Creating capabilities: The human development approach.* Harvard University Press.

Peters, S., & Wals, A. (2013). Learning and knowing in pursuit of sustainability: Concepts and tools for trans-disciplinary environmental research. In M. E. Krasny & J. Dillon (Eds.), *Trading zones in environmental education: Creating transdisciplinary dialogue* (pp. 79–104). Peter Lang Verlag.

Pfeffer, J. (1998). *The human equation: Building profits by putting people first.* Harvard Business School Press.

Pool, A., & Parker, M. (2017). *Creating futures that matter today: Facilitating change through shared vision.* Executive Savvy.

Prove, C., Kemper, D., & Loudiyi, S. (2018). The modus operandi of urban agriculture initiatives toward a conceptual framework. *Nature and Culture, 13*(1), 17–46. https://doi.org/10.3167/nc.2018.130102

Rowe, G., & Frewer, L. J. (2004). Evaluating public-participation exercises: A research agenda. *Science Technology & Human Values, 29*(4), 512–557. https://doi.org/10.1177/016224 3903259197

Swensen, G., Stafseng, V. E., & Nielsen, V. K. S. (2022). Visionscapes: Combining heritage and urban gardening to enhance areas requiring regeneration. *International Journal of Heritage Studies, 28*(4), 511–537. https://doi.org/10.1080/13527258.2021.2020879

UNESCO. (2017). *Education for sustainable development goals: Learning objectives.* UNESCO.

van der Jagt, A. P. N., Szaraz, L. R., Delshammar, T., Cvejic, R., Santos, A., Goodness, J., & Buijs, A. (2017). Cultivating nature-based solutions: The governance of communal urban gardens in the European Union. *Environmental Research, 159*, 264–275. https://doi.org/10.1016/j.envres.2017.08.013

Wiek, A., & Iwaniec, D. (2014). Quality criteria for visions and visioning in sustainability science. *Sustainability Science, 9*(4), 497–512. https://doi.org/10.1007/s11625-013-0208-6

Wiek, A., & Kay, B. (2015). Learning while transforming: Solution-oriented learning for urban sustainability in Phoenix, Arizona. *Current Opinion in Environmental Sustainability, 16*, 29–36. https://doi.org/10.1016/j.cosust.2015.07.001

Chapter 9
From Prescription to Adaptation in the Future Productive City: Classroom-Inspired Principles for Design and Planning of Urban Agriculture

Deni Ruggeri

9.1 Relevance

Over the past few decades, urban agriculture has become a go-to strategy for sustainable development. Indeed, urban agriculture can potentially induce innumerable positive consequences on several urban systems (Wadumestrige Dona et al., 2021; Lovell, 2010). A new vision is emerging of a city built around publicly accessible, productive landscapes disseminated across the urban fabric and integrated into an interconnected blue-green infrastructure that helps detain water, sequester CO_2, increase biodiversity, activate biophilia, and enhance well-being for human and nonhuman species (Palmer, 2018; Beatley, 2011). Whereas the city of the Modern era privileged efficiency, fast mobility, and the exploitation of natural resources and land, the biophilic, ecologically vibrant city of the future will help deepen humans' connections to the local landscape and encourage stewardship and care while balancing the human needs for housing, jobs, and cultural life with those of nature (Beatley, 2016).

The extent and quantity of benefits urban agriculture produces is a question that researchers have only begun to scratch the surface of. In measuring these benefits, some have emphasized yield over experience (McDougall et al., 2019). Researchers agree that urban agriculture may not significantly impact the food security of the world's urban population, especially in Northern Climates (Goldstein et al., 2016). Others have illustrated the socio-ecological benefits of urban agriculture for ecosystems and communities, where urban agriculture can serve as a tool to connect children and adults to nature and thus reduce their ecoliteracy and experience deficit (Louv, 2012) and instigate new forms of socialization and construction of a shared identity (Ruggeri, 2018). Urban agriculture has allowed marginalized, fragile

D. Ruggeri (✉)
Department of Plant Science and Landscape Architecture, University of Maryland,
College Park, MD, USA
e-mail: druggeri@umd.edu

© The Author(s) 2024
B. Sirowy, D. Ruggeri (eds.), *Urban Agriculture in Public Space*, GeoJournal
Library 132, https://doi.org/10.1007/978-3-031-41550-0_9

communities to reclaim their right to landscape, repair environmental injustices (Alomar, 2018) and practice landscape democracy (Egoz, 2018). This entitlement goes beyond the mere possibility of accessing and experiencing the landscape. It includes the opportunity to participate in new practices of democratic life, cultivate and activate human capabilities, and empower all individuals to reach their full potential (Nussbaum, 2011).

While urban agriculture's positives vastly outweigh its negatives ensuring that it unleashes its full benefits is a challenge for designers, planners, and organizers. Actual conflict exists between densification, a necessity for a sustainable city, and the demands for easily accessible open spaces to grow food and community. Studies show that greater residential densities harm the quantity and quality of our cities' public realm (Murphy et al., 2022; Lin et al., 2015). Urban agriculture's long history as a tool for social justice, empowerment, community redevelopment, and reparation continues to be alive and thrive in many contemporary urban agriculture sites, particularly those in marginalized communities (Lawson, 2005). Urban agriculture is expanding into place and culturally-informed practices that restore and construct identities, celebrate diversity, and serve as arenas for the practice of democratic life (Hou, 2017). This is not without challenges, as this identity-affirming role might conflict with the prescriptive, top-down, and place-neutral policies and planning efforts around the idea of a compact city (Abelman et al., 2022). Similarly, a 'critical geography' of urban agriculture is emerging (Chap. 13; Tornaghi, 2014), which challenges the creativity, cultural sensitivity, and agency of all involved by questioning the benevolent image of a practice that may be contributing to socioeconomic inequalities, gentrification, and caters to mainstream lifestyles and aesthetics over the real needs of the working poor, differently abled and marginalized (Reynolds, 2017). Urban agriculture is not immune to conflict, and that is particularly true in public space, where the interests of farmers may be at odds with those of the nearby residents and occasional users. Urban agriculture may sometimes public access. Designing urban agriculture spaces that serve as common ground for the daily negotiation and renegotiation of individual and public claims will be a critical factor in their long-term resilience and strength as food and community-building systems (see Chap. 4 in this volume).

9.1.1 Urban Agriculture in Public Space: Technique Versus Experiences?

Urban agriculture's idiosyncratic, far-reaching impacts on human and ecological systems make it a 'wicked problem' that defies standardized solutions and replicable strategies (Rittel & Webber, 1974). Yet, designers' and planners' responses have

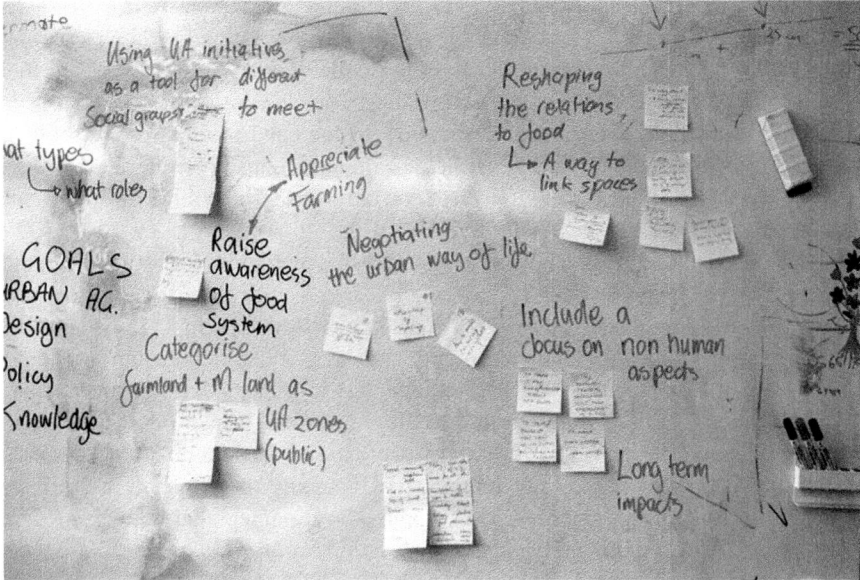

Fig. 9.1 The multifaceted nature of urban agriculture in compact-city development emerged from a brainstorming by the Cultivating Public Space project participants (image by the author)

been simplistic, envisioning an urban agriculture made of small, individual plots of land, rather than a system of city landscapes collective food production. At the onset of the, the Cultivating Public Space (CPS) project partners discussed at length how to integrate urban agriculture into everyday life starting with the city's public spaces (Fig. 9.1). They made recurring references to the monotony and pervasiveness of the planter box, which became a metaphor for the tension between urban agriculture as a standardized, uniformly distributed function in the urban landscape—from rooftops to balconies, from vacant lots to utility easements, from inner courtyards to semipublic commercial spaces—and urban agriculture as a retrofit and adaptation of public space to renew social bonds or construct new shared identities across socioeconomic and cultural divides.

9.1.2 Cultivating Public Space Through a Critical Pedagogy

The CPS project wanted to engage students as partners in action research and discussed at length the kinds of experiences and knowledge needed to design and plan for urban agriculture that could advance systemic change across as many of the 17 United Nations Sustainable Development Goals (UNSDGs) as possible (United

Nations General Assembly, 2015). Framed as a Participatory Action Research effort, the CPS project sought to tackle many of the above issues through a partnership between academia, nonprofits, and the public. By engaging students in their research, CPS partners and researchers wanted them to experience a critical pedagogy by questioning personal and professional biases and assumptions as tools for domination (Reynolds, 2017, 55) and letting them imagine how future urban agriculture could help heal past injustice and cultivate democratic discourse and social equity.

This chapter reflects on a few pilot educational experiences for which the author served as main or co-instructor, deliberately crafted to explore the CPS research goals and questions through a design-as-research process. The first pilot course was a studio taught in 2017 for landscape architecture master's students at the Norwegian University of Life Science (NMBU), entitled *"LAA341, the Urban Landscape as a Social Arena."* This was followed in the Fall of 2019 and Winter of 2020 by a continuing education course targeting activists, professionals, and policymakers interested in urban agriculture. After joining the University of Maryland in 2022, the CPS project theories, practices, and findings were integrated into *"LARC151 Designing Transformative, Productive Urban Agriculture Landscapes"* a general education course offered in the Spring and Fall of 2022 and LARC748, a landscape architecture capstone studio for third-year graduate students. Collectively, these education-based case studies offer a unique window into the evolution of urban agriculture and its adaptation to the unique socio-cultural and ecological contexts.

9.1.3 Pedagogical Questions

How can resilience and landscape democracy-affirming urban agriculture be better integrated into the city's public realm? What unique strengths, weaknesses, opportunities, and threats can those designing, planning, implementing, and managing these productive spaces leverage for positive change? How transferable might urban agriculture models be across urban environments and types of communities? And what practices, strategies, and tactics may be needed to ensure that urban agriculture sites are ready to improve the lives, health, and personal capacities of the individuals they touch? The students and the perspectives of the communities they partnered with in their education shed light on many of these questions and helped test the relevance of the academic reflections and theories guiding the work of the CPS partners. Through the students' interactions with urban farmers, it became clear that no urban agriculture site in public space could be successful without a meaningful integration and celebration of the uniqueness and specificity of each locale. Rather than a universal toolbox for urban agriculture, the students translated what they learned into design principles, strategies, actions of spatial, sociocultural, and ecological landscape transformations communicated in the form of richly-illustrated stories of change and adaptation.

9.2   Case Studies

9.2.1   Case Study 1: LAA341: Urban Agriculture as a Social Arena for New Citizenry

In Fall 2017, the CPS project inspired 11 landscape architecture graduate students to enroll in *"LAA341-The Urban Landscape as a Social Arena"*, a design studio for master's students at the Norwegian University of Life Sciences (NMBU). Over 17 weeks, they would partner with the urban agriculture community of Losæter in Oslo to help shift perceptions and physical barriers that keep lower-income families of the nearby neighborhood of Gamle Oslo (Old Oslo) from participating in its activities. Losæter is a 4.6-acre site above a large tunnel built in 2010 to bury a freeway and re-connect the city to its waterfront. The southern access to the tunnel featured a large opening in the ground and two tall concrete ventilation shafts. At the base was a ruderal space that a small community of artists, led by local activist Beate Hovind, began to occupy in 2012 with the vision to make it a hub for artistic expression, biophilia, healing, and food production (Fig. 9.2).

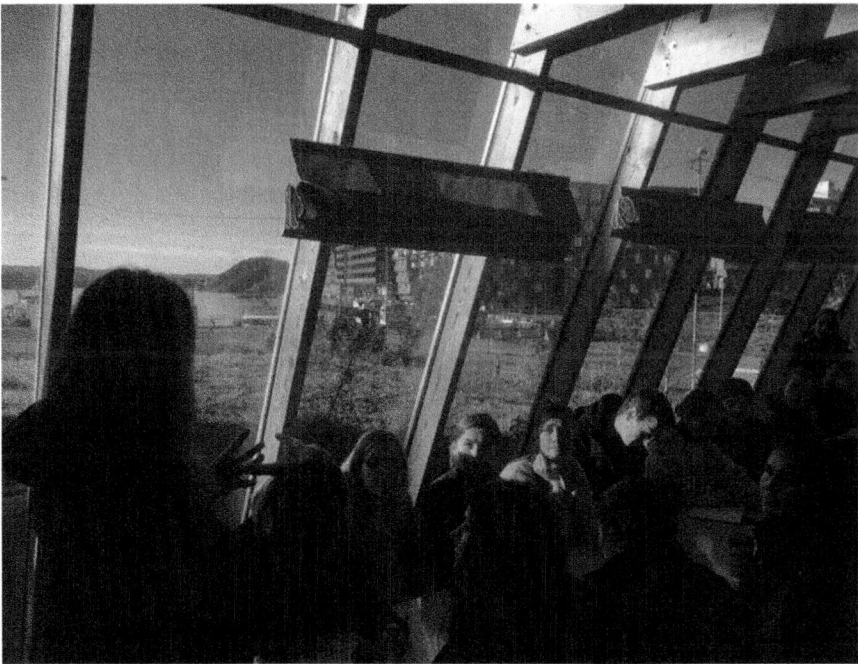

Fig. 9.2 LAA341 students in Losæter's baking house, listening to Beate Hovind's stories about the project's roots (image by the author)

NMBU students began with a deep listening activity that involved Losæter's variegated communities of practice: the Future Farmers Flatbread Society/baking house users, early-dementia patients, elementary school children, and immigrant women enrolled in a language course. NMBU students co-created a metaphorical "recipe" for the future of Losæter as an educational, health, and community-building neighborhood open space. They argued for a change in the city's plans to replace Losæter with a traditional public park, advocating that its permanence would provide a much-needed place for an evolving and adaptable commons to become a sacred space for the new and old citizenry.

The participatory process involved an inventory of landscape and community assets, resources, and shortcomings, and an extensive phase of listening to the many stories of self (Ganz, 2011) connected to Losæter. The students heard about the 2001 temporary art installation that planted the first seed and the other meaningful milestones in its evolution to what Losæter is today (Fig. 9.3). In the focus groups and interviews, they learned about the Flatbread Society. With the opening of an outdoor baking oven, this community of practice could link to the immigrant groups, using the metaphor of the flatbread as a shared platform to bring together Norwegian and foreign residents in a celebration of bread. This work also set the foundation for a series of cultural events, like the 2015 procession that brought soils from across Norway to the garden, and the construction of the public Baking House in 2016. Co-creating a timeline of the core story of Losæter was the opportunity to reveal and celebrate its living history. It was a much-needed moment of awareness that this story would need to become co-owned to be resilient and harness its full potential as a transformative landscape.

The resulting "recipe" for a more inclusive Losæter sought to remove physical and perceptual barriers to the site. It imagined safer pedestrian connections from Gamle Oslo to the waterfront, the reuse of an unused viaduct as a linear urban agriculture space, and a new streetscape designed to slow traffic and allow animals and humans to reach the sea easily. As to the site, an expanded and redesigned Losæter

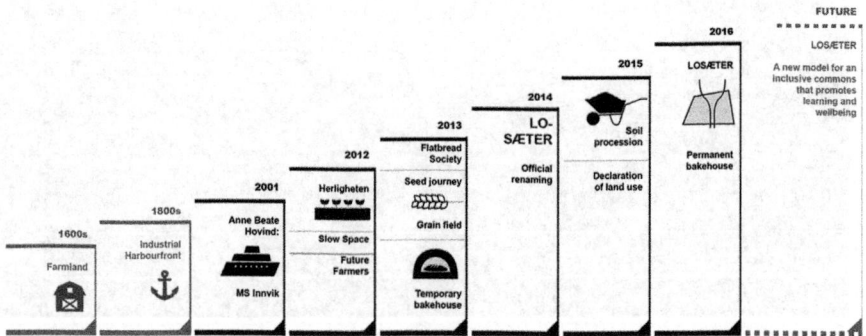

Fig. 9.3 Co-creating a timeline of the core story of Losæter was the opportunity to make all users a part of its living history project (Image by Åse Holte, Kristin Sunde, Kjersti Børve Skjelbreid, Andrea Haave Jenssen, Maren Helgerud Gynnild, Hanne Tveter Åmdal, Betina Øvstaas Amundsen, Martha Kvalheim, Annie Hedger, and Thomas Crowe)

would offer more affordances for passive recreation, environmental education, and healing. The site would also extend into the Oslo Fjord, with floating gardens as stepping stones for biodiversity and pollinator-friendly habitats.

9.2.2   Case Study 2: SEVU Continuing Education: Making Urban Agriculture Between Policy and Practice

The second educational experience from the CPS project activities was a continuing education course offered through NMBU's Center for Continuing Education (SEVU). The post-professional course open to planners, designers, activists, and lifelong learners enlisted CPS project partner Arild Eriksen and the author as instructors of an intense hybrid course, during which students worked collaboratively through remote and in-person group activities to co-create a vision of how urban agriculture functions may be integrated into five notable sites in central Oslo: the vacant land situated in the waterfront development area known as Sukkerbiten, the Royal Palace Garden, the Tullinløkka urban void, and the mixed-use district of Vollebekk.

Students attended three weekend-long intense workshop sessions, supplemented with online lectures by international experts in landscape architecture, ecology, planning, and development and by CPS partners (Fig. 9.4). Field trips took students

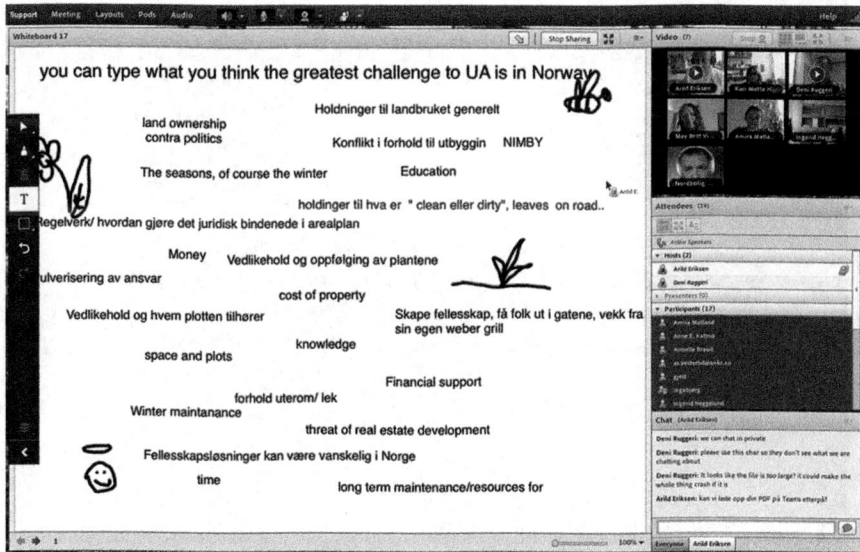

Fig. 9.4 The 2019-2020 SEVU Continuing Education course at NMBU was a hybrid class involving lectures by project partners and urban agriculture experts, interactive online sessions, and in-person workshops (image by the author)

to urban agriculture sites in the Oslo region and helped them reflect on the similarities and uniqueness of each community. Throughout the course, they were to collaborate in analyzing, synthesizing, conceptualizing, and co-designing urban agriculture interventions that would challenge the status quo and offer new suggestions to policymakers and city planners as to the productive functions they could introduce into the existing public urban spaces of the city functions typically relegated to private or semi-private spaces.

During the course, students formed interdisciplinary teams to develop strategies for urban agriculture integration in the Oslo city center public spaces. Rather than a kit-of-parts, four typologies of urban agriculture emerged from the engagement of post-professional learners. Their vision for the Royal Palace Park, "At the King's Table," re-imagined this iconic cultural landscape to showcase Norway's tangible and intangible agricultural heritage and the contemporary city's needs for greater environmental sustainability and multiculturalism. The students, with their diverse backgrounds as municipal planners, designers, activists, and public servants, brought innovative ideas to the table. They imagined the zoning of urban public spaces and cultural landscapes based on their heritage value, visibility, and potential for eco-literacy and education (Fig. 9.5). Their vision transformed the Tullinløkka site from a void in the historic city fabric into a technologically-advanced recycling, re-use, soil, and energy production center, with interconnected living machines to process wastewater. On the east side of Oslo, one of the teams proposed an eco-district with housing, parking, and commercial uses integrated into

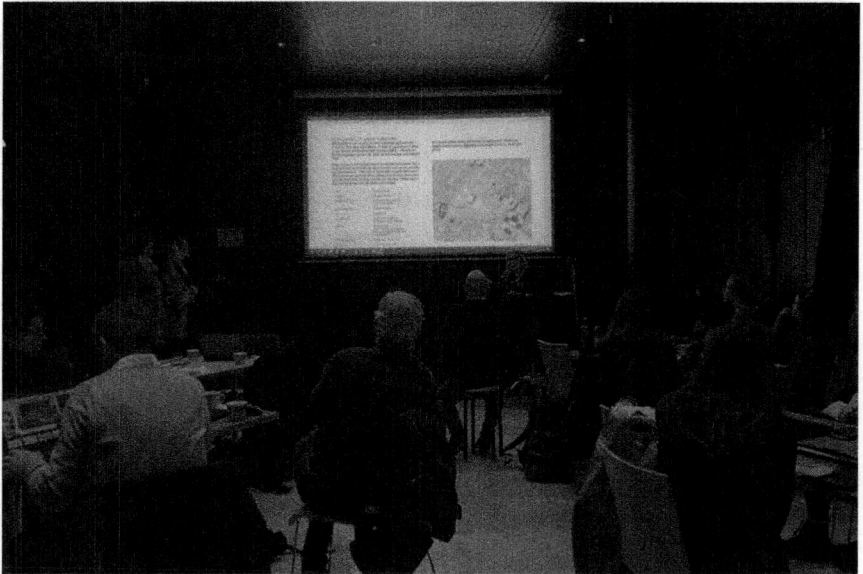

Fig. 9.5 In the vision of one of the continuing education student teams, entitled "At the King's Table", the Oslo Royal Palace Park became a case study for a policy instrument to guide the integration of urban agriculture in cultural landscapes (image by the author)

south-facing, energy-efficient buildings designed to maximize sun exposure and private terraces, and shared plots for the neophytes and less abled in public space. Another team offered a new vision for Sukkerbitten, the only vacant site along the Oslo waterfront as a public 'Commons' integrating wetlands, edible forests, and a rich ecotone for plants, fish, and other species. They described it as a nonjudgmental space where everyone could find shelter from the rain available without a charge.

9.2.3 Case Study 3: Designing Transformative, Productive Urban Agriculture Landscapes

In the Spring and Fall of 2022, at the University of Maryland, the author had the opportunity to design an "I" series course LARC151 *"Urban Agriculture: Designing Transformative, Productive Landscapes."* 'I'series courses are intended to be experimental and applied to real-life, wicked problems to prepare students to engage with ambiguity, uncertainty, and change. Course enrollment is open to university students in any major. In designing the course, many of the experiences and knowledge created within the CPS project—readings, remote lectures, and case studies—were folded into the syllabus and assignments. Over two semesters, 200 LARC151 students were encouraged to become citizen scientists and agents of sustainable change by envisioning design transformations for existing urban agriculture sites in Washington, DC, and Baltimore, Maryland.

LARC151 students began exploring their chosen urban agriculture community through site visits, research, interviews and participant-observation. One of the biweekly course meetings was devoted to workshops during which students formed groups to discuss a topic, brainstorm an idea, and share knowledge. They also attended a weekly section where teaching assistants offered guidance and inspiration to perform seven assignments, which would collectively merge into a landscape plan to add greater sustainabilty and strengthen their resilience in the face of uncertainty. The 17 United Nations Sustainable Development Goals provided a foundation for the student's work, beginning with crafting a personal "manifesto" to visually represent their visions for urban agriculture's future. The course included a site inventory and mapping phase, where students represented the physical infrastructure, social life networks, and community resources. This information was then used for a strategic SWOT analysis, leveraging their unique strengths and external opportunities against weaknesses and threats. The students also engaged in power mapping, critically examining disparities in resources and opportunity within society, and brainstormed new partnerships that could challenge these disparities by redistributing power to grassroots and community-based organizations. They were encouraged to integrate strategies from international case studies selected from those studied by CPS researchers. These efforts culminated in an equation of change (Cady et al., 2014) a model that envisioned a future scenario based on a series of strategic actions (Fig. 9.6).

A critical discussion within the course revolved around failure and adaptation. The class began with viewing a video telling the story of the South-Central Farm, a

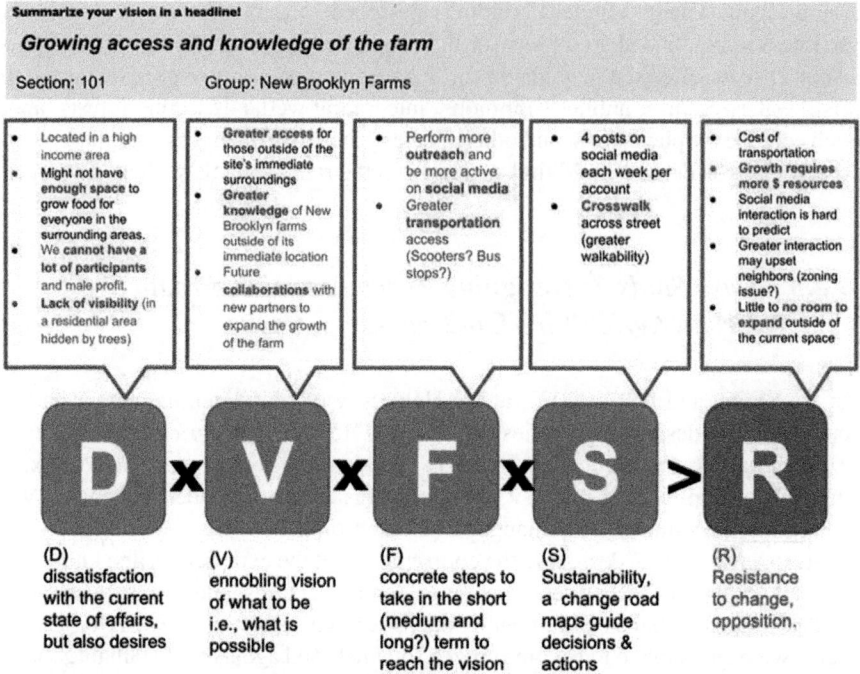

Summarize your vision in a headline!

Growing access and knowledge of the farm

Section: 101   Group: New Brooklyn Farms

• Located in a high income area • Might not have enough space to grow food for everyone in the surrounding areas. • We cannot have a lot of participants and male profit. • Lack of visibility (in a residential area hidden by trees)	• **Greater access for** those outside of the site's immediate surroundings • **Greater knowledge** of New Brooklyn farms outside of its immediate location • Future **collaborations** with new partners to expand the growth of the farm	• Perform more **outreach** and be more active on **social media** • Greater **transportation** access (Scooters? Bus stops?)	• 4 posts on social media each week per account • Crosswalk across street (greater walkability)	• Cost of transportation • Growth requires more $ resources • Social media interaction is hard to predict • Greater interaction may upset neighbors (zoning issue?) • Little to no room to expand outside of the current space

$$ \mathbf{D \times V \times F \times S > R} $$

(D) dissatisfaction with the current state of affairs, but also desires

(V) ennobling vision of what to be i.e., what is possible

(F) concrete steps to take in the short (medium and long?) term to reach the vision

(S) Sustainability, a change road maps guide decisions & actions

(R) Resistance to change, opposition.

Fig. 9.6 Envisioning the future of a landscape is no small feat; it requires strategic, purposeful action and vision. The Equation of Change helped students imagine change as the interplay of dissatisfactions (D), vision (V), first steps (F), and sustainability (S) against resistance (R) (image by the author)

15-acre urban agriculture site in Los Angeles established in 1994 and demolished in 2006 among the protests of residents and environmental activists. During the first week of the course, the class engaged in a post-mortem assessment and reflection of what went wrong for this specific urban agriculture community. Still, it reflected on the transiency and impermanence of these landscapes. One of the communities they partnered with was Temperance Alley, a temporary community garden established in 2020 on a ¼ acre vacant lot in the U Street/ Cardoso neighborhood through a collaboration between the U Street Neighborhood Association, University of Maryland (UMD) students, and other local partners in Washington, DC (Fig. 9.7). Through their interactions with Temperance Alley founders and urban agriculture activists Josh Morin and Aaron Lewis, they were encouraged to think beyond present conditions and accept the temporary nature of the site, and imagine a strategy that would allow to re-locate the garden's pollination and community-building functions to the neighborhood's rooftops, vacant spaces, and rights-of-way at the end of their lease.

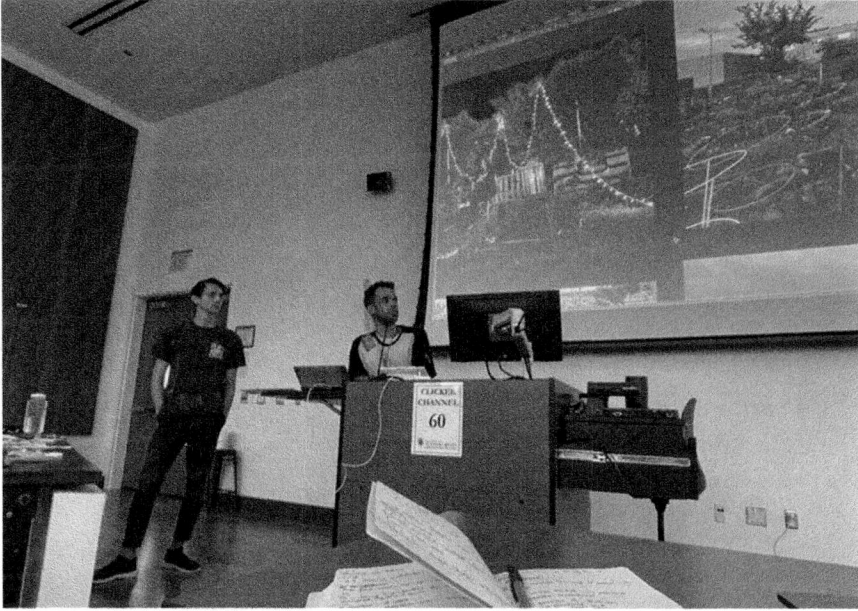

Fig. 9.7 LARC151 included many opportunities to engage the experience of urban farmers. Among them are Josh Morin and Aaron Lewis of Temperance Alley in Washington, DC, a temporary urban farm that grows food nnd community (image by the author)

9.2.4   Case Study 4: Plantation Park Heights: From Urban Agriculture to the Agrihood

During the Fall of 2022, the "*LARC748 Capstone Studio*" at the University of Maryland involved third-year Landscape Architecture graduate students in co-designing and prototyping an *Agrihood* for the Park Heights neighborhood of Baltimore. The urban farm, called Plantation Park Heights (PPH) leases and owns two acres of land, divided into four plots. Park Heights is a neighborhood undergoing a slow but tangible transition from decline to regeneration. In the vision of its founder, Richard Francis (known in the city as Farmer Chippy), the *Agrihood* would use food production to build human capacity, job security, and a virtuous circular economy within a nonjudgmental new public space. Through day-to-day food production, weekly farmers markets (Fig. 9.8), and the distribution of community-supported agriculture (CSA) boxes to hundreds of families on food aid, the Agrihood would attract the youth and inspire in their landscape and community stewardship.

Plantation Park Heights' name references Baltimore's history of racial segregation, social injustices, and neglect. Rather than continuing to adhere to models of community that did not fit the needs of his Trinidadian American community, (Farmer Chippy) Francis wanted to create a new place that would empower the human capabilities of younger generations by exposing them to culturally and

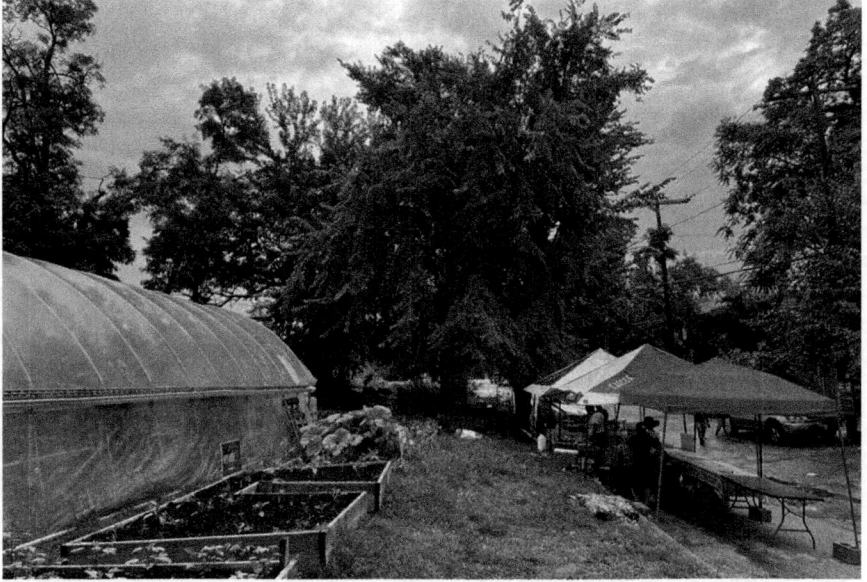

Fig. 9.8 Plantation Park Heights volunteers prepare for the traditional Saturday Farmers' Market, with booths selling spices, veggies, fried shark, and a basil team, part of the Trinidadian gastronomic heritage (image by the author)

experientially rich urban farming activities as a low-threshold entrée into the responsibilities of community life. He also wanted to reclaim the identity and ethnic roots of many residents in Caribbean culture, choosing to grow staple foods, spices, and flavors that would connect them to their original homeland. At their weekly Farmer's Markets, fried shark and fish peppers[1] became opportunities to rediscover long-forgotten traditions that could be re-integrated and woven into a new story to guide the site's future.

Through their direct engagement with the PPH community, landscape architecture students understood the need to think beyond traditional urban agriculture aesthetics and definitions. They also understood the need for participation to be driven and negotiated with them rather than imposed by the needs of academia. While picking peppers, they listened to their stories, and learned firsthand about PPH's challenges, its successes, and their future visions (Fig. 9.9). University of Maryland students went beyond the need to be sustainable by asking their designs to perform across a range of UNSDGs. To do so, they looked for help in transdisciplinarity by researching and incorporating strategies borrowed from across many fields—organic farming, food science, planning, community development, energy, and health, to mention a few and see their designs as accountable to changes in ecology, community, and livability. To communicate the potential synergies in benefits, a group of students produced a

---

[1] This site discusses the Fish Pepper's centrality in the lives of enslaved communities in North America and beyond. https://www.preservationmaryland.org/maryland-food-history-the-fish-pepper/

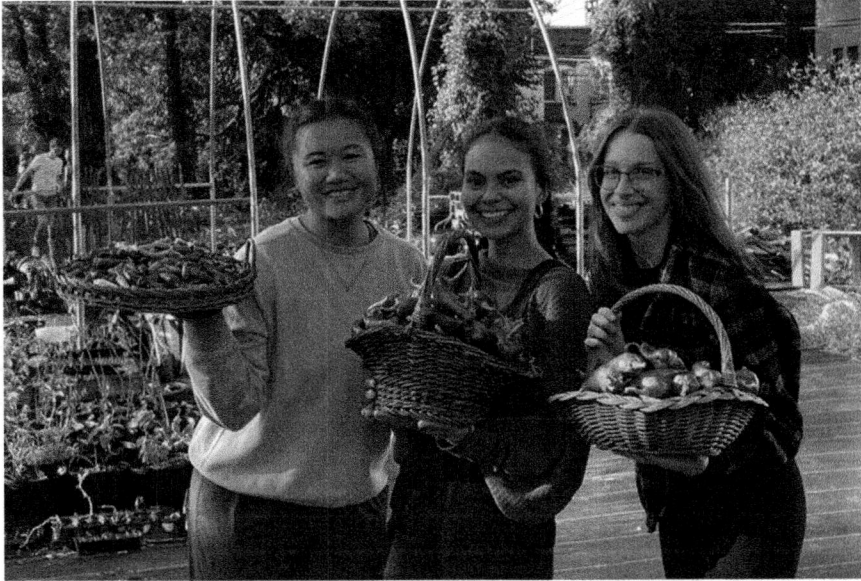

Fig. 9.9 While picking peppers, landscape architecture students learned about the fish pepper, a staple food in the Baltimore African American community (image by the author)

pattern language of physical and socio-ecological transformations in the long-, medium-, and short-term. In contrast, others sought to translate these patterns into interventions to improve PPH's circular economy, making their new visions accountable to concrete stormwater management, biodiversity, health, and livability benefits.

9.3 Discussion: From One Toolbox to Six Emergent Principles for Future Urban Agriculture

To some designers and planners, it feels empowering to think of people-in-place practices like urban agriculture as a series of cause/effect relations that can be shaped or altered by design to achieve certain behaviors. Yet in the classroom experiences described earlier, as in daily work of the urban farmers they collaborated with, the students learned that growing food and community is a wicked problem that defies standardized, sectorial, or piecemean solutions, and requires activation and education. Programmatic elements and objects are only affordances that require peoples awareness of their benefits, require investment, and stewardship to continue to perform their magic (Fig. 9.10).

In the intent of the CPS project partners, students would translate their research scientific findings into a toolbox of physical designs that would illustrate how to better integrate urban agriculture into the public realm of Norwegian and other world cities. It was enlightening and humbling for students and researchers to partner with existing urban agriculture communities and to listen to their stories

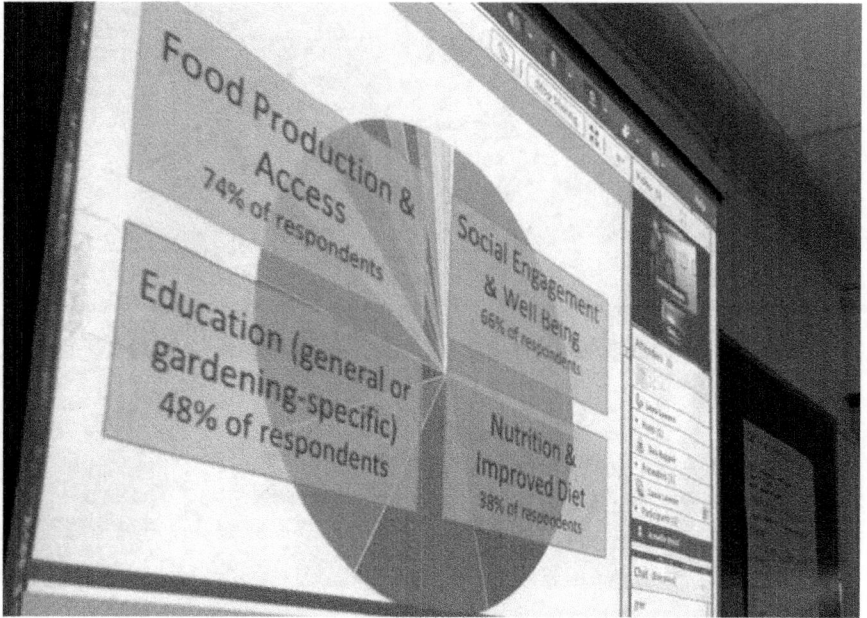

Fig. 9.10 Laura Lawson, Dean of the School of Agriculture at Rutgers University shared her reflections on the perceived benefits of urban agriculture from the point of view of underserved communities (image by the author)

of success, failure, persistence, and hard work. They understood that a thriving urban agriculture needs to be rooted in individual and shared stories of the unique circumstances of their creation. The narratives and values they discovered while engaging with urban farmers taught them that in addition to yielding food, urban agriculture sites are grounds for resolution of conflicting visions of sustainable and resilient change, the cultivation of new shared identities, and the promotion of collective stewardship. Rather than offering a transferable toolkit, this chapter reflects on a few emergent principles that can guide future urban agriculture projects in public space, serving as a point of departure or contrast for future research and practice.

9.3.1 Principle 1: Urban Agriculture Is a Multidimensional Ecology of Actions and Counteractions

They endeavored to impact as many sustainability goals as possible by leveraging synergies and imagining cross-systemic changes. Linking their work to the UNSDGs, the students strived to make their designs accountable to more than just creativity and intuition. Connecting the classroom to the transdisciplinary work of nonprofits and start-ups involved in implementing the same goals leads to mutually beneficial opportunities to learn from each other. It leads to innovative, out-of-the-box thinking and solutions. An essential contribution to education came from the CPS project's extensive documentation of Norwegian and international case studies, which served as a source of inspiration and reflection for students' visions.

Implementing and sustaining the transformations that the UNSDGs demand requires permeating urban agriculture processes in people's lives and the spaces where their stories unfold. These systemic changes required students to think beyond the physical infrstructure and design the flows of energy, money, and resources needed to activate them. Designing these flows required being strategic about which ones to prioritize and be involved in to achieve the changes desired by the community (Fig. 9.11). To synthesize their knowledge of their chosen urban agriculture sites, students developed a SWOT (strengths, weaknesses, opportunities, and threats) analysis to select which strengths and opportunities they would tackle in counteracting weaknesses and strategize against external threats. Power maps helped them be tactical in identifying which processes to target in their visions and which partners to involve.

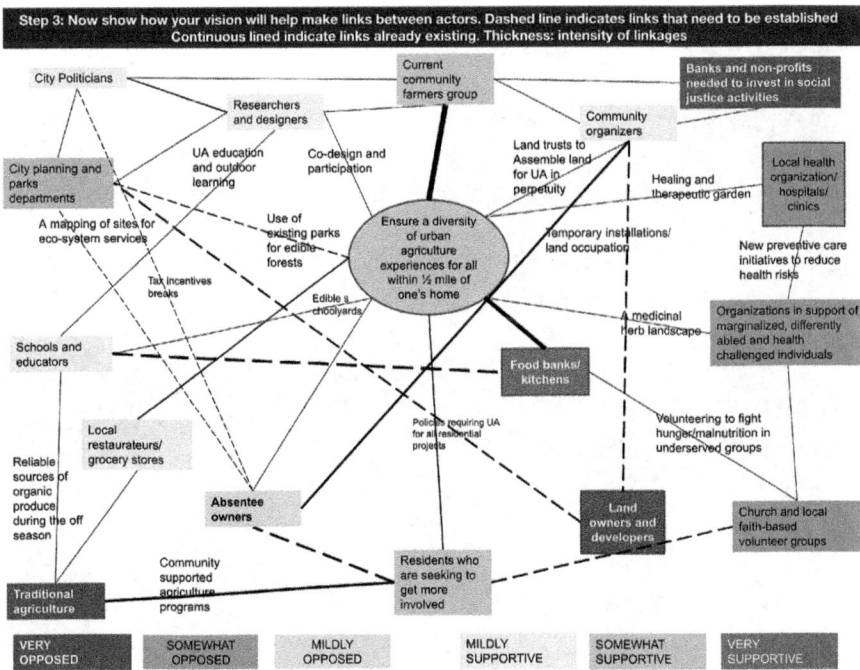

Fig. 9.11 Power mapping helps us identify processes having the greatest potential to achieve the changes needed to fully make urban agriculture benefit society (image by the author)

9.3.2   Principle 2: Successful Urban Agriculture Demands Bountiful Partnerships and Cooperation

No single source of knowledge can fully capture the multitude of considerations, dimensions, and scales involved in designing for transformative urban agriculture. For designers, this means being open and prepared to engage across fields of knowledge, professionalism, and value systems and to be transformed by this engagement. During day-long project meetings, Cultivating Public Space project partners explored urban agriculture sites and invited representatives of community organizations and nonprofits, private citizens, and public officials to join the discussion and add their perspectives. The stories we heard were documented, and served well the students, giving them a view from the inside of the challenges each community face as it seeks to reclaim their public spaces for food and community production.

Yet, if we think of urban agriculture's future, we must continue operating to ensure its presence in our cities is visible and felt. For urban agriculture to perform its full cultural and eco-systemic benefits, all kinds of landscapes should be included in the city's green infrastructure (Fig. 9.12). This means starting with public landscapes but eventually expanding to include private spaces and rooftops like the "Tak for Maten" rooftop garden created by CPS project partner Nabolagshager.[2] Traditional farmers also have a role to play by reducing their ecological footprint, water

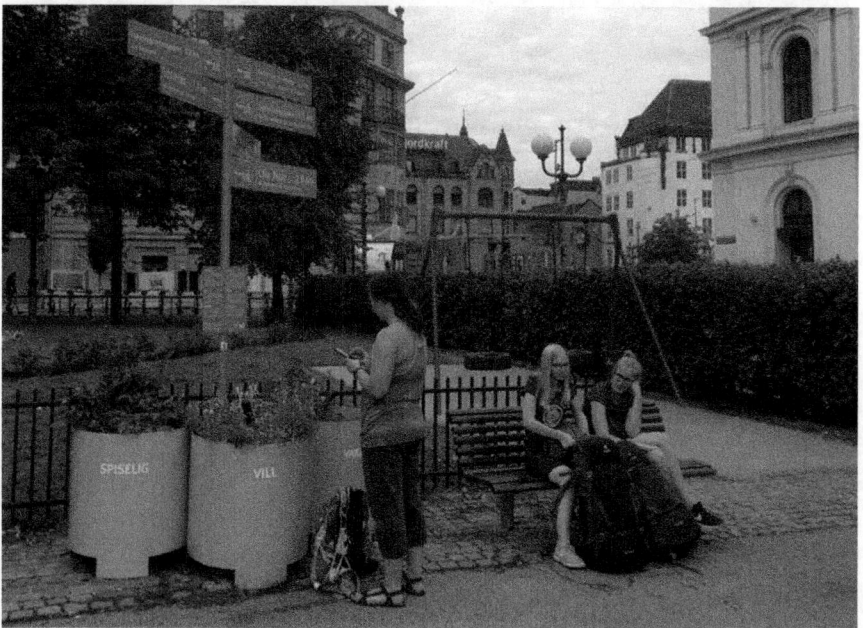

Fig. 9.12 This signage directs visitors to the Oslo center to the city's growingly productive urban landscapes from edible schoolyards to the entire waterfront (image by the author)

---

[2] The "Tak for Maten" was created by the Oslo nonprofit Nabolagshager (www.nabolagshager.no)

consumption, and transportation costs and supplementing local production with organically and locally grown food. Community-Supported Agriculture, vertical and rooftop farming, and cooperative agriculture can easily co-exist and integrate with the smaller-scale community and allotment gardens. They help ensure the resilience, reliability, diversity, and affordability of food supply, particularly for the economically challenged and fragile members of our society.

9.3.3   Principle 3: Urban Agriculture Cultivates a Shared Transformative Experiences

The European Landscape Convention defines landscape as areas "perceived by people, whose character is the result of the actions and interactions of natural and human factors"(Council of Europe, 2000, article 1), which fits the type of urban agriculture project partners and students experienced. In their interactions, they experienced how urban agriculture can help us connect to the natural landscape, make us healthier, more engaged in the community, and more willing to share the collective responsibility to the landscape and each other.

The experiences people share and the feelings they develop toward their community landscape are ideal entry points into their bodily knowledge, perceptions, and visions of the urban landscape, which ultimately shape their actions and interactions.

By integrating these experiences and elevating them into a shared sense of purpose and motivation, we can witness the transformative power and energy to ensure the resilience of all public spaces, especially urban agriculture sites. In Oslo's Losæter community, students discovered an inaccessible community that involuntarily excluded the nearby immigrant populations. They learned about these perceptions from a small group of refugee women enrolled in Norwegian language courses held at the public baking house. To overcome language and cultural barriers, they asked them to bring their favorite vegetables and share their experiences as foreigners and new urban agriculture participants. Afterward, they used the oven to prepare a soup as the ultimate heart-warming, healing activity. Speaking of vegetables, spices, and homemade food created a safe space for individual and group identity expression. The women's words led students to propose design changes that would connect and facilitate access for those who needed it most: the fragile, the differently abled, children, and women.

9.3.4   Principle 4: Connecting Urban Agriculture to People's Lives Requires Storytelling

Sustainable change like the ones urban agriculture can affect in our neighborhoods is not an issue of physical interventions. For change to be resilient, it must be embraced and owned by the communities and individuals it will affect. Landscape Architecture uses drawings, models, and prototypes that tell a story about a community's past, present, and future. In uncovering and co-creating these stories, communities develop an attachment to their landscapes and one another. In times of uncertainty, they can motivate and inspire actions, but only if they represent the diversity of experiences and conditions in our society.

Storytelling, that is, the telling, sharing, and listening to narratives, is also a potent participatory activity and can be instrumental in healing and repairing injustices. These narratives require sufficient time and space to emerge, be shared, and fold into a cohesive and collectively embraced story of us (Ganz, 2011). A similar lesson occurred in Baltimore's Plantation Park Heights, where LARC748 students listened as they picked produce and weeded planter boxes. In the process, they connected with the community with a radical empathy that required hearing and acknowledging. In Washington, DC's Temperance Alley, a story circle takes a prominent place in the site layout and its programming. Every event incorporates the sharing of stories and social capital, shared identity and ecological knowledge production. Still, many more storytelling opportunities abound throughout the garden and serve as physical affordances and prompts that invite visitors and residents to connect, share, and learn on a daily basis (Fig. 9.13).

Similarly, the bricks that once covered the alley of an informal shantytown now mark the edge of planting areas and remind us that the only way for our communities to heal from the injustices and racism of the past is to reveal, confront, and act upon them by co-designing a better future.

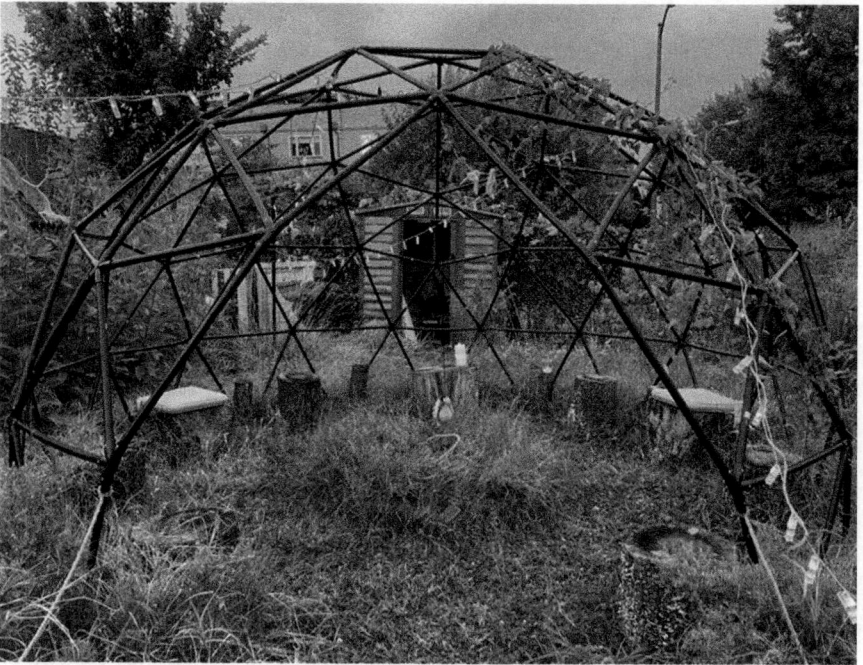

Fig. 9.13 Temperance Alley in Washington, DC, features a story circle. At its center, the community buried the 'founding brick,' an artifact from its past as a slum, and reminder that present and future stories are mindful of past injustices (image by the author)

9.3.5 Principle 5: Urban Agriculture Is Best When it Integrates Form, Function, and Emotions

There is an inherent tension between the work of designers and landscape architects and the realities of urban agriculture. Design is often thought of in artistic terms, positioning the landscape architect as the originator of a concept or idea that seeks to address practical concerns with an overarching vision and inspiration. Urban agriculture is quite the opposite. Its aesthetics often result from functionality and efficiency rather than creative inspiration. The wooden box, a quintessential element in any urban agriculture project worldwide, is the metaphor for a relationship that puts efficiency above the heart when it comes down to it.

In truth, we do not need to choose, as urban agriculture can defy categories and be productive, seductive, transferable, recognizable, practical, and emotional. Norwegian and American students could test new forms and aesthetics of urban agriculture, valuing visual contrast over uniformity and cohesion. In the Continuing Education course, it became clear that the aesthetics of nature and agriculture would be at odds with the aesthetics of the compact city. In the center of Oslo, south of the iconic Opera House, students imagined a biodiverse landscape that, once strengthened, could support fishing, fermenting, and foraging. Not far from it, in the nearby neighborhood of Gamle Oslo, activists imagined new floating gardens for the Vaterlandsparken area along the Akerselva River as a tactical response to the ever-shrinking public space (Fig. 9.14).

9.3.6 Principle 6: Urban Agriculture's Stories of Failure and Uncertainty Are Critical Resources for Adaptation

Urban agriculture sites appear quickly. They can be easy to set up, move, and install elsewhere. Temperance Alley Garden in DC materialized in just six months, despite being years in the minds and ambitions of the U Street neighborhood to regenerate their alleys after the demolition of the informal housing that occupied them in the 1950s and '60s. There is tension in the current urban agriculture between the aim to secure permanently public open spaces in the urban mosaic and a reality of constant change, adaptation, and evolution of many urban agriculture sites. There are also stories of lost urban agriculture, like the South-Central Farm in Los Angeles, evicted in 2006 after 12 years and forced to relocate to other landscapes and other communities, leaving no evidence of its former glory if not for a farmers' market that continues to this day (Fig. 9.15). The CPS project partners learned about lost urban agriculture in the Netherlands, Denmark, and beyond. While no longer active, some of these projects have not stopped producing benefits for their communities. The shared identity and collective capital they generated continue to shape the future cities, offering practical lessons for new urban farmers. They inspire researchers, academics, students, and residents to care and steward their landscapes. If anything,

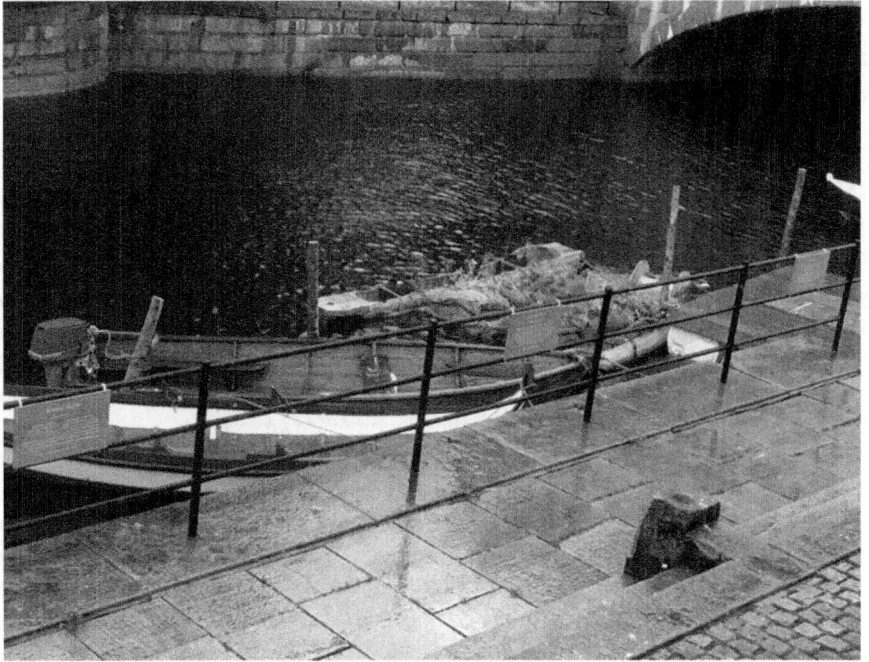

Fig. 9.14 CPS researchers were able to visit and inspired by prototypical urban agriculture installations in Oslo, including the guerrilla urban agriculture site of Gamle Oslo's floating garden, on the Akerselva River (image by the author)

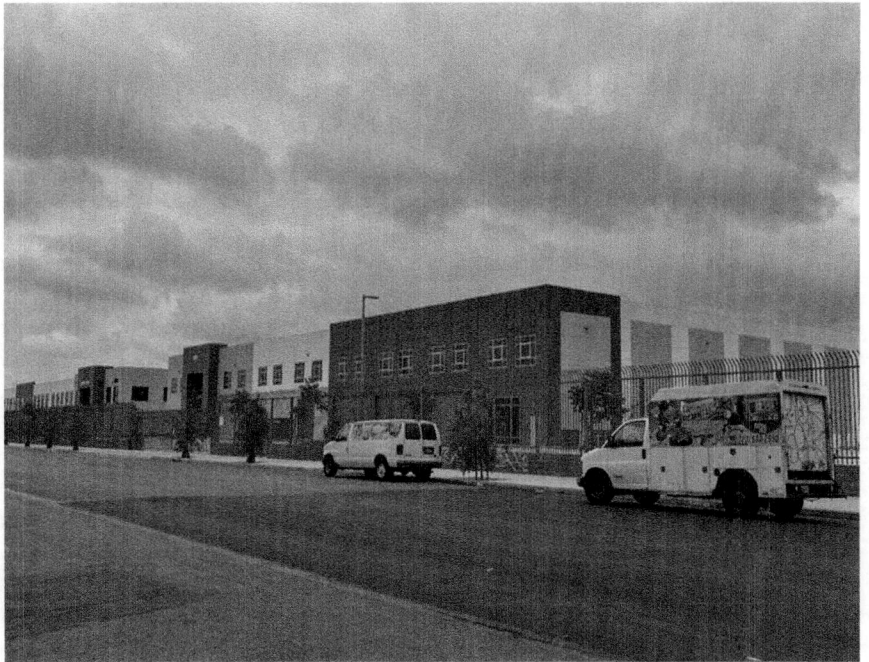

Fig. 9.15 Once a thriving urban agriculture community, Los Angeles' South-Central Farm (1994–2006), the northwest corner of East 41st and South Alameda Street is now occupied by warehouses. While it has moved to other community places, its story lives on (Photo: Deni Ruggeri)

they should motivate us to work harder and envision new policies, plans, and actions to help them sustain communities in the transition toward a new civic practice of urban agriculture.

While seeing images of thriving civic engagement and shared purpose in successful urban agriculture sites is reassuring and comforting, failure may be just around the corner. Yet, this realization should not hold us back. There is no such thing as a failed urban agriculture site. Stories of dismissed or dormant community gardens demonstrate the ecological necessity for the decline and re-organization of our ecosystems to adapt and regenerate (Allen & Holling, 2010).

9.4 Conclusions

The CPS wanted to shed light on the workings of urban agriculture in contemporary development in Norway and develop a unique toolkit of actions that could instigate urban agriculture transformations in urban neighborhoods. We discovered that local success required researching stories and experiences of on-the-ground urban agriculture activists and entrepreneurs worldwide. The project partners folded their research findings recognizing the invaluable role of design and planning students in challenging traditional urban agricultures. Their collaborative efforts aimed to create a systemically performing urban agriculture, where growing food became an opportunity to advance biodiversity, circular economy, energy efficiency, and regenerative management practices.

Undoubtedly, it takes more than a few case studies to derive a theory or universal toolkit for practice. Rather than focusing on explaining and synthesizing improbable standards, CPS researchers and students directed their efforts to listen, observe, and analyze these sites through a human capabilities lens, trying to understand them as engines of systemic, sustainable *local* change. Within the classroom, these reflections became new stories and visions for a future urban agriculture adapted to the uniqueness of a place and able to advance human capabilities for all members of their ecosystems, particularly the most fragile. Through the educational experiences discussed in this chapter, we planted a seed in university students that their classroom work, connected to active communities, could be genuinely transformative and impactful for all involved. Students challenged traditional urban agriculture conceptions in Norway as in the United States, making food growing one of many systemic actions and practices for cultivating a better society.

More case studies are needed; more stories should be documented, reflected upon, and disseminated broadly. I hope others might find something in these stories that will resonate with them.

Bibliography

Abelman, J., Chang, C. Y., Chang, S. E., Hou, J., Hung, S. H., Lai, P. H., & Pryor, M. (2022). Reimagining urban agriculture for sustainable urban futures: Education, health, and urban commons. In *The Routledge handbook of sustainable cities and landscapes in the Pacific Rim* (pp. 155–163). Routledge.

Allen, C. R., & Holling, C. S. (2010). Novelty, adaptive capacity, and resilience. *Ecology and Society, 15*(3), 24.

Alomar, R. (2018). Invisible and visible lines: Landscape democracy and landscape practice. In *Defining landscape democracy* (pp. 96–105). Edward Elgar Publishing.

Beatley, T. (2011). *Biophilic cities: Integrating nature into urban design and planning*. Island Press.

Beatley, T. (2016). The urban nature diet: The many ways that nature enhances urban life. In *Handbook of Biophilic city planning and design* (pp. 33–40). Island Press.

Cady, S. H., Jacobs, R., Koller, R., & Spalding, J. (2014). The change formula. *OD Practitioner, 46*(3), 32–39.

Egoz, S., Jørgensen, K., & Ruggeri, D. (Eds.). (2018). *Defining landscape democracy: A path to spatial justice*. Edward Elgar Publishing.

Ganz, M. (2011). Public narrative, collective action, and power. In *Accountability through public opinion: From inertia to public action* (pp. 273–289). World Bank Publications.

Goldstein, B., Hauschild, M., Fernández, J., & Birkved, M. (2016). Testing the environmental performance of urban agriculture as a food supply in northern climates. *Journal of Cleaner Production, 135*, 984–994.

Hou, J. (2017). Urban community gardens as multimodal social spaces. In *Greening cities* (pp. 113–130). Springer.

Lawson, L. J. (2005). *City bountiful: A century of community gardening in America*. University of California Press.

Lin, B., Meyers, J., & Barnett, G. (2015). Understanding the potential loss and inequities of green space distribution with urban densification. *Urban Forestry & Urban Greening, 14*(4), 952–958.

Louv, R. (2012). *The nature principle: Reconnecting with life in a virtual age*. Algonquin Books.

Lovell, S. T. (2010). Multifunctional urban agriculture for sustainable land use planning in the United States. *Sustainability, 2*(8), 2499–2522.

McDougall, R., Kristiansen, P., & Rader, R. (2019). Small-scale urban agriculture results in high yields but requires judicious management of inputs to achieve sustainability. *Proceedings of the National Academy of Sciences, 116*(1), 129–134.

Murphy, M. A., Parker, P., & Hermus, M. (2022). Cultivating inclusive public space with urban gardens. *Local Environment, 28*, 1–18.

Nussbaum, M. C. (2011). *Creating capabilities: The human development approach*. Harvard University Press.

Palmer, L. (2018). Urban agriculture growth in US cities. *Nature Sustainability, 1*(1), 5–7.

Reynolds, K. (2017). Designing urban agriculture education for social justice: Radical innovation through farm school NYC. *International Journal of Food Design, 2*(1), 45–63.

Rittel, H. W., & Webber, M. M. (1974). Wicked problems. *Man-made Futures, 26*(1), 272–280.

Ruggeri, D. (2018). Storytelling as a catalyst for democratic landscape change in a modernist utopia. In S. Egoz, K. Jørgensen, & D. Ruggeri (Eds.), *Defining landscape democracy* (pp. 128–142). Edward Elgar Publishing.

Tornaghi, C. (2014). Critical geography of urban agriculture. *Progress in Human Geography, 38*(4), 551–567.

UN General Assembly. (2015). *Transforming our world: the 2030 Agenda for Sustainable Development*, 21 October, A/RES/70/1, available at: https://www.refworld.org/docid/57b6e3e44.html. Accessed 13 Jan 2023.

Wadumestrige Dona, C. G., Mohan, G., & Fukushi, K. (2021). Promoting urban agriculture and its opportunities and challenges—A global review. *Sustainability, 13*(17), 9609.

Urban Agriculture Case Studies Mentioned

Losæter, Oslo (Norway).
59.9030981946685, 10.758825533094264
Nabolagshager.
59.90974283842508, 10.765620526212082
Plantation Park Heights, Baltimore, MD.
39.33254211507427, -76.66063079613899
Temperance Alley, Washington, DC
38.91659621262728, -77.02874788146833
Vaterlandsparken, Oslo.
59.91317716077654, 10.75708949457558
Sukkerbiten, Oslo (Norway).
59.90503859637613, 10.753559126219534
Royal Palace Garden, Oslo (Norway).
59.91769803404384, 10.730769977624519
Tullinløkka, Oslo (Norway).
59.916923903897775, 10.73754380076
Vollebekk, Oslo (Norway).
59.93645386098382, 10.828277616977035
South Central Farm, Los Angeles.
34.00811090026115, -118.23949921362394.

Chapter 10
Urban Agriculture and the Right to the City: A Practitioner's Roadmap

Arild Eriksen, Deni Ruggeri, and Esben Slaatrem Titland

10.1 An Increasingly Commercial City

In the contemporary city, municipalities often rent or sublet public space for the benefits of commerce and private profit. Oslo municipality rents street ground and green areas to both commercial and non-commercial organisations. In 2022, during the COVID-19 epidemic, the Oslo Municipality decided to make public space available for free to bring back city life and attract citizens isolating at home to local businesses. The municipality also initiated various tactical urbanism projects, including the temporary closure of streets in the inner-city districts of Grønland and Gamle Oslo, where it installed trees and created temporary hay meadows. For a few summer months, Oslo residents saw how the city's public spaces could be transformed to include cultivation and urban nature. They also observed some of the benefits to commerce in and around these spaces, improved safety perceptions, and streets made more livable by the newly planted small but leafy vegetation.

Today, many municipalities operate both as commercial property developers and managers. Various public enterprises must deliver profits to the municipal coffers, and this means that residents must pay to use the city's public spaces. In Oslo, it is the

It is an Open Access publication, available here (in Norwegian): https://oa.fagbokforlaget.no/index.php/vboa/catalog/book/38.

A. Eriksen (✉)
Partner and general manager, Fragment AS, Oslo, Norway
e-mail: arild@fragmentoslo.no

D. Ruggeri
Department of Plant Science and Landscape Architecture,
University of Maryland, College Park, MD, USA

E. S. Titland
Oslo, Norway

© The Author(s) 2024
B. Sirowy, D. Ruggeri (eds.), *Urban Agriculture in Public Space*, GeoJournal Library 132, https://doi.org/10.1007/978-3-031-41550-0_10

Agency for Urban Environment that rents streets and public spaces. If a district wants to run an urban agricultural initiative or other noncommercial project on public land, it must pay a rent. Securing a reasonable rent is often dependent on finding a municipal worker who is knowledgeable and supportive of community-oriented initiatives.

A recent example of Oslo municipality's support for noncommercial purposes is the 2022 *Selvbyggeren* (Self-builder) art project realized in the district of Økern by the *Kunstnerboligforeningen* (Artists' Housing Association). The project consists of a temporary pavilion, which was realized on a lawn near a local school, on land rented from the municipality on preferential conditions. The pavilion has been functioning as a canteen for local artists and a place for cultural arrangements. The project idea is rooted in the district's historical background as a productive part of the city with industry and manufacturing workshops, which has been gradually erased by private real estate actors. Through joint work, materials, and artistic reflection, the Self Builder has given physical expression to the collective memory of Økern as part of the productive city. It has also inspired a discussion on the right to the city. When urban spaces become a commodity, those who can pay the most will have the first right to define their program and in turn influence both people's imagination and use of urban spaces. Ironically, this results in internal competition between various departments of city government, illustrate by the the Culture Agency in Oslo municipality paying rent to the Urban Environment Agency for the site.

In her 1958 paper "Downtown is for People," North American critic Jane Jacobs criticized modernist urban development and warned of its consequences for the quality and inclusiveness of public space.

> This is a critical time for the future of the city. All over the country civic leaders and planners are preparing a series of redevelopment projects that will set the character of the center of our cities for generations to come. ... What will the projects look like? They will be spacious, park-like, and uncrowded. They will feature long green vistas. They will be stable and symmetrical and orderly. They will be clean, impressive, and monumental. They will have all the attributes of a well kept, dignified cemetery. ... These projects will not revitalize downtown; they will deaden it. For they work at cross-purposes to the city. They banish the street. They banish its function. They banish its variety. (Jacobs, 1958:126)

In today's neo-liberal society, urban development is most often profit-driven, but Jacob's reflections are still valid.

> The remarkable intricacy and liveliness of down- town can never be created by the abstract logic of a few men. Downtown has had the capability of providing something for everybody only because it has been created by everybody. (Jacobs, 1958:130)

Jacobs believed that citizens should be the ultimate experts on urban development and that their involvement and ability to inform the design of cities was necessary to ensure their success in attracting a diversity of users. Her work has inspired today's vision for a sustainable city where people can use public spaces on their own terms, buy locally produced vegetables in public market squares, and participate in city life with a great diversity of other people. In the Modernist city, natural processes were excluded from the urban landscape. Today, we understand that people need access to rich experiences of both wild nature and man-made landscape. They need the scents and colors, a dandelion pushing its way through the asphalt, and the sound of forest birds and pollinators finding their way to the city center from shrub to shrub. To many, this is the main motivation for starting an urban agriculture project. By growing their own food, urban farmers learn that making the city productive requires sweat and tears, and that it is essential to human well-being and happiness. Gradually, they also gain a deeper understanding of climate change and the importance of self-reliance and local economies in counteracting the negative impact of global economics and lifestyles reliant on cheap imports of food, energy, and goods from developing countries.

10.2 From Non-Place to the City's Food Platter

A livable city encompasses a variety of public spaces, from the park of the Royal Palace, a public garden, city's squares, roadside strips, power lines easements, and green spaces along railway tracks. Many of these patches of land have long traditions of agricultural production. During World War II, the park around the Oslo royal palace was used to grow potatoes, and residents and commuters cultivated vegetables on patches of soil along many railway lines.

Today, establishing an urban agriculture project within a well functioning system of productive landscapes must necessarily be supportive of a diversity of users, and it should involve participatory processes. In many places, consideration for other residents (secondary and tertiary users) will require that their design be adapted to the surroundings, which in return will give the urban garden unique character and identity. It will require re-thinking past decisions and choosing radically different ways forward, as governments have done in the past to address changes prompted by global and local events.

In the autumn of 1960, after WWII's rationing policies came to an end, Norway lifted its state-mandated limits to the purchase of passenger cars, starting a rapid increase in the number of registered automobiles. From 1960 to 1964, the car fleet doubled to just over 410,000 cars.[1] Another priority was to create new housing. In many places, it took several decades for municipalities to remedy the post-war housing shortage. At Ammerud, in the Groruddalen district of Oslo, negotiations with landowners began in the late 1940s, but it was not until the mid-1960s that Ammerud was re-zoned as a residential area. Developed as dormitory towns, these new residential districts featured spaces in support of basic human functions, except for workplaces, which were in industrial areas at the bottom of the valleys or in the city center.[2] Public and open spaces were designed functionally, rather than ecologically, and uses were carefully separated. The food system was also designed for efficiency and economic viability.

---

[1] https://www.rablad.no/60-ar-siden-bilrasjoneringen-ble-opphevet/s/5-90-189091

[2] Guttu and Hansen (1998). Fra storskalabygging til frislepp - Beretning om Oslo kommunes boligpolitikk 1960–1989. Byggforsk.

Today, we understand the need for a city to be authentically multifunctional and integrate sites where people can produce most of what they eat locally. Two major challenges exist to advancing this city vision. In urban and peri-urban areas, topsoil has been depleted, and Modernist city district land-use plans lack space for food processing or light industry (see also Chapter 13). This requires the re-zoning of housing districts to include these productive uses, which often finds opposition from politicians or administration.

Several European cities have ambitions to make the city self-sufficient within a few decades. Many cities like Barcelona and Hamburg have joined the Fab City Global Initiative, a network of municipalities working together to help manage production of urban services at the scale of a city's' bioregion, a geographical area defined not by political borders but by ecosystems.[3] Improving urban nature and food production in the city is part of the work needed, but it also requires re-integrating permanent agricultural areas within its limits. It will also become increasingly necessary to regulate coexistence between residents and the urban farming communities. Transportation access, noise, and safety are topics that should be addressed and resolved, and new forms of cohabitation must be explored. How should the urban agriculture transitions take place? What should industry and agriculture look like in the cityscape? Can people in the city help co-create the productive, inclusive city of the future?

10.3   What's Going on in Town: Participation and Form

Temporality is a fundamental premise for urban agriculture in public space and has a visual expression in the familiar planter box, a stackable, replicable building element, easy to assemble, install, and move.

The idea behind temporality has very often been to challenge familiar beliefs about how the city should function and make it possible to imagine other ways of doing things. Today, temporality is often a requirement rather than an opportunity. And many who live in the city are beginning to question the fact that everything that creates joy and a sense of freedom in a city should be temporary. When we participated with the Planning and Building Agency of Oslo's municipality in the preparation of an action plan to increase urban life in the districts of Grønland and Tøyen, inhabitants proved tired of participation and temporary measures and asked instead for investments and lasting improvements. Residents living in disadvantaged communities are frequently targets of extensive participation processes, often without clear consequences for their inclusion. Their engagement often leads to experimental projects and temporary greening installations that fail to motivate their continued involvement and sense of stewardship (see the discussion of our case studies from this area in Chapter 6).

---

[3] https://fab.city/

10.4 Developing an Urban Agriculture Toolbox for Community: The Idea and the Process

When tasked with creating a toolbox for urban agriculture in public space, the authors concluded that toolboxes are worthless if they are merely a collection of objects and solutions, disconnected from the unique physical and sociocultural contexts and practices unfolding within a community. Given the short timeframe of the Cultivating Public Space project, developing a toolbox for agriculture in city squares and parks based on limited knowledge and experiences from pilot projects did not seem to sufficiently acknowledge the diversity of contexts and locations urban agriculture inhabits and grows in. A manual also seemed unhelpful to those who, alone or together with others, are already engaged in urban agriculture and have clear ideas about its aesthetics and performance.

Studying in their investigation of urban agriculture projects both outside and inside of Norway, the authors found copious evidence of the kind of systemic and personal transformations urban agriculture has helped generate, and of the challenges urban farmers face in activating productive landscapes. Over the past few years, the Oslo municipality has become more welcoming and accommodating of urban agriculture, yet public enterprises rarely communicate or join forces to assist urban agriculture growers. Many sites have started as either a leisure activity or a social enterprise, and agreements with the municipality regarding commercial projects on public land do not yet exist. Most recently, a growing awareness of land policy due to climate-neutrality commitments has raised the need for strategic plans to make more public land available for cultivation.

The functional segregation of the modern city does not help local food production. Until now, spatial planning in the compact city has prioritized housing, services, and infrastructural investments for resilience and climate change/emergency preparedness, over food cultivation in public spaces. In Oslo, the redevelopment of the district of Trosterud has been an exception. There, the relocation of an older allotment garden to a new area was a sign that the municipality felt compelled to offer more spaces for urban agriculture and to fulfill its commitment to a more sustainable city. Such initiatives suggest a green shift toward the collective cultivation, harvesting and processing of crops grown in city or peri-urban areas. Today, many urban agriculture projects are either private or run by volunteers in agreement or partnership with the municipality, and the relationship has been managed at the local level, in idiosyncratic ways, but coherently with the community's unique resources and abilities. The authors imagine that in the future, as more people will grow and sell their products locally or outside the cities, uniform guidelines and regulations may be needed to balance public access and private claims.

Many examples of urban agriculture in public space we have encountered during this project have been activism-driven, temporary, self-constructed, and often poorly maintained. Creating a toolbox for agriculture in the city's public space requires considerations of processes, motivations, context, form, and also operation overtime. Understanding a place's sociocultural conditions is crucial, as place identity and people's wishes about the appearance of the physical surroundings will create expectations about the way urban agriculture is designed and how it looks. The wishes and ambitions of neighborhood residents in Ullevål Hageby in Oslo will be very different from those of Grønland Square users, but not necessarily in the way one would expect. Many would think that the residents of Ullevål, a historic Garden City district near the city's largest hospital, would want a conservative design adapted to the buildings, while residents in Grønland might accept a self-built, colorful, and less permanent urban agriculture design. This may well be the opposite.

How can one balance the ownership, commitment, and vision of urban agriculture initiators and society's need for coherence and standardization in the planning, design, and implementation of urban agriculture projects? Both perspectives are important to the future of urban agriculture in the Norwegian city, as in many other places worldwide. We decided to illustrate and share these stories as evidence of the diversity of perspectives values, practices, and visions that underlie the creation of food and community-producing public landscapes in our cities.

We have made our toolbox a graphic novel not only to make it more engaging and accessible for different users but also to give it the colorful and joyful expression of an urban garden. There is no linear guide or a point-by-point form to follow. It's about people and relationships.

Artoonist Esben Slaatrem Titland and the Oslo-based architecture firm Fragment have worked to compile knowledge from Cultivating Public Space research project, reading through and synthesizing findings from literature and interviews of urban farmers in Oslo. Even though as architects we were asked to develop a design manual, or even architectural solutions, it became clear early on that design guidelines and architectural responses might not be a suitable method for facilitating lasting, resilient urban agricultural sites in the diverse neighborhoods of the Norwegian capital.

In 2019, Arild Eriksen and Deni Ruggeri led a continuing education course at NMBU where students helped imagine new cultivation projects in public spaces for four iconic urban areas (see Chapter 9 in this book). The students' urban agriculture in public space should be site-specific and that the formal solutions should also adapt to the sociocultural context of every place. To successfully achieve the goal to grow most of what we consume within the city's bioregional context, urban agriculture must be given a unique and lasting character, tell a rich and compelling story, and be embraced by both municipal agencies and community members, who share the responsibility to steward them.

Conflicts between an urban agriculture project and a neighborhood suggest that it is not just good or bad design that people respond to. For urban farmers, a well established project can appear as a victory and as proof that they can also use the city's public spaces. For others, the project may appear as privatization of public space (see the discussion of publicness of urban agriculture in Chapter 4).

The toolbox (whose excerpts are presented in Figs. 10.1, 10.2, 10.3, 10.4, and 10.5) illustrates both process and form, ideas and ambitions, unique experiences, shared setbacks, and replicable strategies, but it does so in the form of "storied

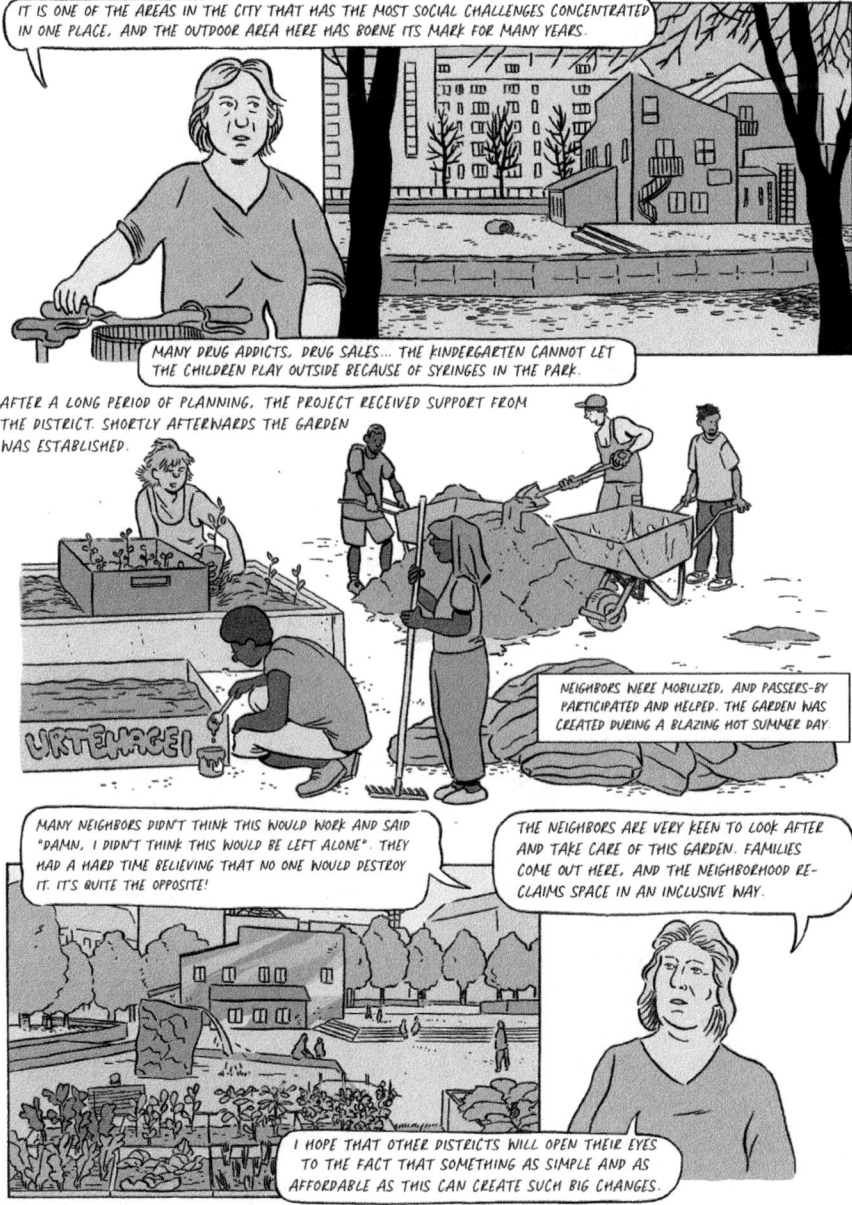

Fig. 10.1 Helene Gallis talks about neighborhood cultivation in public spaces at Grønland, Oslo Page from the cartoon Byens Bønder by Fragment and Esben S. Titland. Fagbokforlaget 2023 (p. 43) [A comment for the publisher: *please use the translated high-resolution versions of all illustrations delivered in a separate folder*]

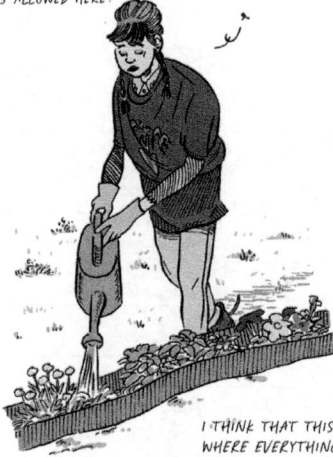

THE TEENAGERS TALK ABOUT THE PRESSURE THEY EX-PERIENCE IN THE "ACHIEVEMENT SOCIETY". TRIAL AND ERROR IS ALLOWED HERE.

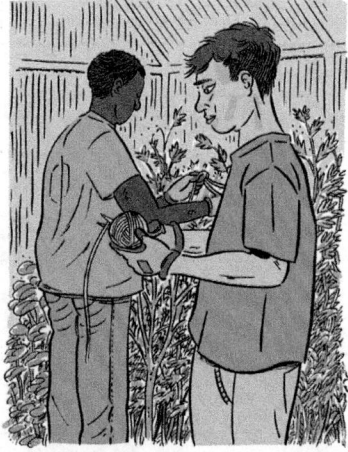

I THINK THAT THIS IS A NICE COUNTERBALANCE TO THE STRESS AT SCHOOL, WHERE EVERYTHING IS ABOUT WHAT HAPPENS THIS MONTH, OR THAT THE EXAM COMES AT THE END OF THE SCHOOL YEAR.

BECAUSE THINGS GO A LITTLE SLOWER HERE. WE PLANT TREES THAT WILL BE BEAUTIFUL IN 20 OR 200 YEARS. IT STARTS A CONVERSATION, AND WE ALLOW OURSELVES TO BE A LITTLE POMPOUS.

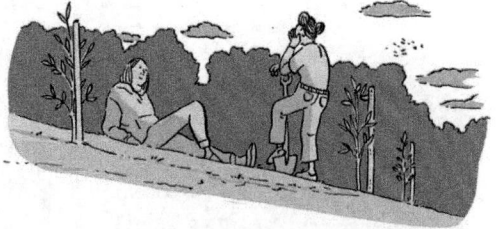

WE HAVE A LOT TO DO BEFORE WE MANAGE TO TAKE OWNERSHIP OF THE PUBLIC URBAN SPACE.

BUT ORDINARY PEOPLE CAN HELP SHAPE THE CITY, AND THE YOUNG PEOPLE EXPERIENCE EXACTLY THAT.

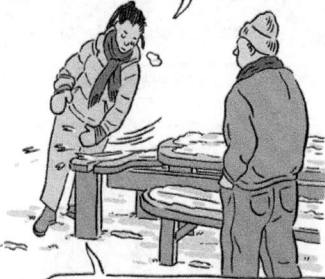

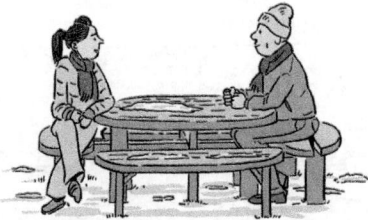

WHEN WE LIVE IN A CITY, WE ARE SO USED TO EVERYTHING BEING REGULATED.

DESPITE THE COMMUNITY THAT ENTHUSIASTS LIKE FROYDIS HELP CREATE, A LACK OF COLLEGIAL DRIVE CAN MAKE THE JOB A LITTLE LONELY AT TIMES. SHE TELLS OF A LOT OF GOODWILL AND ENTHUSIASM FROM THE MUNICIPALITY, BUT FEW EMPLOYEES AND UNCERTAIN FUNDING MAKE THE PROJECT VULNERABLE.

Fig. 10.2 "Because things go a little slower here." Urban agriculture with young people in Oslo's suburbs
Page from the cartoon Byens Bønder by Fragment and Esben S. Titland. Fagbokforlaget 2023 (p. 45)

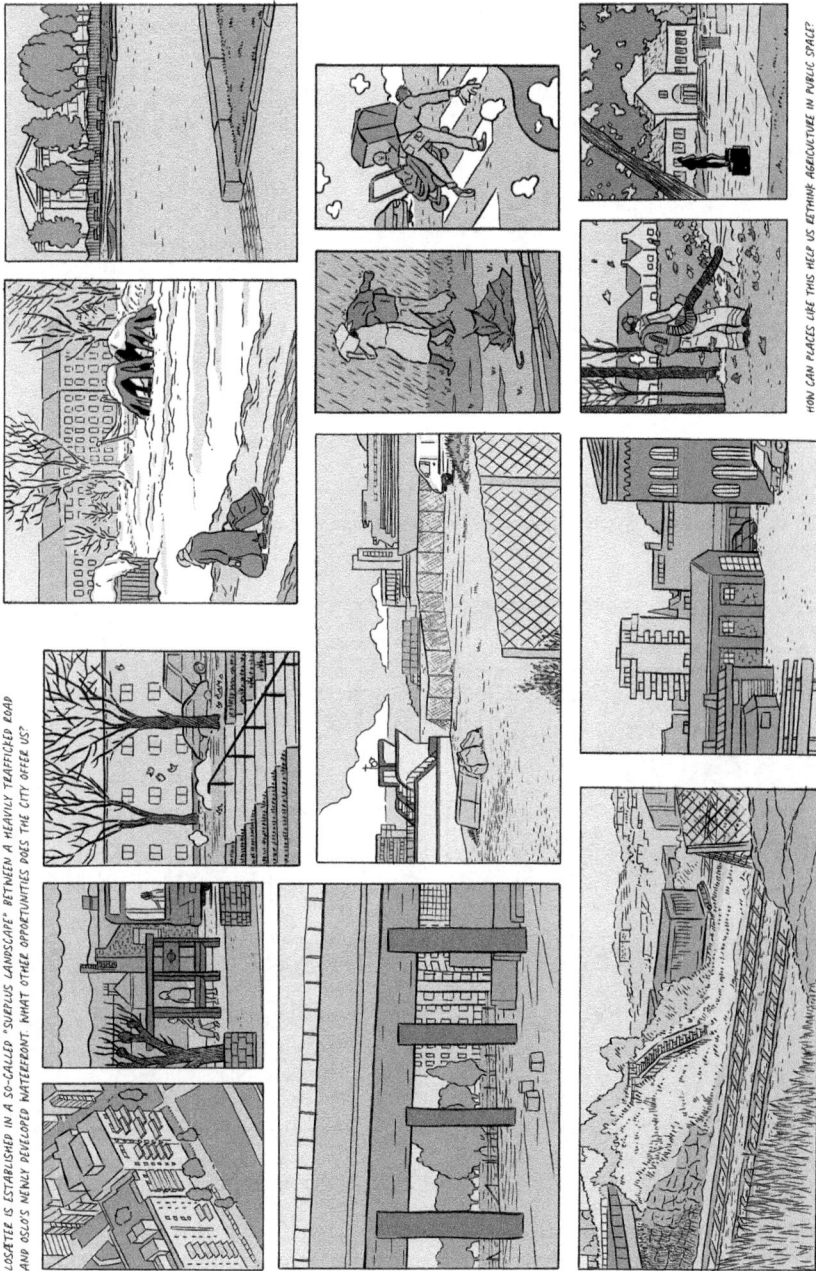

Fig. 10.3 The city has many public spaces that you don't immediately think could be used for the purposes of urban agriculture Page from the cartoon Byens Bønder by Fragment and Esben S. Titland. Fagbokforlaget 2023. (p. 30)

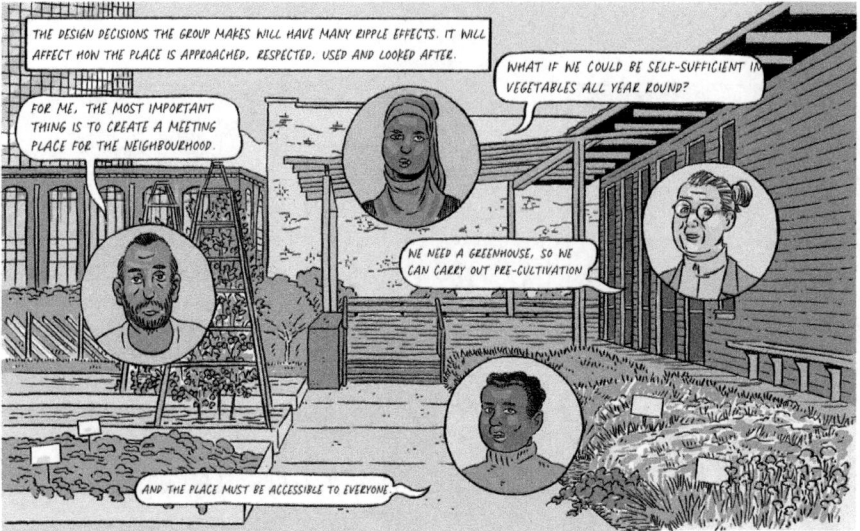

Fig. 10.4 Decisions have consequences
Page from the cartoon Byens Bønder by Fragment and Esben S. Titland. Fagbokforlaget 2023 (p. 66)

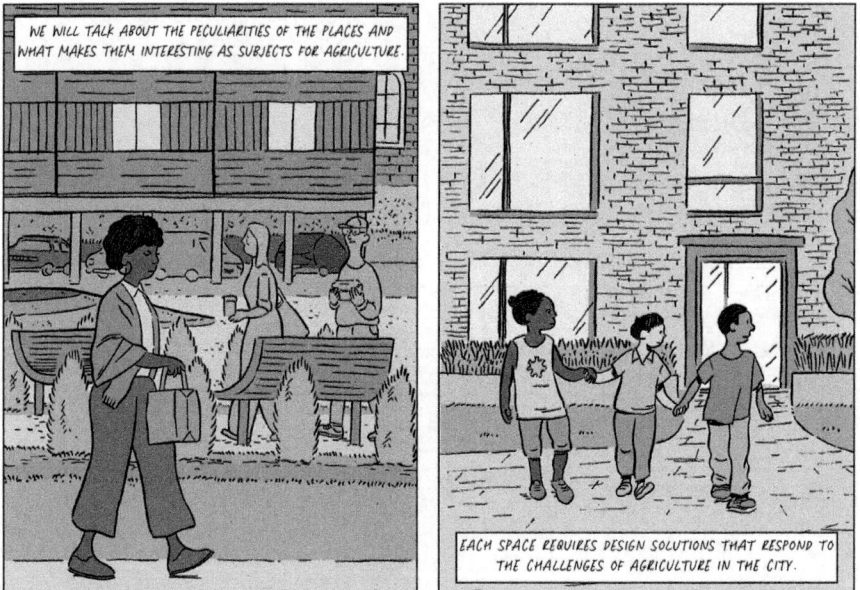

Fig. 10.5 Different places require different solutions
Page from the cartoon Byens Bønder by Fragment and Esben S. Titland. Fagbokforlaget 2023 (p. 35)

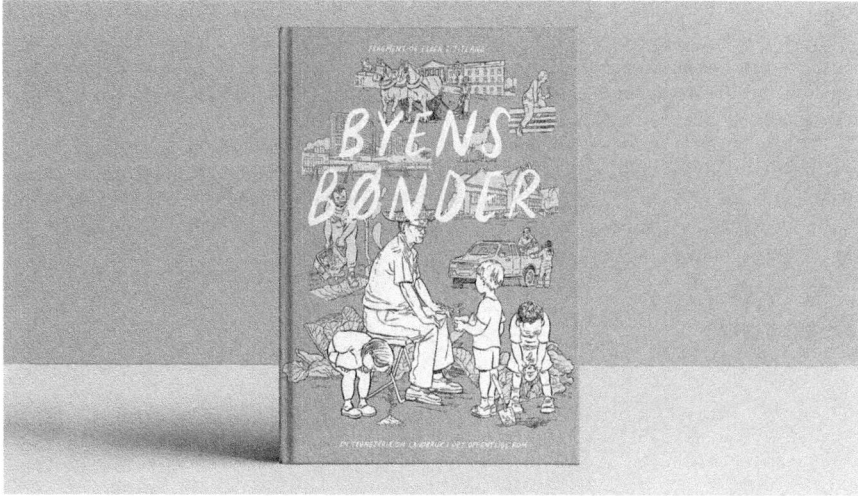

Fig. 10.6 The cover of the published book. (Photo: Fragment)

knowledge"[4] rather than abstraction. These stories have the power to move and motivate people to get involved, something that planning and strategic documents do not.

The toolbox is entitled "Byens Bønder" ("City's Farmers") and was published open access with Fagbokforlaget in May 2023. It is available in the Norwegian version here: https://oa.fagbokforlaget.no/index.php/vboa/catalog/book/38 (Fig. 10.6).

References

Guttu, J., & Hansen, T. (1998). *Fra storskalabygging til frislepp – Beretning om Oslo kommunes boligpolitikk 1960–1989*. Byggforsk.
Handlingsprogram for økt byliv på Grønland og Tøyen. 2021–2027. (2021). *Plan-og bygningse-taten Oslo kommune*.
Jacobs, J. (1958). Downtown is for people. *The exploding metropolis, 168*, 124–131.
Kreiswirth, M. (2000). Merely telling stories? Narrative and knowledge in the human sciences. *Poetics today, 21*(2), 293–318.
Planprogram med veiledende plan for offentlig rom for Trosterud og Haugerud. (2019). *Eiendom-og byfornyelsesetaten Oslo kommune*. p. 58–61.

---

[4] Kreiswirth, M. (2000). Merely telling stories? Narrative and knowledge in the human sciences. Poetics today, 21(2), 293–318.

Part IV
Planning for Urban Agriculture in Norway

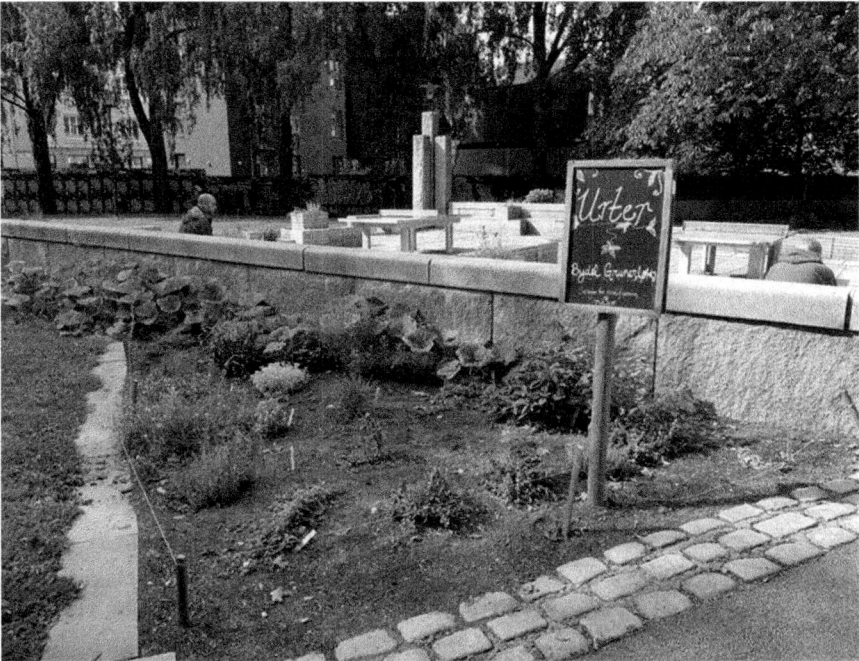

Chapter 11
Motivations for Urban Agriculture Policies: Evidence from Norway's Largest Urban Areas

Inger-Lise Saglie

11.1 Introduction

Urban agriculture has become increasingly popular among citizens in many Norwegian urban areas, and a number of initiatives have been taken by local dwellers, see Chapters 6 and 7. Politicians and public authorities have also become interested in urban agriculture. The aim of this chapter is to describe the emergence of public policies and planning for urban agriculture with a focus on the motivations behind these. Why do Norwegian public authorities develop policies for urban agriculture? Norway is an interesting case, as an example of the Nordic welfare state, and the role urban agriculture can play in this context. The empirical focus is on the three largest cities in Norway, as they are among the earliest examples of public policies for urban agriculture.

More specifically the chapter discusses the institutionalization of public policies for urban agriculture in the three cities. It describes the actors involved, their patterns of cooperation and influence, and the formal and informal rules, measures, and plans they follow.

11.2 Background

From its start, urban agriculture has been based on citizens' initiatives and activities (Buijs et al., 2019; Certomà & Tornaghi, 2015; McClintock, 2014). However, in later years, urban agriculture has also emerged as a domain of public policy. Some Norwegian cities have developed strategic plans for urban agriculture, and the national

I.-L. Saglie (✉)
Department of Urban and Regional Planning, Faculty of Lanscape and Society, Norwegian
University of Life Sciences, Ås, Norway
e-mail: inger-lise.saglie@nmbu.no

© The Author(s) 2024
B. Sirowy, D. Ruggeri (eds.), *Urban Agriculture in Public Space*, GeoJournal
Library 132, https://doi.org/10.1007/978-3-031-41550-0_11

level government has adopted a strategic plan for urban agriculture (Norwegian Ministries, 2021). Given how deeply grounded urban agriculture is in citizens' bottom-up activities, the idea of developing a public planning and policy for urban agriculture may seem counter productive. This chapter seeks to uncover the motivations for public authorities to support urban agriculture and the role of citizen activism in this.

Urban agriculture is a complex phenomenon and most often is driven by several motivations. This is also the case for urban agriculture as a public policy domain. Urban agriculture was early associated with an alternative, transformative, and radical activism (McClintock, 2014; Buijs et al., 2019). It was viewed as a means to increase food justice and secure nutritious, affordable food to people in need. It has also sought to provide an alternative to the dominant food systems through its support of small-scale farming and alternative food supplies systems (Simon-Rojo et al., 2018). Another radical stream has been connected to activism and public space reappropriation to secure the "right to the city," giving everyone access to and actual influence over the cities' public spaces (Certomà & Tornaghi, 2015), Rosol, 2010). Thus, urban agriculture has been closely associated with citizen activism and voluntary work based on local bottom-up initiatives. Rosol (2010) points out that while in the 1980s citizen groups had to "fight for their right to influence green public spaces" (p. 557), such initiatives are now encouraged and supported by politicians and administration, as we will show in this chapter.

However, urban agriculture has also been problematized as being co-opted and in fact serving neo-liberalization interests when stepping in when social security nets have been rolled back (McClintock, 2014). In case studies from Berlin, the acceptance of urban agriculture in public space can partly be explained by limited public funds for the upkeep and management of the urban landscape (Rosol, 2010). Urban agriculture has also been placed within neo-liberal traits in urban development and labelled as a "controlled space" (Brody & de Wilde, 2020 p. 243) and as being both neoliberal and radical (McClintock, 2014; Brody & de Wilde, 2020). On the other hand, a number of studies have tried to uncover the general benefits of urban agriculture, its contributions to integration (Christensen et al., 2019), and its possibility to offer companionship and build community (Firth et al., 2011) and provide locally available food (Simon-Rojo et al., 2018). Such benefits may form the background for the development of public policy.

The emerging policy realm of urban agriculture has been less studied than the actual growing initiatives. However, some studies exist. These underline the importance of local governments and planning authorities' efforts to *integrate* urban agriculture into planning and to *enable* urban agriculture through appropriate regulatory measures (Thibert, 2012). Others have pointed at the importance of combining the top-down urban green space management with citizen activism (Buijs et al., 2019). The nature and quality of the cooperation between local authorities and the citizen's initiatives have implications on the performance of urban agriculture projects. The more the nonprofit organization is included the higher the performance of the collaborative network (Uster et al., 2019).

This chapter contributes to this growing body of literature through an in-depth analysis of urban agriculture policies and plans. We focused on three Norwegian examples: Oslo, Bergen, and Trondheim. It has been noted that urban agriculture including its motivations as well as effect needs to be understood within its specific socioeconomic context (van der Jagt et al., 2017; Rosol, 2010). This is the case also for the motivation of public planning and facilitation of urban agriculture. The empirical emphasis here is within a Nordic context, with a strong welfare state.

We ask: *What are the motivations for developing municipal public policy for urban agriculture in Oslo, Bergen, and Trondheim?*

The focus of this text is on the municipality level, but the empirical investigation will show that all three cities have worked in strong cooperation and networks with the agricultural department of their respective county governors. Municipalities in Norway are responsible for delivering a range of public welfare services, including kindergartens, primary schools, health, integration and social security, and management of green spaces. The county governor is the state representative in the county, ensuring implementation of national policies at a local level. In this case, it has been the department for agriculture of the county governor's that has been involved. The networking between dedicated individuals in these departments across the country has been highly instrumental to the development of public policy for urban agriculture in all three cities, and their motivation for doing so will be addressed further in this text.

11.3   Theoretical Approaches: Policy Programs and Discourses as Motivations for Public Policy

Public policies for urban agriculture can have many different motivations. The motivations are being anchored in particular policy programs and discourses, being one of the four dimensions influencing policy domain (Arts et al., 2006). The other dimensions are the actors and their coalitions, power, and influence over the policy domain. In this chapter, we will investigate the first dimension, the rationale, or the discourses behind interest in urban agriculture as a public policy domain. The other dimensions are discussed in the following chapter.

Policy programs and discourses refer to the views and narratives of the actors influencing a policy domain. Discourses can be understood as an institutionally founded ways to think and communicate (Arts et al., 2006).

On a general level, the municipalities's motivations to support urban agriculture are much the same as growers' motivations. Frequently mentioned is food, and food production, as well as social side of communal growing. Municipalities may also have other motivations, such as knowledge building and social inclusion. The public interest in urban agriculture may also differ from sector to sector depending on their area of responsibility, for example, educational departments are foremost interested in education while social services departments focus on integration or public health.

11.4 Methods

In this chapter, interviews and content analysis of planning documents are the primary methods for an investigation of public policies and planning in Oslo, Bergen, and Trondheim, which are three largest Norwegian cities (Fig. 11.1). In 2019–2020, the researchers interviewed 18 people including municipal urban agriculture coordinators, employees of the county governor, individuals engaged in voluntary movement, repre-semtants of farmers associations, social entrepreneurs, and a developer. The municipal contact persons for urban agriculture in all three cities were the first to be interviewed. The following interviewees have been selected through snowballing method, where the interviewees have suggested further persons to contact. Since urban agriculture policies have been in a continous development over the last years, we conducted fol-low-up interviews in 2021 with the urban agriculture coordinators in the municipalities. Due to Covid-19, two out of three interviews were conducted online, recorded and transcribed.

Interviewees also provided us with documents they considered as critical to a better understanding of the policy linkages of urban agriculture. In Oslo, this included the social element of the municipal master plan, the municipal strategy for urban agriculture, and the strategy for green roofs. In Bergen, this included the municipal strategy for urban agriculture and, in Trondheim, the hearing document for the municipal plan for agriculture. These documents have been analyzed qualitatively, but the strategic plans in Oslo and Bergen have also been analyzed quantitively (Bratberg, 2020). The quantitative analyses show the frequency of mention of concepts within documents. The concepts have been chosen based on a literature review on the multidimensional benefits of urban agriculture. This included the emphasis put on food and food production, social issues, urban development, voluntary activity, social entrepreneurship, and relation to peri-urban agriculture. The researchers also used an "in vivo" model to extract key words and phrases from interviews and the documents as codes, such as innovation and commercial urban growing (Saldaña, 2015).

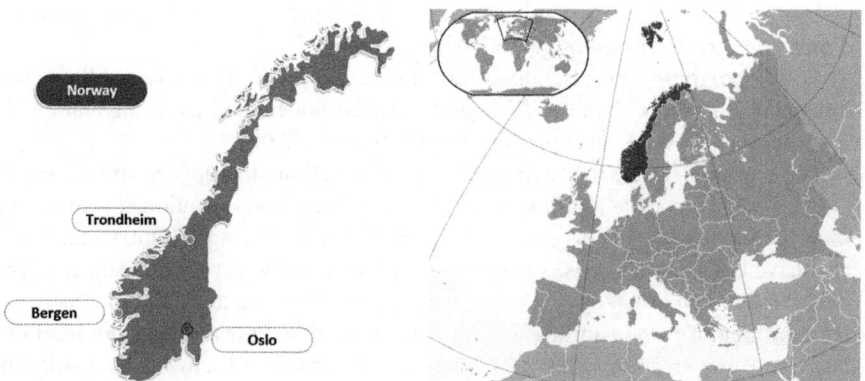

Fig. 11.1 The location of the discussed municipalities of Oslo, Bergen, and Trondheim, in Norway (Source: Wikimedia Commons. The picture is licensed under the Creative Commons Attribution-Share Alike 3.0 Unported license)

11.5   Empirical Studies: Motivations for Public Policy

11.5.1   County Governors

Across Norway, employees in the county governor's departments for agriculture observed the early grassroot initiatives within urban agriculture, and in 2009, they formed a network based on their interest these activities but also on their potential for the wider agricultural sector (Forsberg et al., 2019).

In the beginning, it was not explicitly expressed in their mandate to address urban agriculture, but in some counties, there was an interest in the possibilities it offered. In the network they formed, they worked with this policy field in different ways and with different starting points (Forsberg et al., 2019).

The background for this interest was the production of ecological, local food often on the intersection between peri-urban professional agriculture and the evolving interest in food growing among the urban population. They watched what was happening on a grassroot level and observed the emergence of multiple bottom up urban agriculture projects. For these early initiators of public policy, the reasons for supporting urban agriculture were as follows: urban agriculture could support the reputation of professional agriculture and then indirectly also support the protection of farmland. In addition, the general interest in food production could increase the recruitment of future farmers, an issue of concern within the agricultural sector. In this way, urban agriculture could support traditional agriculture. These arguments need to be understood within the Norwegian agricultural production context. At the national level, only 3% of the land is arable with a topography and a cold climate making agriculture "difficult" and costly and requiring substantial public subsidies. Continued public support for agricultural subsidies is important to the sector. Food security and civil protection are also important, as Norway is dependent on agricultural import. During crisis, lately under WW II, urban agriculture was a necessity, and every possible green space—gardens and parks—and unused land were used for agricultural purposes. So, one of the the arguments was that knowledge about growing would also be important in a civil protection perspective (Forsberg et.al 2019). In addition to these aspects, an argument for engaging in urban agriculture was connected to its benefits to *urban development*, such as enhancing attractiveness and biodiversity of green urban spaces and parks; and having positive impacts on climate change adaptation. Another important argument was related to *health and social effects* of urban agriculture, such as the facilitation of physical activity, creation of social meeting places, and social integration. Arguments related to *economy* emphasized aspects such as the innovation potential of urban agriculture, value creation, and social entrepreneurship (Forsberg et al., 2019).

11.6   The Cases: Urban Agriculture in Three of Norway's Largest Urban Areas

The three cities vary with respect to size and are situated in very different regional contexts and relation to agriculture and food production (Table 11.1).

11.6.1   Oslo

The Social Element of the Municipal Master Plan: "Municipal Societal Plan"—Motivations

Oslo is the only city among the three examined ones that mentions urban agriculture explicitly in the social element of the municipal master plan, further referred to as "the municipal societal plan." The municipal societal plan is a formal high-level strategic planning document that sets out the city's main priorities. For the period 2018–2040, mentions of urban agriculture suggest a clear political signal that urban agriculture is something the city wants to develop. The definition used in the plan is as follows:

> Urban agriculture is animal husbandry and food production in the city—for example, in allotment gardens, private gardens, green lungs, backyards, and window sills, at visiting farms and on roofs. Often, social relations and meeting places, education, health, integration, entrepreneurship, food culture, biological diversity, and protection of farmland and green areas are more important than food production (Oslo municipality, 2019a p. 82).

Table 11.1 Some characteristics of the three cities

	Oslo	Bergen	Trondheim
Inhabitants approx	Approx. 710,000	Approx. 290,000	Approx. 210,000
Landscape	Situated in eastern Norway. Within its borders, there are large woodlands but very limited agricultural land. The areas around the Oslo fjord are well suited to agriculture climatically and also with areas with arable soil. But these areas are not within the borders of Oslo municipality	Mountainous landscape situated at the west coast of Norway. Limited farmland within its border 100–120 active farms	Situated in in mid-Norway one of the primary agricultural regions in Norway, with good farmland also within the municipal borders and 218 active farms
Farmland within municipal borders	2,1%	6,5%	17%

This citation presents a wide spectrum of motivations, and it also states that these may be more important than food production. Urban agriculture can be *a means* to achieve something else, such as health, integration, meeting places, etc. This is also evident in the societal plan, where food and food production are hardly mentioned.

However, urban agriculture and circular resource management are an important part of the discussion on the "green city" (Oslo municipality, 2019a p. 18). In addition, urban agriculture is an important part of the development of "green meeting places," which are "free and can offer peace and stillness are made on the inhabitants' premises and adapted to the values of the local community" (Oslo municipality, 2019a p. 21). So, even if urban agriculture is at its core about cultivation, food production does not appear to be a central argument in the policy. Still urban agriculture is a central part of the development of "the green city" together with many other means to reach environmental goals and to create green meeting places.

At the time of writing this chapter, the formal municipal land-use plan has not been updated, so the effects of the stated interest in urban agriculture on land-use are not yet clear. However, Oslo has developed a separate strategy for urban agriculture and a guide for developers concerning the use of green roofs, addressing the potential for urban agriculture to be housed on rooftops.

Strategic Plan for Urban Agriculture: Motivations

The city councilor commissioned the Agency for Urban Development to produce a strategy for urban agriculture, adopted politically in 2019, emtitled. "Sprouting Oslo – Room for everyone in the city's green spaces. A Strategy for urban Agriculture 2019-2030" (Fig. 11.2).

The strategy follows up on the ideas embedded in the municipal societal plan, with emphasis on the green city and the social aspects of urban agriculture. The first goal in the strategy is *"a greener city"* (Oslo municipality, 2019b p.4). The document acknowledges that there is competition over space and land availability for urban agriculture may be a challenge. However, the general need for green space, including finding green space for growing, is underlined. The second main goal is *"short traveled food"* (p. 9) where urban food production can contribute to national self-sufficiency. Also, commercial urban agriculture is mentioned, that is, hydroponics and possibilities for larger-scale production in connection to professional agriculture. The third goal, *"sprouting meeting places"* (p. 13), underlines the social aspects and the positive effects of urban agriculture for public health. The fourth goal underlines *"green arenas for learning"* (p. 17) in schools and kindergartens, The fifyh goal a *"co-operating knowledge city"* (p. 21), underlines the potentials for urban agriculture related innovations and new technologies for commercial growing, it also points out the objective to maintain and further develop cooperation with entrepreneurs and research institutions.

Oslo

Sprouting Oslo
- Room for everyone in the city's green spaces
A Strategy for Urban Agriculture 2019–2030

Adopted by the City Council in Oslo 13.11.2019
(Proposition 336/19)

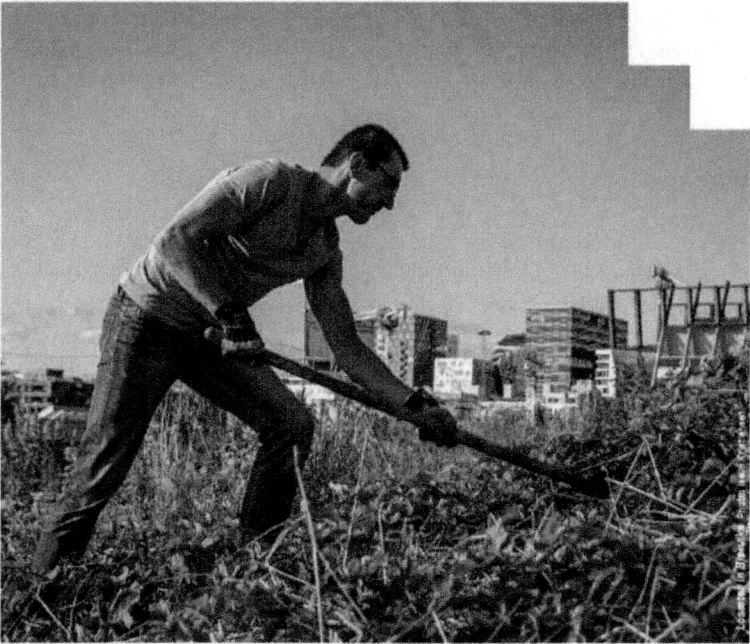

Fig. 11.2 Front page of Oslo's strategic plan for Urban Agriculture. The picture shows Losæter- a center for urban agriculture in Oslo (Source: https://www.oslo.kommune.no/getfile.php/13398183-1614956203/Tjenester%20og%20tilbud/Natur%2C%20kultur%20og%20fritid/Urbant%20land-bruk/BYM_SpirendeOslo_engelsk_A4_digital.pdf)

Green Roofs

The strategy for green roofs in Oslo recently developed by the city's planning and building department (2022) is meant as guidance for developers when proposing new development. The document underlines four functions for green roofs: nature, water, energy, and health (Oslo municipality, 2022). It further elaborates on how green roofs are important for climate change adaptation by retaining water and increasing urban biodiversity, also pointing out that they are areas for renewable energy production, and offer potential spaces for recreation, mostly private but also public. This multiplicity of goals for green roofs reflects the competition for space in cities. Urban agriculture is mentioned as a part of the strategy but plays no big role in it.

11.6.2 Bergen

"Cultivate Bergen-Strategic Plan 2019–2023": Ideas and Motivations for Urban Agriculture

The division for agriculture in Bergen municipality initiated the preparation of this strategic plan (Fig. 11.3). They previously administered a financing scheme for urban agriculture and they saw the need for more explicit political signals for the use of these means (Interview 9). Based on this, they suggested a strategic plan, which was approved politically. The division for agriculture developed the plan in close collaboration with growers, the division of agriculture in the county governor's administration, and farmers' associations. The process involved two well-attended public workshops for interested individuals and organizations (Bergen municipality, 2019). The plan was well received by the politicians and accepted without any changes in the text (Interview 9).

Urban agriculture in Bergen is firmly grounded *within an urban development discourse*. The city council wants Bergen to be "the greenest city in the country" as expressed in their political platform (Bergen municipality, 2019 p. 3). Urban agriculture is among several means to make the city "greener" and more "beautiful." Urban agriculture is also a future-oriented means for reaching goals in climate and environment (ibid.s 3) and an important means to plan for the future smart city and to enable a climate-smart society. The city council's vision is that Bergen shall be an active and attractive city enabling an environmentally friendly lifestyle (ibid. p. 3). The strategy connects urban agriculture to the UN sustainable goals (ibid. p. 5). The vision is:

> *Bergen is a sustainable city that shall be the greenest city in the country through enabling its citizens to cultivate their own food and to increase their knowledge about food production from soil to table.* (Bergen municipality, 2019 *p. 7*)

Fig. 11.3 Front page of
the strategic plan for urban
agriculture in Bergen.
"Dyrk Bergen" (Cultivate
Bergen). (Source: https://
www.bergen.kommune.no/
politikere-utvalg/api/fil/
bk360/4816303/
Dyrk-Bergen-Strategi-for-
urbant-landbruk)

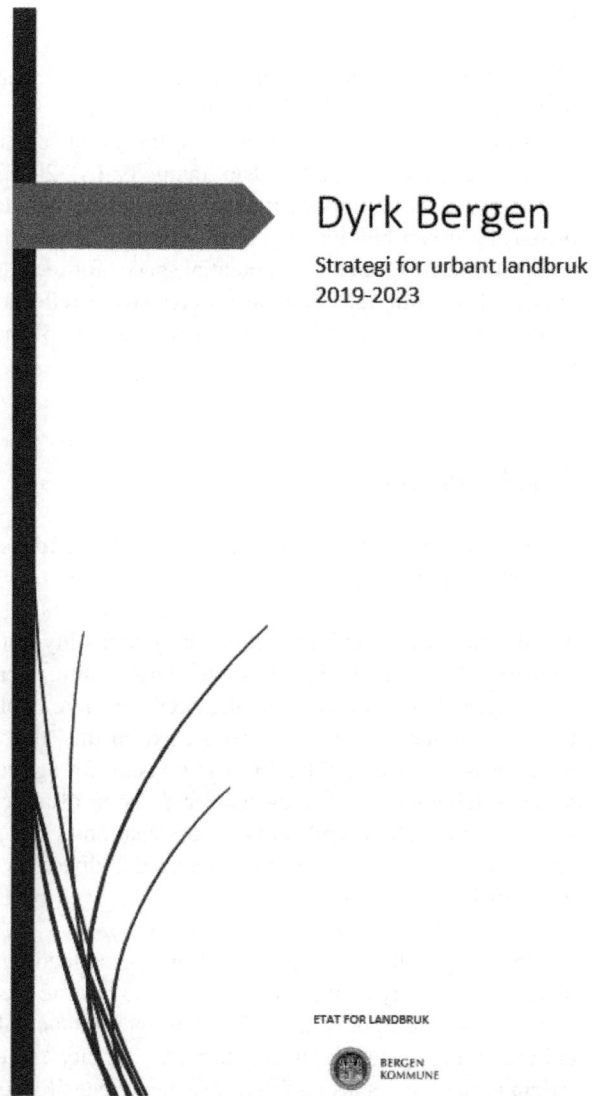

Dyrk Bergen

Strategi for urbant landbruk
2019-2023

ETAT FOR LANDBRUK

BERGEN
KOMMUNE

When moving to more concrete goals for urban agriculture, food and social aspects
become most prominent. The first main goal is that Bergen will protect agricultural
land and improve food distribution systems and also biodiversity (ibid. p. 7). The
subgoals include urban agriculture in parks and public spaces, allotments, pollinators friendly and edible plants in municipal green space management, protecting
farmland, and establishing communal gardening in cooperation with professional
agriculture. The second goal is to create social meeting places across different
groups of the population with a number of subgoals (p. 8).

Urban agriculture is also described as a means in welfare provision, thus *a means to reach internal goals for other departments* in the municipality. The strategy mentions inclusion and language training, institutions dealing within care and social sector, and refers to the goal of improving life conditions in areas with low score on socioeconomic factors.

In addition to the need for political signals, the motivation for the strategy is also *to organize further work.* This includes *"the need to work across the various sectors and departments within the municipality itself, but also to map out how to work with external partners"* (p. 6). It is also acknowledged that cooperation with growers is essential to implement the prioritized actions.

11.6.3   Trondheim

Steering Logic and Choice of Planning Instruments: Networking and Co-Production

The municipality of Trondheim has not adopted a strategy for urban agriculture but has included urban agriculture in their plans and policies for agriculture in general. The interviews we conducted provide insights into the motivations for doing so. Lack of strategic plans has not hindered urban agriculture becoming popular, with a number of initiatives. The steering logic applied by the city is networking and co-production of policies. The main point for Trondheim municipality has been to ask the inhabitants for directions for development of policies and practice in supporting urban agriculture initiatives.

> *Don't think about what the municipality needs, but rather what the inhabitants want. This is not a question of «participation» which in practice is only a meeting. The inhabitants should give directions to policy and practice. The important thing is to elucidate what the inhabitants want, not what is best for the municipality. This strategy has worked very well for us* (Interview 10).

Indirectly there are some underlying goals. Urban agriculture has in its start been connected to inner-city urban space development. However, the experiences are that this has not been the direction urban agriculture has taken. There are hardly any initiatives in inner-city locations in Trondheim. On the contrary, the experience is that people want to grow where they live, in more suburban or indeed peri-urban locations (Interview 10). This also shows in the distribution of support for the financing scheme, where housing cooperatives, housing co-ownership, or neighborhood associations are the main receiver of grants.[1]

---

[1] The receivers of financial support may not be representative of the whole population of initiatives in Trondheim. However, there are good reasons to believe they are fairly representative. The administration work in close relationship with growers and have a good overview of the local situations, and according to them, the figures are representative.

Planning Program for Agriculture

Trondheim is about to develop a thematic municipal plan for agriculture, for the next ten years. The aim is to describe goals and strategies for municipal agricultural policy and the steps to be taken. However, the first step required by the planning law is to make a "planning program" setting out the main purpose of the plan. This "planning program" is meant for public scrutiny, to solicit peoples' views on important elements that should be incorporated in the plan, as well as views on the planning processes. The thematic municipal plan targets ordinary, professional nonurban agriculture. However, it includes urban agriculture under the theme of *Education, communication, and knowledge sharing*. Interestingly, in this "plan-before-the-plan" document, urban agriculture is closely linked to citizen involvement, "co-producing" the city, traditional agriculture and "the green city."

The document states the following goal: *"The co-produced city: to investigate further how to make agriculture more visible through urban agriculture and make Trondheim visible as the green city"* (Trondheim municipality, 2020 p. 9).

Trondheim municipality wants to stimulate cooperation between traditional and urban agriculture for knowledge sharing, promoting, and improving the standing of agriculture. Furthermore, the municipal actors acknowledges that urban agriculture secures social meeting places and spaces for citizen activism. The city has set in motion an initiative called Trondheim 3.0, with the aim to enhance citizen involvement, and urban agriculture is set into this discourse, as seen in the following citation.

> The city council wants an increased citizen involvement. This necessitates new meeting places where allotment and community gardens, natural meeting places and low threshold activities are vital to stimulate the activity in the local community (Trondheim municipality, 2020 p. 9).

The document also calls for the establishment of low-threshold meeting places to enhance interaction and activities between people in the local community. There is also a clear intention to *develop the urban populations' ties with ordinary agriculture.* This could be facilitated through an involvement of urban population in growing initiatives on farms (cooperative farming) or by stimulation of new forms of professional "urbanized" growing (market gardens), which are intensive gardens in or near urbanized areas with the main purpose to sell produce to the city's population.[2]

---

[2] The following is a definition from the EU Innovation Partnership:

"Market gardening" concept "is based on the efficient use of small areas of land using manual labour and simply mechanised equipment. It aims at achieving high yields per hectare and market a wide variety of high-quality vegetables directly. ... Market gardening is about revisiting traditional methods of agricultural production, improving them thanks to recent research results and the sharing of current practical knowledge. It has a focus on the environment, farmers' well-being and income" (The agricultural European Innovation Partnership (EIP-AGRI). https://ec.europa.eu/eip/agriculture/en/news/inspirational-ideas-market-gardening)

The municipality wants small scale production and distribution to develop and identify measures available. (Trondheim municipality, 2020 p. 9).

Availability of land is also an element in the plan program, *with the objective to identify possible areas for cooperative farming and market gardens.* (Trondheim municipality, 2020 p. 9)

11.7   Quantitative Analysis of the Strategic Plans of Agriculture in Oslo and Bergen

We conducted a quantitative assessment of the strategic planning documents where we measured the frequency of appearing of selected concepts. These were chosen from state-of-the-art literature on the multidimensional character of urban agriculture. The analysis revealed an emphasis put on food and food production, social issues, urban development, voluntary activity, social entrepreneurship, innovation and commercial urban growing, and relation to peri-urban agriculture (Table 11.2). However, the content analyses and the interviews clearly indicated that urban agriculture is also considered as a means for achieving goals in other municipal sectors, including education, health, integration, and work training.

Table 11.2 Quantitative analysis of frequency of themes in the planning documents in Oslo and Bergen

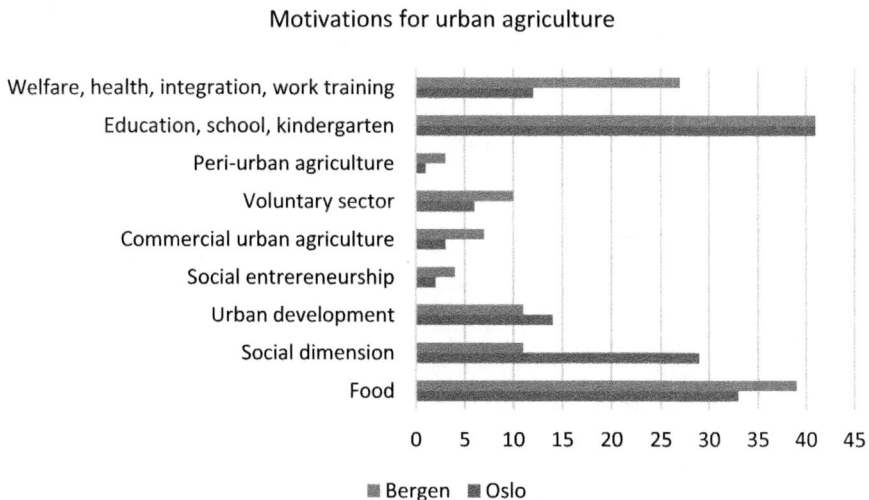

Motivations for urban agriculture

11.7.1   The Content Analysis

The content analysis shows the high number of themes that urban agriculture is connected to (Table 11.3). The *first* clear motivation is that urban agriculture contributes to urban development, more specifically the *Green city* urban development. This is the case for both Oslo and Bergen where this goal figures at the top among all others. However, the quantitative analysis shows that this green city discourse is not mentioned as frequently as others. This seems reasonable since the documents do not discuss urban development per se, but the role urban agriculture plays in urban development. Green city can have a double meaning. On the one hand, *green* means being environmentally friendly, focusing on the provision of ecosystem services such as strengthening biodiversity, increasing the mount of pollinating plants, improving water retention, and general access to green areas. On the other hand, this means also literally "green" and refers to adding vegetation to the city. Since the

Table 11.3 Overview over the main discourses and motivations in the planning documents

Main discourse	Sub-discourses	Oslo Strategy for urban agriculture	Bergen Strategy for urban agriculture	Trondheim Planning program agriculture, section mentioning urban agriculture
Urban development	Greener cities/ nature diversity	Goal 1	Overall goal	Mentioned
Food and food-systems	Food production-contribution to local food supply	Goal 2	Goal 1	Mentioned and to be developed in ensuing plan
	Stronger support for traditional agriculture			Part of motivation
	High-tech production/ microgreens	Goal 2		
	Alternative food distribution channels	Goal 2	Goal 1	Mentioned and to be developed further
Social dimensions-extended welfare	Education	Goal 3/goal 4		
	Health/social work	Goal 3		
	Integration			
	Work training	Goal 3		
	Social meeting places/life quality	Goal 3[a]	Goal 2	Mentioned and to be developed
Active citizenship		Mentioned as a part of social meeting places		Co-producing the city through local meeting places such as urban agriculture

[a]A print error places this as goal 2

Trondheim planning program only concerns agriculture, it is not surprising that urban development is not a topic for discussion.

The second motivation is that all cities also frame urban agriculture within a *food and food systems discourse*, and the quantitative analysis clearly shows this. However, it should also be added that the societal plan for Oslo puts other motivations as perhaps more important. All cities refer to the aim of producing alternative channels of food distribution. However, the strongest connection to ordinary agriculture is found in Trondheim, where an important aim is to enhance the visibility and improve the image of traditional, nonurban agriculture, through the experiences of urban dwellers engaged with their own growing activities.

The third important dimension is urban agriculture as *social meeting places* as shown in the quantitative analysis. This is ranked high among the goals in both Oslo and Bergen. Urban agriculture increases social life in public spaces through providing social meeting places. It is underlined in both strategies that these should be meeting places across diverse groups of citizens.

The fourth dimension *is the extended welfare dimension.* Urban agriculture can also contribute to reach goals for the welfare state, by providing working opportunities for youth, an arena for language training and integration, by reaching goals in education about growing and plants as well as animal husbandry.

A *fifth* dimension is the role of citizens as actors in urban development, in other words, their *active citizenship.* According to Oslo policy documents, urban agriculture means that the inhabitants change their role in public space from being spectators to active participants. The Trondheim documents, in their very short sentences about urban agriculture, clearly say that urban agriculture can also further the politician's ambitions to improve citizen involvement from participation into "co-creation" of the city. Thus, urban agriculture is also motivated by the desire to strengthen active citizenship.

11.8 Conclusion: Multidimensional Motivations for Public Policies for Urban Agriculture

What are the motivations for developing municipal public policy for urban agriculture in Oslo, Bergen, and Trondheim? And which discourses do the motivations expressed in each municipal context connect to? In this discussion, we will focus on Oslo and Bergen, since they have clearly expressed their motivations in urban agriculture-centered strategic plans that have been adopted by the respective city council. Trondheim has not formulated a clear strategy, but their "planning program" for a thematic municipal master plan gives some indications for their motivations. There were differences also between Oslo and Bergen's policies. Oslo's strategy does not include references to specific measures, focusing instead on setting broader goals, while Bergen's included both aims and actions.

The analysis of the policy documents shows that support for urban agriculture has several motivations, following from the multidimensional character of urban agriculture: (i) urban "green" development, (ii) food production and food systems, (iii) social meeting places, (iv) means to attain goals in municipal welfare services, and (v) active citizenship. Despite limitations due to the differences across municipalities, our study shows that the motivations are the same, with some different weighting.

Urban agriculture is clearly embedded in a discourse about *future city development*, and this is particularly evident in Oslo and Bergen. In their strategies, it is the first goal (Oslo) and the whole framing for discussions of urban agriculture in Bergen: *Bergen as the "greenest" city*. A "green" city in this context can have different interpretation, "green" as environmentally friendly or "green" as enhancing the presence of vegetation in built environments, either as green structure or as integrated in buildings. The discussion in the strategies shows both interpretations, but particularly Bergen underlines the advantage of bringing more vegetation in the city, particularly in existing gray areas, also for aesthetical reasons (*Grønnere og skjønnere* (Greener and more beautiful)). This theme is also present in the strategy for green roofs in Oslo.

By definition, urban agriculture is about *food production,* and this forms an important part of the discourse on urban agriculture in cities. This is less evident in Oslo's "Societal Plan," which discusses whether other motivations may be more important. The food emphasis in urban agriculture is strongest in Trondheim. Here, the relationship to food production is a clear motivation for urban agriculture. As urban agriculture is a part of a plan of agricultural production more generally, this is not so surprising. Yet this also reflects the city's location in one of Norway's main areas for agricultural production. This also reflects the active role that farmers organizations play as providers of knowledge and the existence of financial mechanism in support of peri-urban agriculture.

All three cities are concerned with the *social side* of urban agriculture with emphasis of its role as a meeting place across groups, such as in Oslo with the emphasis on "green meeting places" in their strategy. Oslo, Bergen, and Trondheim have also been concerned with extending urban agriculture *in the provision of municipal welfare services*, in care facilities, in integration, or in the form of knowledge and education. This is shown not only in the planning documents but also in projects and to some degree in financial mechanisms (see Chapter 12).

Urban agriculture is also set into an ongoing discourse about *co-creating the city*, as shown particularly in Trondheim.

Most of these motivations are known from earlier literature, but it is interesting to note the emphasis on strengthening welfare service and on urban development. The municipalities are responsible for providing welfare services, as well as the wider urban development, and they clearly see a role for urban agriculture in these tasks. The activist element in urban agriculture is also appreciated in the form of enabling active citizenship and co-creation of the city.

References

Arts, B., Leroy, P., & van Tatenhove, J. (2006). Political modernisation and policy arrangements: A framework for understanding environmental policy change. *Public Organization Review, 6,* 93–106. https://doi.org/10.1007/s11115-006-0001-4

Bergen municipality. (2019). *Dyrk Bergen. Strategi for urbant landbruk. 2019–2023* (Cultivate Bergen. Strategy for urban agriculture 2019–2023).

Bratberg, Ø. (2020): *Tekstanalyse for samfunnsvitere.* Cappelen Damm Akademisk (Analyzing text for social scientists).

Brody, L. S., & de Wilde, M. (2020). Cultivating food or cultivating citizens? On the governance and potential of community gardens in Amsterdam. *Local Environment, 25*(3), 243–257. https://doi.org/10.1080/13549839.2020.1730776

Buijs, A., Hansen, R., Van der Jagt, S., Ambrose-Oji, B., Elands, B., Lorance Rall, E., Mattijssen, T., Pauleit, S., Runhaar, H., Stahl Olafsson, A., & Steen Møller, M. (2019). Mosaic governance for urban green infrastructure: Upscaling active citizenship from a local government perspective. *Urban Forestry & Urban Greening, 40,* 53–62.

Certomà, C., & Tornaghi, C. (2015). Political gardening. Transforming cities and political agency. *Local Environment, 20,* 1123–1131. https://doi.org/10.1080/13549839.2015.1053724

Christensen, S., Malberg Dyg, P., & Allenberg, K. (2019). Urban community gardening, social capital, and "integration" – A mixed method exploration of urban "integration-gardening" in Copenhagen, Denmark. *Local Environment, 24*(3), 231–248. https://doi.org/10.1080/1354983 9.2018.1561655

Firth, C., Maye, D., & Pearson, D. (2011). Developing "community" in community gardens. *Local Environment, 16*(6), 555–568. https://doi.org/10.1080/13549839.2011.586025

Forsberg, E. M., Dagsrud, E., Panman, A., Lindén, F., Holm, K. M., & Pflüger, A. (2019). *Hvorfor er urbant landbruk viktig for Fylkesmannen? Innlegg på Konferanse om urbant landbruk. Arrangert av landbruks- og matdepartementet.* 18/11–2019 (Why is urban agriculture important for the county governor? Presentation at the conference on urban agriculture arranged by the Ministry for Agriculture and Food. 18.11.2019) https://www.regjeringen.no/contentassets/a633d684a2d947ca9d8f0011850325d1/0950-oppsummering-hvorfor-er-urbant-landbruk-viktig-for-fylkesmannen%2D%2D-innspillskonferansen-2019.pdf

McClintock, N. (2014). Radical, reformist, and garden-variety neoliberal: coming to terms with urban agriculture's contradictions. *Local Environment, 19*(2), 147–171. https://doi.org/10.108 0/13549839.2012.752797

Norwegian Ministries. (2021). *Norwegian strategy for urban agriculture. Cultivate cities and towns.* strategi-for-urbant-landbruk-engelsk-web.pdf (regjeringen.no)

Oslo Municipality. (2019a). *Vår by, vår framtid. Kommuneplan for Oslo 2018. Samfunnsdel med byutviklingsstrategi. Visjon, mål og strategier mot 2040.* Vedtatt av Oslo bystyre 30.01.19 (sak 6). Our city, our future, Municipal masterplan for Oslo 2018. The social element of the municipal master plan with strategy for urban development. Visions, goals and strategies towards 2040. Adopted by Oslo city council 30.01.19 (item 6) https://www.oslo.kommune.no/getfile.php/13324093-1572596131/Tjenester%20og%20tilbud/Politikk%20og%20administrasjon/Politikk/Kommuneplan/Vedtatt%20kommuneplan%202018/Kommuneplan%20Oslo%20–%20%20utskriftvennlig.pdf

Oslo Municipality. (2019b). *Sprouting Oslo – Room for everyone in the city's green spaces. A Strategy for Urban Agriculture 2019–2030* Adopted by the City Council in Oslo 13.11.2019 (Proposition 336/19) https://www.oslo.kommune.no/getfile.php/13398183-1614956203/Tjenester%20og%20tilbud/Natur%2C%20kultur%20og%20fritid/Urbant%20landbruk/BYM_SpirendeOslo_engelsk_A4_digital.pdf

Oslo municipality. (2022). *Strategi for grønne tak. 2030 grønne tak og fasader i 2030 Sak 160/22 – vedtatt av bystyret 25.05.2022* (Strategy for green roofs. 2030 green roofs and facades in 2030. https://www.oslo.kommune.no/getfile.php/13452654-1654694941/Tjenester%20og%20til-bud/Plan%2C%20bygg%20og%20eiendom/Byggesaksveiledere%2C%20normer%20og%20skjemaer/Strategi%20for%20gr%C3%B8nne%20tak%20og%20fasader.pdf

Rosol, M. (2010). Public participation in post-fordist urban green space governance: The case of community gardens in berlin. *International Journal of Urban and Regional Research, 34*(3), 548–563. https://doi.org/10.1111/j.1468-2427.2010.00968.x

Saldaña, J. (2015). *The coding manual for qualitative researchers.* Sage publications.

Simon-Rojo, M., Bernardos, I. M., & Landaluze, J. S. (2018). Food movement between autonomy and coproduction of public policies. Lessons from Madrid. *Nature and Culture, 13*(1), 47–68. https://doi.org/10.3167/nc.2018.130103

Thibert, J. (2012). Making local planning work for urban agriculture in the north american context: A view from the ground. *Journal of Planning Education and Research, 32*(3), 349–357. https://doi.org/10.1177/0739456X11431692

Trondheim municipality. (2020). Forslag til planprogram. *Landbruksplan for Trondheim kommune.* (Proposal for a planning programme. Agricultural plan for Trondheim municipality).

Uster, A., Beeri, I., & Vashdi, D. (2019). Don't push too hard. Examining the managerial behaviours of local authorities in collaborative networks with nonprofit organisations. *Local Government Studies, 45*(1), 124–145. https://doi.org/10.1080/03003930.2018.1533820

van der Jagt, A. P. N., Szaraz, L. R., Delshammar, T., Cvejić, R., Santos, A., Goodness, J., & Buijs, A. (2017). Cultivating nature-based solutions: The governance of communal urban gardens in the European Union. *Environmental Research, 159*(2017), 264–275.

Chapter 12
The Development and Institutionalization of Urban Agriculture Policy: Emerging Governance Models in Three Norwegian Cities

Inger-Lise Saglie

12.1 Background

While urban agriculture has been very much based on citizens' activism, public policies for urban agriculture have also been developed. While much research has been focused on specific urban agriculture initiatives, we know less about the public policies that have emerged over time, particularly in Norway. The aim of this chapter is to fill this gap, through a case study investigation of Norway's three largest cities, Oslo, Bergen, and Trondheim (Fig. 12.1). Norway provides an interesting context for urban agriculture public policies, being an example of a strong welfare state, often referred to as the Nordic model (Knutsen, 2017).

In Chapter 11, the author described the rationales and motivations for developing an urban agriculture public policy in these three cities. This chapter describes and analyzes the establishment of policy measures for urban agriculture. This process will be described through the concepts of institutions and institutionalization (Olsen, 2007; Arts et al., 2006), which can help us understand both the formal and informal ways a policy develops.

The measures for support/plans for urban agriculture are developed within the existing municipal institutional setting, including the organization of the administration and its norms and values (Olsen, 2007). This existing institutional setting thus influences the choice of steering logics and planning instruments. The main focus of this text is the municipal level, as this level is closest to the citizens. But as we shall see, the regional level may also play an important role in urban agriculture policy development.

The chapter seeks to answer the following questions: "How have public policies for urban agriculture emerged and got institutionalized? And which models for

I.-L. Saglie (✉)
Department of Urban and Regional Planning, Faculty of Lanscape and Society, Norwegian University of Life Sciences, Ås, Norway
e-mail: inger-lise.saglie@nmbu.no

© The Author(s) 2024
B. Sirowy, D. Ruggeri (eds.), *Urban Agriculture in Public Space*, GeoJournal Library 132, https://doi.org/10.1007/978-3-031-41550-0_12

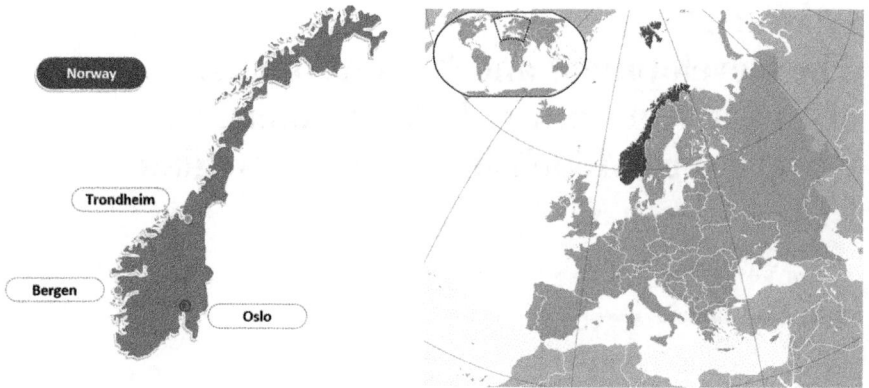

Fig. 12.1 The location of the discussed cases. (Source: Wikimedia Commons. The picture is licensed under the Creative Commons Attribution-Share Alike 3.0 Unported license)

organization of the urban agriculture policy domain are emerging and to which extent are growers involved?

12.2 The Perspectives on Institutionalization of Urban Agriculture as a Policy Field

The development of public policies and planning for urban agriculture can be studied as any other public policy field. A specificity of this policy field is its start as a voluntary, bottom-up activity. But the interplay between public policies and voluntary activism is a specificity shared with many other activities/policy fields such as sports, cultural heritage, health etc.

An institution has been defined by Olsen (2007 p. 3) as "*an enduring collection of rules and organized practices, embedded in structures of meaning and resources that are relatively invariant in the face of turnover of individuals and changing external circumstances.*" The related institutionalization concept refers to the process whereby individual's or group's loose, fluid actions over time begin to show patterns (Arts et al., 2006). These patterns then turn into more solid and established structures, which in turn structure people's behavior in later stages. In public policy, this means that relatively stable definitions of the phenomenon emerge and that gradually responses or solutions to the phenomenon are found. This leads to organization of tasks in particular ways, and interaction between actors is structured through more or less fixed rules and systems (ibid). Institutionalization is thus well suited to describe the development of public policy for urban agriculture. This perspective also means that public policy can adjust in response to changes and stabilize for certain periods (Arts et al., 2006).

The focus of this chapter is on the analysis of the emergence of public policies of urban agriculture and its subsequent institutionalization. The chapter describes five phases of development, suited to urban agriculture.

- The first phase is the fluid phase, with the emerging phenomenon of citizens activism.
- The second phase is a definition of urban agriculture as a public policy field and emerging policy measures.
- The third is structuring and organizing of the policy field and policy measures.
- The fourth is refining the measures and expanding the field of urban agriculture.
- The fifth is the formalization of urban agriculture in the planning system.

These phases follow a timeline, yet they also overlap, coexist, and interweave in the process as definitions, structures, organizations, and measures may change and different formal and informal practices may occur.

The institutionalization of urban agriculture leads to particular forms of organization of the policy domain, which may show local variations of models since they are is developed in particular institutional contexts. The development of urban agriculture policy takes place between particular actors, such as politicians, administration, and voluntary sector.

Arts et al. (2006) introduced a framework for policy domains that can be useful for urban agriculture analyses. This framework, called the Policy Arrangement Approach, includes four dimensions (see Fig. 12.2). The first refers to *actors and their coalitions*. This means that certain actors are important in developing a policy and that they also may form coalitions and thus influence over policy.

The second is the division of *power and influence* between these actors where "power refers to the mobilization, division and deployment of resources, and influence as to who determines policy outcomes and how" (Arts et al., 2006 p. 7). The third is *the rules of the game* currently in operation, both in terms of formal procedures for pursuit of policy and decision-making and, importantly, also informal and more or less structured patterns for political and other forms of interaction. The fourth is the current *policy programs and discourses* where discourses refer to the views and narratives of the actors.

Fig. 12.2 Visual representation of the four dimensions in a policy domain (Source: Arts et al., 2006: 90)

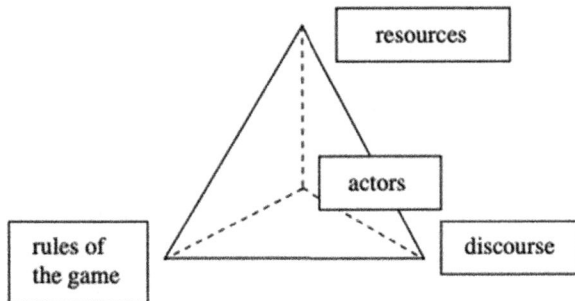

These four dimensions are linked together so that changes in one dimension will influence the others. Differences in "rules of the game" may change the flows of power and influence which actors might get involved. Discourses are important because they also define who the relevant actors may be and thus also their possibilities for power, influence, and outcome in the form of policy programs and measures. A way of applying this analytical tool to the policy domain of urban agriculture in this chapter will be to systematically look for the role of a particular actor, the growers, because of the important role of citizens' initiatives. A particular focus will be to investigate whether they are, or to which degree they are, among the actors and how this influences the other dimensions.

The outcome, the actual policies pursued by each municipality, may also show differences across the cases investigated. As shown in the preceding chapter, urban agriculture is pursued by a number of reasons, so it may be expected that also the actual policies emphasize different aspects. These concerns are as follows:

- First, *the municipal support* mechanisms for *urban agriculture*
- Second, *urban agriculture as a means to reach welfare goals*
- Third, *the relation of urban agriculture to professional urban agriculture* in its new and traditional form
- Fourth, *the connection of urban agriculture to food and food systems*
- Fifth, *the relationship of urban agriculture to public space, civic* participation and co-creating the city

12.3 Methods

In our study, we selected the three largest cities in Norway, which have also been among the most advanced in developing urban agriculture policies. They represent different local contexts for urban agriculture in size, climate, topography, and availability of farmland (Table 12.1).

Table 12.1 Overview of some characteristics of the three municipalities

	Oslo	Bergen	Trondheim
Inhabitants approx.	Approx. 710,000	Approx. 290,000	Approx. 210,000
Landscape	Within its borders, there are large woodlands but very limited agricultural land. The areas around the Oslo Fjord are well suited to agriculture climatically and also with areas with arable soil. But these areas are not within the borders of Oslo municipality	Mountainous landscape situated at the west coast of Norway. Limited farmland within its border 100–120 active farms	Situated in one of the primary agricultural regions in Norway, with good farmland also within the municipal borders and 218 active farms
Farmland	2.1%	6.5%	17%

The methods used in this study included interviews and analysis of planning documents. In total, we interviewed 21 people including municipal urban agriculture coordinators, administration at the county governor, voluntary movement, farmers' associations, social entrepreneurs, and a major developer (see Appendix 1). Since urban agriculture policies have been continuously developed over the last years, follow-up interviews have been made with the urban agriculture coordinators in the municipalities. The interviewees have been selected through snowballing method, where the interviewees have suggested further persons to contact. Two third of the interviews have been conducted online due to Covid-19, most recorded and transcribed. The planning documents have also provided information about how they have been produced and who the main actors have been in the formulation of the planning documents. Also, the municipalities' websites have provided important information about the policy instruments used, such as funding mechanisms, recipients of funding, courses available, contact points, etc. Observation and participation in an internal workshop in Oslo municipality provided information of efforts to expand urban agriculture as a means to obtain goals in their respective field of responsibility. Official political statements are other important sources of information.

12.4 Empirical Studies

12.4.1 The Emergence of Public support for Urban Agriculture

Like in many cities around the world, there has been an increasing interest in food growing in Norwegian urban areas. In private gardens and in allotments, there has been an unbroken history of growing but with varying intensity over years. Growing is thus not new, but the locations where this recent wave of growing started were unusual. These locations included inner-city sites such as public spaces, parks, rooftops, or gray areas such as urban squares, with the intent to produce locally grown and often ecological food. These initiatives were often connected to ideas of transition to a more ecologically friendly and sustainable development, like the example of "Bærekraftige liv" (Sustainable lives) in Bergen, but also to more socially concerned initiatives to improve living conditions and employment opportunities for youth in inner city locations (Interview 1). Motivations also included social meeting places and community building in addition to production of food, as described in the cases studied in Chapters 6, 7 and 8.

As described in Chapter 11 on motivations for public policy on urban agriculture, the county governors were early initiators for development of such policies. In 2009, they formed a network among county governors nationally, but they were also closely involved in networks with cities in their respective regions. Some of the early financial mechanisms were initiated at a county level. While the county level actors early observed these trends, the national agricultural authorities later also established urban agriculture as a policy domain. In 2019, they initiated the work on a National Strategy for Urban Agriculture, recently published (Norwegian Ministries, 2021).

Oslo: Political Initiatives and Administrative Implementation

Oslo is characterized by early initiatives for urban agriculture within inner-city locations, also in highly visible urban spaces, see also Chapters 6 and 7. An example is Losæter an urban garden that was initiated in 2011 as an art project in a former harbor area undergoing transformation. More than 2000 inhabitants competed for space to grow when the opportunity arose (Interview 2). Agriculture in this location was in a stark contrast to the new high-rise and high-end development. This initiative got a massive press coverage, becoming close to an icon for urban agriculture, and by far the most well-known initiative in Oslo. Several social entrepreneurs were also established, working with urban agriculture. Some city districts, particularly inner-city districts, supported these early initiatives.

In the county of Oslo and Akershus,[1] the county governor started early to give financial support to urban agriculture projects under a budget post for ecological agriculture (Interview 1). They started to use the term "urban agriculture" since they wanted to emphasize the particularity of agriculture in the city and to make visible the importance of agriculture for the urban population in the capital (Forsberg et al., 2014 p. 8). A "think tank" for urban agriculture was established in 2013 to give input and share experiences of urban agriculture (Forsberg et al., 2014 p. 8). This group included experienced growers and initiators of urban agriculture. With financial support under the budget post "rural development," the county governor initiated a project resulting in a report with the aim to clarify the content of the concept "urban agriculture," what this could mean for the population of Oslo and which themes and measures should be taken in the future (Forsberg et al., 2014 p. 8) (Fig. 12.3). The county governor organized a group of stakeholders to feed into the report with representatives from Oslo municipality (from urban green space management, agriculture, and planning departments), growers, and initiators. This report increased the understanding for urban agriculture within the agricultural sector and represented an important step in making urban agriculture a policy domain for the county governor with dedicated budget post. Thus, the county governor was able to support early initiatives for urban agriculture in the region.

The politicians in Oslo have also been important actors in developing urban agriculture policies in the municipality. The city council commissioned the administration to work on a program for urban agriculture in 2013, reworked by a new elected city council and adopted in 2015 (Press release: The city council presents an urban agriculture program for Oslo. 8.9.2015.).

---

[1] Akershus merged together with Buskerud and Østfold to Viken county 1.1.2020.

Urbant landbruk –
Bærekraftig, synlig og verdsatt

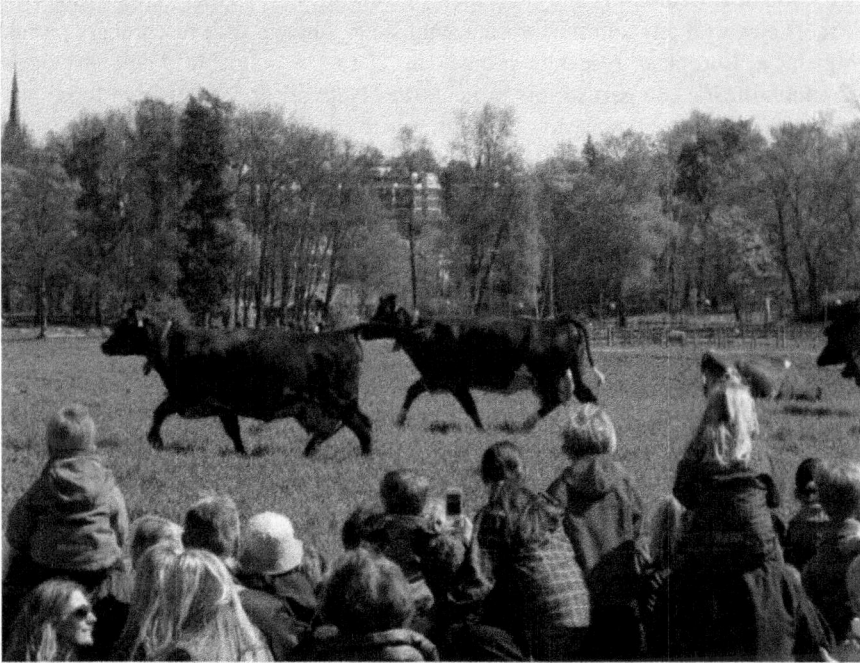

Rapport nr. 1/2014

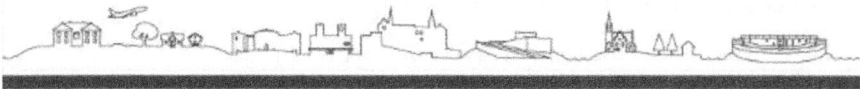

Fig. 12.3 The county governor's report "Urban agriculture-sustainable, visible and valued" (Source: https://www.statsforvalteren.no/siteassets/fm-oslo-og-viken/landbruk-og-mat/naringsut-vikling/dokumenter/rapport%2D%2Durbant-landbruk-barekraftig-synlig-og-verdsatt-nr.1_2014.pdf)

"The city council wants Oslo to be ahead as an internationally leading environmentally friendly city, also within urban agriculture and sees the program for agriculture as an important part of a comprehensive policy to create a green and modern city" says city councilor Guri Melby (Liberal Party) (Oslo municipality, 2015a).

The politicians also initiated a center for urban ecology. Yet, the policy field was so new that it needed to mature. The municipality needed to ask themselves what urban agriculture is and what their role could be in its facilitation (Interview 15). The central city administration established contacts with researchers partaking in a European research project in 2015 "Sustainable Food in Urban Communities." As a part of this project, the "Network for sustainable food" was established by the municipality. The aim was to connect actors engaged in sustainable food and urban agriculture. Urban agriculture had in many ways been a long tradition in the Oslo region including growing in school gardens, private gardens, and allotment. Nevertheless, the recent initiatives situated largely in public spaces, represented something new, and the administration did not quite know how they should connect to this new wave of activities. These were pursued by many different actors, without involvement from the municipality, at least not in an organized way (Interview 2).

In 2017, another political initiative was taken by the new city government. The city administration got another commission from the city councilor to work further with urban agriculture, and a funding scheme was established. They were also asked to further develop urban agriculture as a policy field and to develop a strategy for urban agriculture. As described in the preceding chapter, the strategy discusses why urban agriculture is important for the city and what the city wants to achieve by supporting it. The city strategy was adopted in 2019, and the administration is now working on a follow-up action plan (Interview 2).

The political support for urban agriculture has been strong in Oslo. The new city council after the 2019 election was formed by three parties, and they negotiated a political platform for their work. In this platform, a section is dedicated to urban agriculture, where they declare that their policy is to continue the support of urban agriculture as shown in the quotations below.

"Urban agriculture contributes to more green meeting places that makes Oslo more pleasant for both people and animals. It increases the understanding of where the food comes from and is good both for public health and integration. The city council will take care of the city's colony gardens, allotment gardens and school gardens, transform grey areas to green urban spaces for urban cultivation and strengthen the policies for urban agriculture." Oslos by rådserklæring 2019–2023 (2019).

(continued)

"The city council wants

- Continue the financial support for urban agriculture and facilitate more allotment gardens
- Ensure better access to school gardens when building new schools and facilitate urban cultivation in more school yards and kindergartens
- Facilitate arenas for locally produced food, for example green neighborhood kitchens and markets in connection to cultivating projects in the city"

Oslos by rådserklæring 2019–2023 (2019).

Developing knowledge about urban agriculture has been important for the municipality. In addition to supporting initiatives for urban agriculture, the municipality also supports research and development projects. They have also initiated an evaluation of their schemes. In addition, they have been frequently approached by research organizations to partake in research and are now connected to several projects (Interview 1). In 2017, the politicians decided to establish a funding scheme for urban agriculture, where everybody could apply, but because of a large number of applications, housing cooperatives and housing co-ownerships were prioritized. The rules of this programme were formalized as a Provision of the Local Government Act (a legal act relating to municipalities and county authorities) (https://lovdata.no/dokument/LF/forskrift/2017-03-29-463). The administration saw that the rules did not address the diversity of initiatives and suggested changes (Interview 15). In 2018, the administration received many good proposals including small start-up businesses such as growing fungi on used coffee grains, and these were funded too. For the administration, food production and professional urban agriculture are important. So is knowledge about food production and the origin of food as well as the social aspects of urban gardening (Interview 15). As one interviewee points out,

We try to find the balance where food production is important, while at the same time include the other side effects (interview 2)

The early initiatives for urban agriculture were much centered around inner-city locations. The administration wanted to encourage urban agriculture also in less central locations (Fig. 12.4) as it had an ambition to increase the volume of the production, not just the number of single pallet boxes. Thus, one of the focus areas were the long abandoned farms in the fringes that now serve as farms to visit, social meeting places, or museums (Interview 2). One of them is now the location of an incubator scheme for people wanting to develop market gardens as a way of living. Such initiatives are run by county governors and department for agriculture in several counties (Satser på markedshager| Statsforvalteren i Oslo og Viken). Market gardens are highly intensive cultivation projects in small plots, producing vegetables for sale to the urban population.

In addition, the city also established a pioneer funding scheme directed particularly toward other sectors in the municipality including schools, kindergartens,

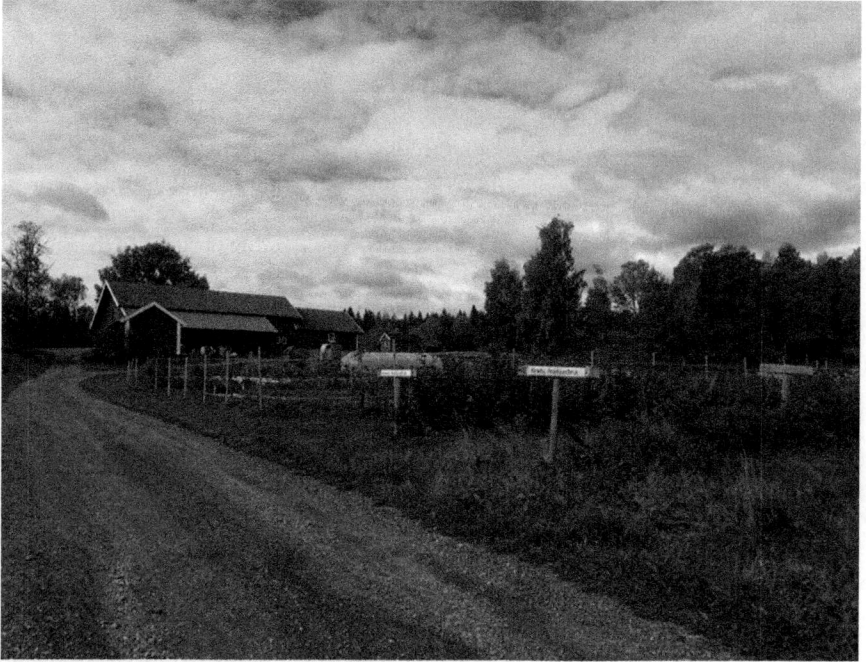

Fig. 12.4 Cooperative farming (*Kirkeby andelslandbruk*) on Kirkeby farm in the urban periphery just outside Oslo's building zone (Photo: author)

health institutions, and cultural institutions (Interview 1). Eight projects received funding, and an external evaluation team followed these activities. The findings were that *social meeting places* were the main driver for the municipal sectors that took part in the scheme, being important for solving their public mandate. The public role varied greatly, from just offering financial support to actually running the initiative (Skorupka & Pålsrud, 2019). In the latter case, the task of the public sector also included the recruitment of growers, what turned out to be difficult to fulfil in a few places. This was particularly the case when the initiative owner did not have potential growers, for example, a museum. The attractivity of the place itself and additional attractive elements seemed to be important for the interest in growing. An important lesson learnt was that to succeed in the long term, the organizators of the growing initiative need to secure maintenance through the season, including summer holiday weeks. In addition, agricultural knowledge needs to be coupled to the initiatives. As establishing a social meeting place was an important motivation, additional capacity to run the area as a meeting place is important to fulfil this function. Not all initiatives succeeded in fulfilling their objectives, for example, establishing connections with NAV (the Norwegian Labour and Welfare Administration) to initiate work schemes for youth. Other noticed that the cultivation itself did not succeed very well (Skorupka & Pålsrud, 2019). The general experience was that a particularly dedicated individual in an organization was necessary to make the initiative work. These experiences also showed the inherent problems in public intentions depending on voluntary work. The municipalities' administrative unit for implementing urban agricultural policy has further worked internally in the municipality, for example, by organizing a workshop to get input to the action plan they are currently working with.

The administration is currently working with different aspects of urban agriculture facilitation. This includes the following:

(i) Launching a survey *to map the urban agriculture iniatives* (Interview 15). There was also a need *to categorize the initiatives*, not the least because the formal "path" to receive approval will be very different as the initiatives vary greatly from commercial enterprises located indoors to local volunteer driven projects using public space. The initiators of urban agriculture projects may be sent from one municipal department to another when dealing with formalities – including issues related to formal zoning of the land, water quality, health, safety, and environment. The municipality hopes to simplify the procedures to obtain the necessary permits (Interview 15).

(ii) *Securing access to land* to grow including *mapping potential areas for cultivation* (Interview 15) to help the public to identify the locations where they can establish a new urban agriculture projects or join an existing one. This mapping also includes an evaluation whether a certain plot should the taken as a land for growing, or whether it has other important biological functions. The municipal actors are aware that they need to develop a more participatory approach when plots are taken for cultivation. This may include involving city districts and local community organizations (Interview 15). In addition, they also are working to *establish a system to identify the owner/manager of a plot*. Initiators for urban agriculture on a particular location need to show an agreement from the owner/manager to use that land for agriculture if they are to receive financial support. The municipality may own the land, but it may be managed by a number of different municipal sectors, including central park management, city districts, department of schools and kindergartens, health care departmen, burial ground, etc. (Interview 2).

(iii) *Connecting resources* between, for example, institutions that own land and organizations that want to grow, or between organizations seeking opportunities for summer jobs for youth and urban agricultural schemes; establishing connections between central level of green space management and the city districts (Interviews 21.1.19 and 16.2.21).

(iv) *Facilitating professional urban agriculture such as projects integrated in buildings or market gardens*. The integration of agriculture in buildings can stumble on bureaucratic hindrances in the planning and building act, regarding zoning and building regulations. It is not possible for the municipality to change the law, but they intend to work with the relevant ministries on this (Interview 15).

Development of market gardens is an initiative from the county governors, and all three case cities are involved in this initiative.

12.4.2   Inclusion of Urban Agriculture in Plans

Since urban agriculture was a clear part of the city council's political ambitions, this policy domain was also included in central formal planning documents. The planning law requires the municipalities to prepare a "societal plan" for the development of the municipality, setting out long-term goals and strategies as a point of departure for other plans (pbl § 11–2). This should be done every fourth year by the newly elected council to set out their priorities. In the 2018 plan, urban agriculture became a part of this strategy, even if not detailed to any extent, as reflected in the following quotation:

> We want a sustainable city with green cultivation and climate friendly buildings- and the inhabitants need to get more knowledge about environmentally friendly living in the city. Urban agriculture, green roofs and roof gardens make the city greener and more friendly for people, animals and plants (Oslo municipality, 2019 p. 21)

In addition, also in land-use plans, visions of urban agriculture began to appear. Thus, not only the urban agriculture unit but also the land-use and planning departments became increasingly involved. The idea of "greening" Oslo has also resulted in a "guidance" report on use of roofs, developed by the planning and building department. The idea is that roofs need to be used for "green purposes" including water retention, recreation, and urban agriculture. These guidelines serve as an informal steering tool directed toward private developers when they plan and construct new buildings.

The cooperation between the urban agriculture unit in the Agency for Urban Environment and the Agency for Planning and Building Services has evolved over time. Lately, urban agriculture unit has been invited into the development of the green space in Hovinbyen, the largest transformation area in Oslo. There is a wish to include urban agriculture in the strategic plan that is developed for the green structure in this area (Fig. 12.5), but the plan is still vague about how urban agriculture should be developed (Interview 15).

Bergen: Networking, Grassroot Initiatives, and Idealists in the Municipal Administration

There has been a long-standing interest in urban growing in Bergen, and a number of initiatives have been taken. A grassroot transition movement, "Sustainable lives," has played an important role. Their idea was to implement actions in the local community in order to reach a more sustainable development.

Like in other regions, these bottom up processes were observed by the county governor as well as the municipality. Networks between public departments and voluntary associations were formed and have been important in developing urban agriculture as a policy field in Bergen. In 2015, a project for agriculture was initiated by dedicated individuals in the city administration and the county governor (Bergen municipality, 2019). This joint project arranged two well-attended workshop open to everyone that showed the magnitude of the general interest for urban agriculture. The project was financially sponsored by county governor and by in-kind contribution from the city. The steering group consisted of the farmers'

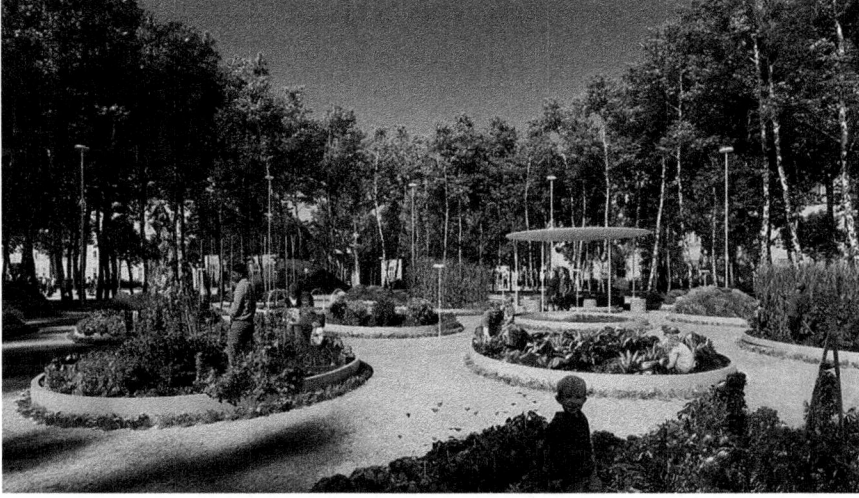

Fig. 12.5 Urban agriculture as an element in visions for the "green ring," a major urban planning idea on the development of Hovinbyen. Hovinbyen is the major new transformation area in Oslo (Source: https://magasin.oslo.kommune.no/byplan/den-gronne-ringen-blir-tydeligere#gref)

association, the small-scale farmers' association, the county governor, and Slow Food Bergen. The working group consisted of representatives from the county governor's department for agriculture, Bergen municipality's department for agriculture, and "Bærekraftige liv Bergen" (Sustainable Life Bergen). The latter is a movement focusing on the actions that a local neighborhood can take to reduce the ecological footprint without compromising life quality, including reduced consumption, circular economy, and ecological thinking. In Bergen, there are several such local initiatives. (Interview 17).

As a part of the project, a survey of potential of municipal land for urban agriculture was conducted, resulting in a map showing potential sites for cultivation, providing information on their suitability for growing such as sun and soil conditions. Courses in growing were given, and a handbook for growing is published online. The politicians in Bergen have been very positive, and a financial scheme for urban agriculture has been in place since 2017. This was due to lobbying to politicians by citizen organizations when the budget was adopted politically. This scheme is limited to joint growing and gives priority to initiatives that benefit children and young people. They support expenditure for buying equipment and also for courses in cultivation (Bergen municipality, 2019). The scheme has so far not been amended (Interview 15).

This scheme of financial support is coordinated by an employee in the department of agriculture, but the coordination of urban agriculture activities is only a small part of the position. Yet, the civil servant has good contact with the growers and acts in practice as a contact point for initiatives. A common question is about land ownership, and she has been able to help people with this. When handling the financial scheme, the administration saw the need for strategic thinking about the use of the financial resources, its place in wider urban development, and the internal organization around urban agriculture in the municipality. The development of a strategy was suggested by the administration and approved by the politicians. The strategy was developed in cooperation with the voluntary sector, Sustainable Lifes (Bærekraftige Liv), and the county governor, integrating also inputs from well-attended, open workshops. The strategy was adopted in 2019.

Lately, other initiatives have emerged. A "city-farmer" has been appointed through a joint initiative in the network, where the municipality, the county council, the county governor, and the farmers' association pay the salary. The farmer's association is the employer. This is a conscious choice, enabling the city-farmer to be free-standing. This also creates a link between urban agriculture and the ordinary agriculture (Interview 15). This has affected the standing of urban agriculture among farmers and also facilitated food distribution schemes (Interview 15). The city-farmer is located in a former so called "lystgård," the Norwegian term that can be translated as leisure farm. This location was a summer residences for well-to-do Bergen citizens, popular in the period 1750–1859. "Lystgården" is now a center for the "sustainable life" movement and its diverse activities including growing. As we can read on the centre's website,

> "*Lystgården is a kind of hotspot for sustainability, quality of life and fellowship*" (Fig. 12.6) (https://www.lystgarden.no/).

Another project is the incubator program, "market gardens," which is also placed in Lystgården. A leader for this program has also a task of finding land for other prospective market gardens. Which involves networking with farmers. This initiative is a part of the wider network that Oslo and Trondheim also are involved in. This network stretches internationally, connected to market gardens in Malmö, Sweden. The partners involved in Bergen are the municipality, the city-farmer in Bergen, Vestland county council, and Vestland county governor, as well as partners working with the ordinary professional agriculture such as Norsk landbruksråd-givning, a company being a link between research and practice in farming.

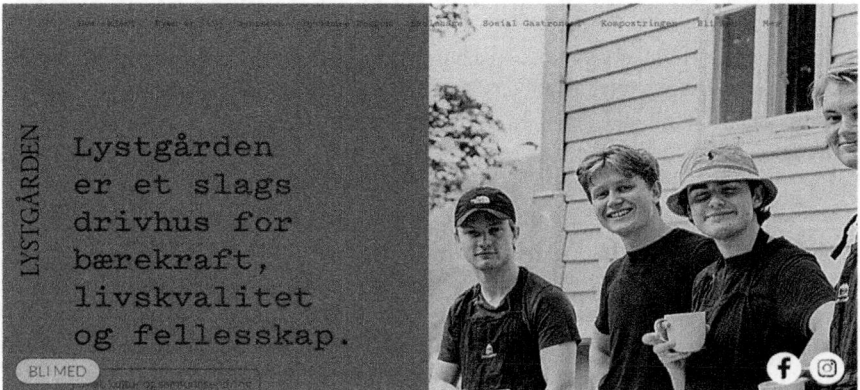

Fig. 12.6 Screenshot from the website of Lystgården: "A hotspot for sustainability, quality of life and fellowship" (Source: https://www.lystgarden.no/ Accessed 3.11.2022)

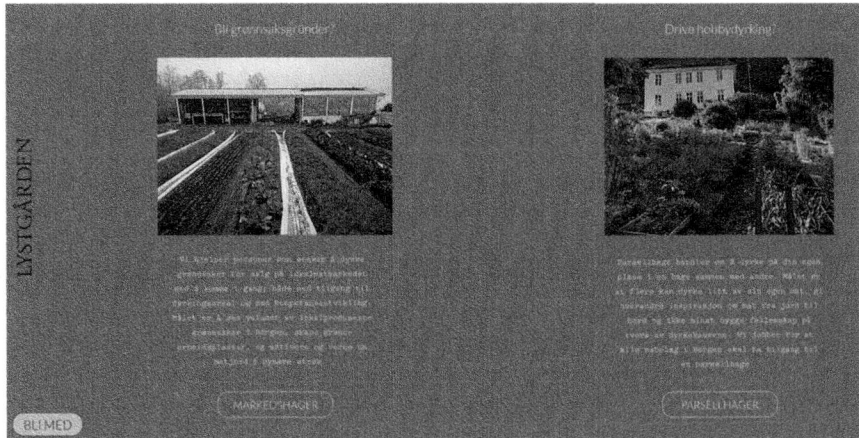

Fig. 12.7 Screenshot from the homepages of Lystgården explaining the difference between market garden and allotment garden (Source: https://www.lystgarden.no/dyrkbarebergen Accessed 3.11.2022)

The text in Fig. 12.7 explains the difference between a market garden (left) and an allotment garden (right) and what Lystgården can offer in terms of support. Market gardens: "We help individuals that want to grow vegetables for sale on the local produce market to get started, both in terms of accessibility to areas for growing and developing necessary competences. The aim is to increase the volume of locally produced vegetables in Bergen, create green workplaces and activate and protect arable land near urban areas." Allotment gardens: "Allotment Garden is about cultivating your own area in a garden together with others. The aim is that more people can grow their own food, give each other inspiration about food from soil to table, and not the least build fellowship across the pallets. We work to secure that all neighborhoods in Bergen have access to an allotment garden."

Trondheim: Co-creation of Policies

In Trondheim, urban agriculture or the local name "cultivating in the city" (dyrking i by), emerged as a policy domain in spring 2015. An initiative was taken for a strategic work connected to urban agriculture in Trøndelag region where Trondheim is situated. The background was a number of grassroot initiatives from urban farmers, community gardens, and cooperative agriculture projects, strategies taken by the municipality and interest from several cross disciplinary research organizations. The county governor coordinated the work together with the municipality.

A seed for Trondheim municipality's financing of urban agriculture was planted through the contribution from university students. The municipality has a long-standing relationship with the Norwegian University of Science and Technology. In 2015, a course called "experts in teams" asked students to design ideas for three sites in the city. Their proposals illustrated how urban agriculture could be integrated into the design of urban places. The city's department of environment prepared a brief advising local politicians to finance the establishment of urban agriculture in these sites. The politicians liked the idea very much, and the cultivation projects were put into practice, and in addition, a general financing scheme was established. The financial scheme was continued in 2016.

Also in 2015, agroecology students from the Norwegian University of Life Sciences held workshops with growers to learn how the municipality could facilitate urban agriculture as a voluntary activity (Finnegan et al., 2015). The growers expressed the need to be physically and digitally connected and learn from each other. They also asked for easy access to knowledge about growing and for help in the transport of pallets, soil, and compost. A common message was that they wanted to spend more time on growing activities, rather than organizing the initiative. An important result was a Facebook group, visits between the gardens, and yearly physical meetings for exchange of experiences and interaction with the municipality. For the municipality, these meetings have been important for further policy development, for example by deciding on how to allocate the financial resources available, or how to provide urban farmers with practical help. Another result was the decision to work closely together with the professional agriculture, not outside it. This includes, for example, making use of the professionals' knowledge of growing in courses and use the farm owned by the farmers' association as the center for urban agriculture activities, Voll farm. The concept *"the green food city"* later became what was termed "the Trondheim model" (Interview 10). The basic idea is that the citizens themselves know where they prefer to grow, how they want to grow, and can best advice the municipality to tailor their help toward their needs.

There is an internal working group in the municipality including city planning, infrastructure, public space management, land ownership, and agriculture. Urban agriculture is also beginning to find its way into formal plans according to the Planning and Building Act. The municipality intends to propose a thematic municipal master plan for agriculture and urban agriculture (Interview 16). This shows the close connection that the municipality wants to establish between urban agriculture and peri-urban traditional agriculture. The farmers' organization has from the beginning seen urban agriculture as a positive development, making the urban population more aware of knowledge about food production, appreciative of local food, and develop direct food channels between producers and the urban population. They cooperate closely with the municipality through visits to urban farms and use of knowledge centers for professional agriculture also for knowledge sharing to nonprofessional urban agriculture growers. In the outskirts of Trondheim, Voll farm has become a center for urban agriculture with high competence in growing (Fig. 12.4). In addition, the farmers' organization has financed the hiring of a city farmer, thus showing their interest in strengthening the ties to urban agriculture.

Voll farm (Fig. 12.8) is both a visiting farm and a center for urban agriculture, the latter presenting itself as follows on its website: "The competence center for urban agriculture is a source for knowledge and inspiration for growing of own food in and

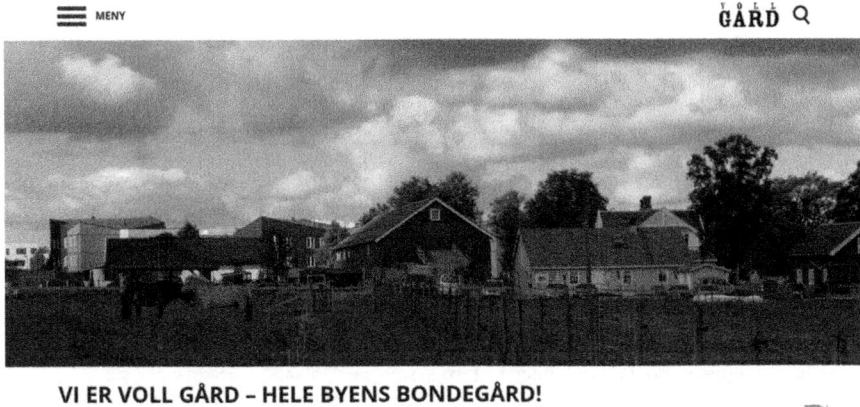

VI ER VOLL GÅRD – HELE BYENS BONDEGÅRD!

Fig. 12.8 Voll farm. The text says: "We are Voll farm- the whole city's farm". Screenshot form its website (Source: http://vollgard.no/om-garden/vi-er-voll-gard-hele-byens-bondegard/ Accessed 3.11.2022)

around Trondheim city. The competence center is a part of Trondheim municipality's program for encourage urban agriculture in the city. Growing your own food is a contribution towards a more sustainable future and enhances stronger ties between people and our life foundation."

All three cities have established a scheme for financial support. The table below (Table 12.2) shows the main aims with the schemes, who can apply and for what purposes. The reasons for the mechanisms are quite similar: to support initiatives involving urban agriculture, increase knowledge about food production, and contribute to community building. But there are differences. Bergen only supports joint growing, while individuals can receive funding in Oslo. Oslo supports commercial activities, and Trondheim supports initiatives in traditional peri-urban agriculture intending to develop ties to the urban population.

12.5 Analyzing the Institutionalization of Urban Agriculture as a Policy Domain in Oslo, Bergen, and Trondheim

The development and institutionalization of urban agriculture as a policy domain in the cities we studied can be synthesized into several phases from an initial fluid state of activities to gradually more established informal and formal patterns of interaction across actors to highly formalized "rules of the game." The development in the three cities can be divided into (1) fluid state of grassroot activism; (2) the initiating phase definition and emerging policy measures; (3) structure, organization, and policy measures in municipalities; (4) expanding and refining policy measures; and (5) urban agriculture in the planning system. The phases we describe below build on

Table 12.2 Overview over financial support schemes in Oslo, Bergen, and Trondheim

	Oslo[a]	Bergen[b]	Trondheim[c]
Aim	The financial support shall contribute to increased knowledge development and more urban agriculture activities in Oslo, through support for initiatives such as developing joint gardens, pallet boxes, beehives, and hen houses	The aim is to increase the inhabitants' knowledge about food production and to facilitate a greener city, good neighborhoods, and attractive meeting places that facilitates activities across age, gender, and origin	Trondheim municipality wants to arrange for growing food in the city. Food production is not only positive for climate and environment, but may also increase life quality for the individuals and also increase unity in the local community
What can be financed	It is desirable that the initiative do not last longer than two years We emphasize that the initiative: Supports one or several of the following points: environment, climate, public health, participation, integration, or entrepreneurship Supports ecological production or/either contributes to increased knowledge about ecological agriculture Is open for broad participation We do not support initiatives supported from other financial mechanisms in Oslo municipality with similar aims We do not support maintenance (ongoing costs for wages in the organization, rent and electricity, maintenance, etc.)	Equipment like planting boxes, soil, seed, plants berry-bearing shrubs, fruit-trees, beekeeping Courses in growing and use of food plants and useful plants, beekeeping Establishment of allotment gardens Growing in roof top gardens Growing in shared city gardens *Priority:* Joint growing such as allotment gardens and initiatives for children and youths	Priority: Start-up costs shared equipment infrastructure (not hothouse) arranging open courses free of charge for participants from Trondheim other activities may be considered Not prioritized: ordinary running costs personal equipment courses/seminar participation deficit guarantee commercial enterprises closed membership organizations activities in private gardens build-up capital (balanced budgets)
Who can apply	Everybody as long as it is carried out in Oslo; for example: housing cooperatives, public entities, commercial enterprises, voluntary organizations, green and social entrepreneurs, persons with private address in Oslo	Associations, organizations, institutions, housing cooperatives and co-ownerships wanting to use land for edibles or beekeeping	Associations and organizations and municipal entities in Trondheim

[a]https://www.oslo.kommune.no/tilskudd-legater-og-stipend/tilskudd-til-urbant-landbruk/ accessed 29/3-2022
[b]https://www.bergen.kommune.no/innbyggerhjelpen/kultur-idrett-og-fritid/fritid/lag-og-foreninger/tilskot-til-urbant-landbruk-i-bergen accessed 29/3- 2022
[b]https://www.trondheim.kommune.no/tilskudd/dyrking/ accessed 29/3-2022

each other, but they may also exist in parallel to one another, depending on contextual factors and motivations distinguishing each locale.

12.5.1 Phase One: The Fluid State of Grassroot Activism

Citizen activists were the early initiators, and some of the activities became highly visible as many appeared in public spaces in inner-city locations, as discussed in the Chapter 6 where projects in Oslo are presented. In Bergen grassroot transition movements have been important initiators of urban agriculture (Bærekraftige liv[2]). In Trondheim, early initiatives combined growing with systemic transformation intent, such as in the urban ecology pilot area of Svartlamoen.[3] There was also a pronounced interest among the public for growing in allotment gardens. D*evelopers* have also been important actors, particularly in Oslo, where they have been instrumental in establishing the "Losæter," an iconic urban agriculture site nestled in the high profile waterfront redevelopment area of the former Oslo harbor.

12.5.2 Phase Two: The Initiating Phase-Definition and Emerging Policy Measures

In the initiating phase urban agriculture is defined and policy instruments are emerging. County governor's employees in the agricultural departments clearly influenced the definition of urban agriculture and the establishing of urban agriculture as a policy domain. They were also important for local initiatives in their regions. In Oslo, the county governors' contact with well-known growers running flagship food growing initiatives also led to a dialogue between municipal actors and farmers' associations representatives. It was at this stage of the process that *definitions, motivations, and financial schemes* for urban agriculture were established. These were important first steps in the institutionalization of urban agriculture policies. In Oslo, city district administrations spearheaded their own urban agriculture initiatives, with funding from the county governor.

In Bergen, a *network* formed between the county governor, municipality, and the voluntary sector was instrumental in establishing urban agriculture as a domain for policy and planning. They initiated a common project in order to identify measures to support urban agriculture. This network-based developing policy approach has continued to characterize policy for urban agriculture in the city. The voluntary sector played an active political role, through the lobbying of local politicians, which resulted in establishing the financial mechanism in Bergen.

---

[2] https://www.barekraftigeliv.no/

[3] https://en.wikipedia.org/wiki/Svartlamone

Also in Trondheim, networking between local actors was important. In the spring of 2015, the county governor and the municipality coordinated the strategic development work connected to urban agriculture in Trøndelag. Early involvement of municipality administrations as partners in national research projects led by universities and research organization has been particularly important in the policy developments for Oslo and Trondheim, linking the development to knowledge and international discourses on urban agriculture.

12.5.3   Phase Three: Emerging Structures, Organization, and Policy Measures in Municipalities

While the early phases were very much the same in the three cities, the next phases showed clear differences (Table 12.3). In Oslo, the administration became involved quite early in the networks organized by the county governor; *political initiatives* were also important in this phase. The city's vice mayor for environment and transport was one of the key actors, especially when instructing the Agency for Urban Environment to develop urban agriculture further. The agency created a unit dedicated to the support of urban agriculture and initiated the development of a strategy. The vice mayor's initiative resulted in a financing scheme. It is in this phase that "rules of the game" (Arts et al., 2006) were established.

Clear rules for applications for financial support were developed, including who could apply for funding for which activities. There were also formal requirements such as the need to register every urban agriculture initiative as an organization in the national register and to confirm the right to use the land for agricultural purposes. Also, in Bergen and Trondheim, these formal requirements apply.

In *Bergen,* the municipality's unit for agriculture played an important role in policy development, within a financial scheme established through lobbying by activists and associations. Like in other cities, rules for who could or could not apply were developed. The scheme favored communal gardening, which also meant that no individual applicant would be able to access the funds.

The administration needed political signals for use and prioritization of the financial support scheme and suggested the development of a strategy for urban agriculture to intersect these political signals. The initiative from the administration was received very well by the politicians. The strategy was developed very much as a bottom-up process, where the network already in place played an important role as well as inputs from the open, well-attended workshops (Interview 9). The strategy suggested further development of cross-sectorial cooperation also within Bergen municipality. There is a cooperation forum within the municipality, but the cooperation could be better, and the situation has been described as "silos" within the administration (Interview 9). The Bergen strategy suggested the creation of a coordinating council with the goal to enhance cross-sectoral cooperation in the municipality. Due to the Covid-19 pandemic, cooperation efforts have been delayed (Interview 15).

Table 12.3 An overview over the phases in institutionalization

Phase 1 *Fluid*	Growing initiatives – citizen and social entrepreneur driven		
Phase 2 *Definition* *Emerging* *solutions*	Regional networks: county governors, municipalities, growers, farmers association Oslo: report/funding at county governor, research projects Bergen: project/handbook how to grow(initiatives) map Trondheim: Research and students' project		
Phase 3 Structures Organization Solutions	Oslo	Bergen	Trondheim
	Political initiative Dedicated administrative unit	Administration "nudging" politicians Lobbying from organized voluntary sector	Administration "nudging" politicians Informal cooperation within municipality
	Administration commissioned to develop strategy Financial scheme	Strategy with action plan developed through networks continued from phase 2 Financial scheme established through lobbyism	Continued network from phase 2. Conscious choice not to develop strategy Incremental development in cooperation with growers in yearly reports to city council Financial scheme
Phase 4 Solutions: expanding and refining measures	Pilot scheme for expansion of growing in other municipal sectors. Action plan for urban agriculture under development "Roadmaps" for handling a variety of initiatives	Formalized municipal cross-sectoral coordination not yet developed. Continued external networking Project "outsourced" to voluntary sector and farmers' organization (center for agriculture, city farmer)	Continued informal internal cooperation and external networking. Deepening contact with peri-urban agriculture
Phase 5 Planning according to planning law	Incorporation of urban agriculture within Municipal plan – Societal plan with land use strategy Green roof strategy		Urban agriculture a part of "planning program" for municipal plan for agriculture

In *Trondheim*, the green sectors of the administration were important actors in policy development. They advised politicians to actually realize students' projects in three public spaces where urban agriculture would be showcased, and politicians reacted positively with the implementation of a financial scheme to support urban agriculture.

The city has a strategic approach to base the development of urban agriculture on citizens bottom-up initiatives, since the citizens themselves know best where they would like to grow, favoring locations close to home. To ease access, the property division was mandated to assist initiatives to check ownership to land.

The Trondheim model that emerged from this phase is based on a bottom-up approach grounded in extensive networking and incremental policy adjustments. Trondheim did deliberately choose *not* to develop a strategy. The policy is directly built on the growers' needs, through yearly meetings with the growers' network to gather their experiences and feedback. On average, 30–40 people meet with a few representatives from the largest urban gardening projects, housing cooperatives, volunteers' organizations, beekeepers, schools, and professional farmers interested in cooperative agriculture. Their input feed directly into the administration's yearly report to the politicians on results and use of financial support. This report further suggests policy changes, leaving it to the politicians to set priorities.

When the growers' pointed out that their greatest bottleneck was not financial but related to their lack of knowledge about how to grow, the policy response resulted in prioritization of courses, made available at low cost. On the other hand, top-down policy changes also occurred, like the decision not to prioritize their own municipal schools and kindergartens in their policies originated purely by a political discussion.

12.5.4 Phase Four-Solutions: Expanding and Refining Measures

In *Oslo*, the urban agriculture unit also worked to expand growing activities as a means to achieve goals in other municipal sectors, and a pilot financial scheme was put in place targeted to stimulate other municipal sectors to engage in such activities. Oslo's city council also commissioned an action plan to follow up the strategy, where, for example, land availability was raised as a main point. The latter is important in Oslo, due to the fragmented system of land management between levels of government, sectors, and maintenance systems making it difficult for local initiatives to access land for growing. The priorities in the financing scheme changed and included also small start-up business initiatives.

In *Bergen*, the networking efforts across urban agriculture stakeholders have also been instrumental in establishing new initiatives, including the appointment of the city farmer. Similarly, the engagement of the voluntary sector played an important role in the establishment of *Lystgården*, a center for urban agriculture and the location for the city farmer.

In *Trondheim*, cooperation and networking with the county governor and the farmers' association has led to municipal support for the ordinary commercial agriculture. The aim is to strengthen ties between producers of food and consumers in the city, facilitating the production of "short-traveled" local food.

In all three cities, the county governors have initiated incubator for market gardens.

12.5.5 Phase Five-Urban Agriculture in the Planning System According to the Planning and Building Act

In *Oslo*, urban agriculture was early given attention in the most important planning documents in the municipality, showing the important role of politicians.

In *Bergen*, urban agriculture has to a limited extent been integrated in plans according to the planning and building act.

In *Trondheim*, a "planning program" for municipal plan for agriculture has been developed, where urban agriculture is a part.

Table 12.3 shows an overview over the different phases.

12.6 Analysis: Which Models for Organization of the Urban Agriculture Policy Domain Are Emerging and to Which Extent Are Growers Involved?

The three cities show clear differences in policy arrangements and a few consistent aspects. Our analysis shows that while similarities are common in the initial phase, the organization and further development of policy within the local contexts lead to variations. In Oslo, the public policy evolved initially from political initiatives followed by implementation by the administration. In Bergen and Trondheim, policy development is characterized by a bottom-up and networking approach, which politicians embraced at a later stage. An overview over the characteristics is shown in Table 12.4.

12.6.1 The Effect of Rules of the Game: Inclusion of Growers

A clear difference between our case study cities concerns the way growers are included in the design of public policy. In Trondheim, their inclusion is strong, and the policies and bottom-up approach ensure that the measures are tailored to grower's needs. The inclusion can be described as participatory or indeed co-creational, as growers are invited to contribute directly to policymaking. Trondheim's approach seems particularly well suited to initiatives where urban agriculture is grounded in volunteerism, and public policy needs to nurture such citizen initiatives. Similarly, professional farmers are also able to make contribution, as illustrated by the ongoing work to ensure the funding for a city farmer. In Bergen, the voluntary sector has also been strongly involved, not only in terms of participation but also in lobbying toward politicians in and carrying out initiatives as joint projects. In Oslo, growers are less directly involved in policymaking, but there are channels for information such as Facebook groups. Participatory methods such as workshops and public inspection were used when preparing the strategy for urban agriculture.

Table 12.4 An overview over rules of the game, actors, influence, and discourses in the urban agriculture policy domain in Oslo, Bergen, and Trondheim

Oslo	*Rules of the game*: Strong political leadership and implementation by the administration *Actors*: Politicians, municipal administration in public space management Strong *discourse* on the green city and on social and environmental concerns, increasing emphasis on food production *Influence:* Politicians, administration in public green space management

Bergen	The Bergen model of governance is characterized by:
	    Rules of the game: Strong emphasis on *networking* between municipality, voluntary sector, and county governor. *Political lobbyism* from voluntary sector, limited internal coordination within municipality, "outsourcing" of projects to voluntary sector and farmers' organizations
	    Actors: Strong early role of the *administrations* both at municipal and county level, early strong role of *voluntary sector* involved in transition movement, farmers' organization increasingly involved, politicians increasingly involved
	    Discourse: strong discourse of "green city" central in political platform – but also transformative practices to reach sustainable goals in local communities and in agriculture and food delivery systems
	    Influence: Administration in agriculture at municipal and regional level, voluntary organization, and politicians

Trondheim	*Rules of the game: networking and co-creation* as mode of governance and close collaborations with growers to adjust policies, conscious choice of no strategy but incremental yearly adjustment of policy, close internal municipal cooperation, and close ties with professional agriculture *Actors*: municipal administration in green space management and agriculture, growers, and farmers' unions; close ties with the professional agriculture, shown in urban agriculture's support to professional agriculture and urban agriculture's inclusion in municipal plan for agriculture *Influence:* municipal administration, politicians, strong influence of growers particularly on financial mechanism and farmers *Discourse*: strong emphasis on co-creation and that the growers themselves know best, emphasis on food production "green food city"

12.7   Conclusion

How have public policies for urban agriculture emerged and been institutionalized? In Norway's largest cities, institutionalization of urban agriculture policies has followed the same pattern including the important role of county governors as early initiators. Yet there are clear differences, which relate to: (1) the role of voluntarism groups and bottom-up and top-down processes, (2) the degree of networking, (3) the relationship to ordinary peri-urban agriculture and new forms of urban agriculture, and (4) the implementation of urban agriculture in plans according to the planning and building act.

Oslo policy development was politically driven and implemented through traditional participatory methods with limited engagement of traditional agriculture but guided by a vision for urban agriculture as a social activity in green/urban spaces and as new ways of professional production of food in dense urban areas.

In Bergen, the role of voluntary sector has been strong, and public policy has developed through networking. Voluntary sector has also played a direct political role through its lobbying of politicians for support and received positive response from them. The connection to transformative ideas and new food production and food distribution networks is strong in the voluntary sector.

In Trondheim, the inclusion of growers is also strong, indeed they were co-producing policy together with the administration. Connections to ordinary peri-urban agriculture including the farmers' association are particularly strong in this city. While Oslo and Bergen have created plans for developing urban agriculture, Trondheim has consciously chosen not to do so. Their incremental policy is co-produced with the growers each year based on their experiences.

Which models for organization of the urban agriculture policy domain are emerging and to which extent are growers involved? The Trondheim "bottom-up" model has consciously chosen not to make a strategy for urban agriculture, but to develop their policy incrementally in a dialogue between growers and administration, and finally get it approved by politicians. An important contextual factor is the fact that Trondheim is located in some of the best areas for agriculture in Norway with farms in operation both within the municipal borders and in the neighboring municipalities. Integral to the Trondheim model is the close cooperation with the peri-urban agriculture and the goal is to improve the image and recognition of both urban agriculture and the professional agriculture. This is also a part of branding Trondheim's food city image that also required strengthening alternative food distribution channels. The networking between the municipality, the agricultural division at county governor, the farmers' associations, growers, and research institutions has been important.

Bergen is also an example of strong influence of a self-organized movement of a large number of growers playing an active role as co-creators of policy through political activism and participation in strategy development. Like Trondheim, *networks* between the voluntary movement, the agricultural division at county governor, and farmers' association have been important. The administration early nudged the politicians to support agriculture, but this has gradually been institutionalized, so that the center for urban agriculture, a result from the work of the voluntary movement, has become a fixed item on the municipal budget. Another goal was to establish cross-sectoral ties within the municipality through a cooperation forum.

The Oslo model is an example of political top-down efforts to support urban agriculture and strengthen the initiatives already in place. For the administration, the task was to establish ties to these initiatives and develop a strategy for political decision-making. The Oslo model is politically driven using statutory planning and usual channels for participation through workshops and public hearings, in addition to a Facebook channel for information sharing. This political top-down model in urban agriculture policy meant incorporating urban agriculture into broader strategies for the development of Oslo. The strategic document and the societal part of the municipal master plan linked urban agriculture to urban development, emphasizing attractive, multifunctional green urban spaces, and the vision of the "green city."

Appendix 1 List of Interviewees

Interviewee	Time	Number of interviewees	Interview number
Employee county governor	November 2018	1	1
Urban agriculture municipal coordinators	November 2018	3	2
Social entrepreneur	November 2018	1	3
Social entrepreneur	November 2018	1	4
Developer	December 2018	1	5
City district	December 2018	1	6
Chief of planning department	November 2019	1	7
Case handler planning department	March 2020	1	8
Urban agriculture municipal coordinator	April 2020	1	9
Urban agriculture, municipal coordinator	April 2020	1	10
Urban agriculture city district coordinator	November 2020	1	11
Follow-up interview urban agriculture coordinator municipality	November 2020	1	12
Member of board, local neighborhood association	November 2020	1	13
Follow-up interview municipal coordinator	March 2021	1	14
Follow-up interview municipal coordinator	February 2021	2	15
Follow-up interview municipal coordinator	March2021	1	16
Volunteer organization	March 2021	1	17
Farmers' association	March 2021	1	18
Total		21	18 4 follow-up interviews, 2 group interviews

References

Arbeiderpartiet, Miljøpartiet De Grønne, Sosialistisk Venstreparti. (2019). *Plattform for byrådssamarbeid mellom Arbeiderpartiet, Miljøpartiet De Grønne og Sosialistisk Venstreparti i Oslo 2019–2023.* Oslos byrådserklæring 2019-2023.pdf (Platform for co-operation in City Council between Labour party, Green party, and Socialist Left-wing party in Oslo 2019–2023).

Arts, B., Leroy, P., & van Tatenhove, J. (2006). Political modernisation and policy arrangements: A framework for understanding environmental policy change. *Public Organization Review, 6,* 93–106. https://doi.org/10.1007/s11115-006-0001-4

Bergen municipality. (2019). *Dyrk Bergen. Strategi for urbant landbruk. 2019–2023* (Cultivate Bergen. Strategy for urban agriculture 2019–2023).

Finnegan, L., Perrreux, A., Underdal, M., & Vouters, M.. (2015). *Urban agriculture in Trondheim: Growing the roots of a community.* Course report: Agroecology, NMBU Norwegian University of Life Sciences.

Forsberg, E. M., Tollefsen, K.-R., Leisner, M., & Leivestad, P. (2014). *Urbant landbruk – bærekraftig, synlig og verdsatt,* Fylkesmannen i Oslo og Akershus, Landbruksavdelingen, rapportnr.1/2014 (Urban agriculture- sustainable, visible and appreciated) County Governor Oslo and Akershus, Department of agriculture.

Knutsen, O. (red.). (2017). *The Nordic Models in Political Science: Challenged, but Still Viable?* Fagbokforlaget. ISBN 978-82-450-2175-2. 296 s.

Norwegian Ministries. (2021). Norwegian strategy for urban agriculture. *Cultivate Cities and Towns.* https://www.regjeringen.no/contentassets/4be68221de654236b85b76bd77535571/strategi-for-urbant-landbruk-engelsk-web.pdf

Olsen, J. P. (2007). *Understanding institutions and logics of appropriateness: Introductory essay.* ARENA Centre for European Studies; University of Oslo. Working Paper No. 13, August 2007 https://www.sv.uio.no/arena/english/research/publications/arena-working-papers/2001-2010/2007/wp07_13.pdf

Oslo kommune. (2015a). *Press release: The city council presents an urban agriculture program for Oslo.* 8.9.2015.

Oslo kommune. (2015b). *Kommuneplanens arealdel. Smart, trygg, grønn. Kommuneplan* 2015 Oslo mot 2030 DEL 2. Vedtatt av Oslo bystyre 23.09.2015 (sak 262) (Muninical Master Plan. Land-use part. Smart, safe, green. Municipal plan 2015. Oslo towards 2030).

Oslo kommune. (2019). *Kommuneplan for Oslo 2018. Vår by, vår framtid. En grønnere, varmere og mer skapende by med plass til alle. Visjon, mål og strategier mot 2040.* Vedtatt 30/1–2019 (Municipal Master Plan for Oslo 2018. Our city, our future. A greener, warmer and more creative city with room for everyone. Visions, goals and strategies towards 2040).

Skorupka, A., & Pålsrud, M. (2019). *Erfaringsinnhenting: Forbildeprosjekter innen urbant landbruk i regi av Oslo kommune, 2019 Hovedfunn og anbefalinger.* Rodeo arkitekter AS i samarbeid med Growlab Oslo og Andreas Capjon (Experiences: Model projects in urban agriculture conducted by Oslo municipality 2019. Main findings and advice.) https://www.oslo.kommune.no/getfile.php/13370468-1591077746/Tjenester%20og%20tilbud/Natur%2C%20kultur%20og%20fritid/Urbant%20landbruk/Utforsk%20det%20spirende%20Oslo/Erfaringer%20fra%20kommunale%20forbindeprosjekter.pdf

Part V

A Way Forward for Urban Agriculture in Cities and Communities

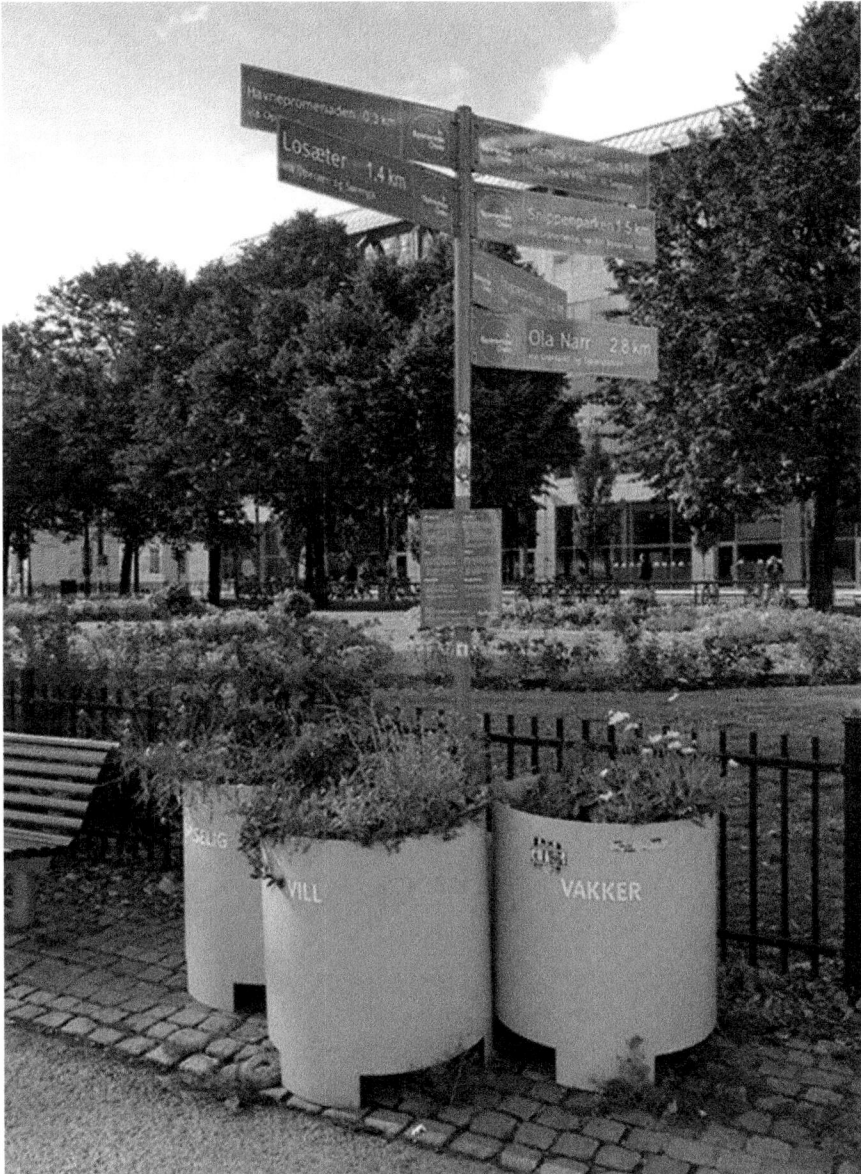

Part 6
Why Care about Peri-urban agriculture:
Cities and Conurbations

Chapter 13
Raising the Ambition of Urban Agriculture in Public Space: Nurturing Urban Agroecology and More-than-Human Health

Chiara Tornaghi

13.1 Introduction

In the last 20–25 years, urban agriculture has been variously embraced by public authorities, NGOs, research agencies, scholars, and civil society actors, across cities of both, the Global North and South. By 'embracing' I refer to a range of approaches: from a simple tolerance of grassroots, semi-illegal, activities such as guerrilla gardening and street verge planting in public space, to the endorsement, pro-active encouragement, direct funding, or even celebration and regulation, with national days[1] and specific local strategies.[2] Urban agriculture is today one of the most multidimensional and multipurpose activities, with all the criteria and features to become the panacea par-excellence of the new century to tackle the many problems of urbanisation. Given that many of these problems relate to environmental damage, food production footprints, climate change and food-related health diseases, urban agriculture is in many ways closely related to each of them. Urban agriculture is claimed to improve urban resilience to heath waves, floods and climate change through its many ecosystem 'services'[3] (Ebissa & Desta, 2022; Maassen & Galvin, 2021; Dubbeling, 2013; Dubbeling et al., 2019; Piacentini et al., 2016), to promote environmental education (Scheromm & Javelle, 2022); to contribute to biodiversity;

---

[1] For example the National Day of Urban Farming, in the Netherlands, instituted in 2012.

[2] See for example Rotterdam's (Netherlands), Ghent's (Belgium) and Barcelona's (Catalunia, Spain) urban agriculture strategies.

[3] Such as the absorption of excess rainfalls, the mitigation and stabilisation of environmental temperatures due to the air cooling effects of vegetation, and the reduction of greenhouse gas emission, when organic urban waste is used a natural fertiliser, instead of chemical fertilisers and landfill of urban waste.

C. Tornaghi (✉)
Centre for Agroecology, Water and Resilience (CAWR), Coventry University, Coventry, UK
e-mail: Chiara.tornaghi@coventry.ac.uk

© The Author(s) 2024
B. Sirowy, D. Ruggeri (eds.), *Urban Agriculture in Public Space*, GeoJournal Library 132, https://doi.org/10.1007/978-3-031-41550-0_13

to tackle urban malnutrition and food security (Hammelman, 2018); to promote food justice (Alkon & Agyeman, 2011; Gottlieb & Joshi, 2010), food sovereignty (Heynen et al., 2012) and food literacy; to promote reconnection between consumers and producers (Lyson, 2004) to increase social inclusion and community cohesion (Nordahl, 2009; Petit-Boix & Apul, 2018); to improve mental health (Ambrose et al., 2020), urban diets and general well-being (Wakefield et al., 2007; Ribeiro et al., 2015; Graham et al., 2018), to diversify urban aesthetics (Lindemann-Matthies & Brieger, 2016); to raise real estate values (Vitiello & Wolf-Powers, 2014); and to be at the forefront of new urban green economies, urban regeneration and sustainable food systems (Hou et al., 2009; Lovell, 2010). And I have surely forgotten more. The good news is that, to some extent and in certain conditions, urban agriculture can contribute to all the above. The bad news is that in many cases it either does not (Tornaghi, 2017), or it may cause harm (Engel-Di Mauro, 2012, 2018, 2021b; Nabulo et al., 2012).

In the last decade, the literature illustrating these practices has grown exponentially, providing examples from every corner of the world illustrating how it works. Less prolific has been the literature illustrating when urban agriculture is not fulfilling its promises: when it does not deliver, when it is mobilised with regressive goals or results, when it is instrumentalised as a tool to disempower indigenous communities or grassroots groups claiming for land access and resource sovereignty, when it is used to justify cuts to welfare state structures and social health spending in the context of austerity politics, when it is explicitly used to promote gentrification and people's displacement and when it is the only existing way to access basic food, but it is carried out on polluted soils and generally when the problems outweigh the benefits. Fortunately, while less extensive, there is a solid body of literature in this field too, which provide tools for political and practical orientation, self-reflection and critical policy development (Richardson & Kingsbury, 2005; Pudup, 2008; Rosol, 2010; McKay, 2011; Meenar & Hoover, 2012; Galt et al., 2014; McClintock, 2014; Tornaghi, 2014; Weissman, 2014; Cadieux & Slocum, 2015; Reynolds, 2015; Walker, 2016; Tornaghi, 2017; Horst et al., 2017; McClintock, 2018; Sbicca, 2019; Lal, 2016, Engel-Di Mauro, 2018, 2021a, b, etc.).

Over the past 15 years, I have navigated the groups above, moving from the first (the ones we could call 'the advocates') to the second ('the critics'), and in between, I have been elected chair of the AESOP's 'Sustainable Food Planning'" group, a community of academics and practitioners affiliated to European schools of planning and/or engaged in researching and theorising sustainable food planning and territorial food systems. Through both, my personal and academic experience across these groups, I have come to understand the advocacy attitude as a direct representation of the degree to which food growing has been alienated from people's lives and have been absent from the discourses and research in planning. The greater the alienation and the understanding of its multidimensional ramifications, the greater the enthusiasm and hopes for its reconquering, for remediation and for building a different world. The practice of urban agriculture is cathartic; it reconnects us to our ancestors, and it brings wonders to the fore. The magic of seeds sprouting, the scent of fertile soils, the incredible and forgotten taste of freshly picked food. The joyous colours and shapes of nature, taking shape in front of us. Their nourishing power on bodies and souls is palpable. It is hard not to dream of urban agriculture everywhere: of getting children pulling up carrots and joyfully picking berries and of turning streets and parks and people's gardens into cornucopias of delights. Food growing reconnects us to our roots, ancestors, intuitions and facilitates a deeper sensory engagement with the natural elements of our environments and their healing properties.

On the other hand, I have come to understand the degree of criticism also present in the field as a direct representation of people's first-hand engagement with the making of urban agriculture and with a practice-based understanding of the structural and systemic obstacles to overcome to make it work in a way that is socially, ecologically and economically just. The lost food growing knowledge, the polluted lands and waters, the ambiguous, double-binary approach of public institutions to land rents and soil testing (not at the service of grassroots food growing), the ongoing undervaluing of soil care, the omnipresent use of legal harmful substances such as pesticides and herbicides commonly in use in community gardens, allotments and public parks, the expectations of vulnerable people's ability to grow their own food in the face of exploitative working and housing conditions, the unfair and inequitable institutional support for unsustainable food systems, alongside a benevolent acceptance of urban agriculture as 'hobbyist' (and related lack of financial investment). The list of contradictions and obstacles is long and enraging and effectively disabling people's ability to build food sovereignty.

From a scholar-activist or socially engaged scholarship perspective, moving from the first group (the advocates) to the second (the critics) is surely a necessity. While positive and promotional discussions around urban agriculture can be generative of innovative ideas and endeavours, the day-to-day functioning of business as usual, social marginalisation and capital accumulation often create barriers and reinforce their negative impacts through the very unfolding of urban agriculture itself (Tornaghi, 2017).

Given the great flexibility with which urban agriculture is mobilised and used in society and policy today and the often highly contradictory outcomes, it is important to enter this field with clear positioning and a clear awareness of both, the pros and cons of certain types of urban agriculture, forms of support and policy frameworks.

The discussion I offer in this short contribution is built from the perspective of a specific type of urban agriculture: urban agroecology.

Urban agroecology is a politically, socially and ecologically positioned segment of urban agriculture (Deh-Tor, 2017; Tornaghi & Dehaene, 2021; for other accounts of urban agroecology, see also Bowen-Siegner et al., 2020 and Nicklay et al., 2020). The defining features of urban agroecology are the principles that govern its social and ecological choices, which are rooted in agroecology. Agroecology is simultaneously a movement, a science and a practice (Wezel et al., 2009), rooted in indigenous and traditional ways of knowing and cultivating soils that were passed down through generations (Mendez et al., 2016; Rosset et al., 2019). Ecologically, it is based on resource conservation and regeneration, biodiversity preservation, care for more-than-human life above and below ground, circular closed-loops farming system and planetary health. Socially, it is based on valuing, celebrating and defending cultural diversity and social equity, on territorially grounded ways of knowing and doing, on food sovereignty and on promoting feminist, anti-patriarchal, anti-colonialist, anti-capitalist and anti-heteronormative practices (Milgroom, 2021).

An 'urban' agroecology therefore differs from a more general urban agriculture in the sense that it makes clear how it stands towards certain choices to be made when engaging in the cultivation of urban soils. For example, urban agroecology will embrace soil-based agriculture for its benefits to soil life and biodiversity and its acknowledgement of the relationship between plants' health and their environment, rather than being open to, or even promoting, energy intensive, soil-less and chemical-dependent vertical farming. It will mobilise companion-planting, natural predators and deeper understanding of the web-of-life to manage 'weeds' and 'pests' (which will be recognised as having their own role in the ecosystem), rather than using oil-based and soil-polluting pesticides and herbicides. Socially, urban agroecology will promote inclusive and equitable forms of producing and sharing food that value farmers dignified livelihoods and celebrates their diverse knowledge, over market-based, exploitative, profit-oriented new 'green' capitalist economies.

Choosing urban agroecology versus urban agriculture means celebrating the mutual interdependency between planetary/ecosystem/more-than-human health, people's well-being and plants' happiness, rather than adopting an anthropocentric perspective based on short-term, selective and exclusive social gains. While many urban agricultural practices will happen to be aligned to urban agroecology values, it is important to develop a discerning capacity, to be able to make informed practical and policy choices that do not – intentionally or unintentionally – end up producing harmful outcomes to the landscapes and the people living in it.

Looking at urban agriculture from the perspective of urban agroecology, in this chapter I aim to contribute to the development of planning policy for the promotion of agroecological food growing in public space. In Section 13.2, after an overview of key challenges of current urbanisation and their intersection with public space and urban agriculture, I will offer a selection of illustrative cases of urban agriculture in public space promoted by local authorities, which offer some space of reflection about their social and ecological limitations.

In Section 13.3, I will then offer a few considerations to guide policy development for urban agroecology in urban public space, with particular attention to its health enhancing dimensions.

13.2   Food Growing in Public Space: Intersection with Key Contemporary Urbanisation Challenges

Processes of (western) urbanisation are known to be unsustainable and a major contribution to social and ecological crisis. Exponential growth of world population and its concentration in urban centres pose the question of who will grow the food for this multitude, particularly given the growing trends in the consumption of non-local and resource-hungry crops and meats; the long food miles and fossil fuel-based agriculture contribute to a fast progressing climate change, with recurrent and more frequent impact on droughts and floods; land and soil loss due to pollution, deforestation and overdevelopment/soil sealing pose the question of how to maintain a fragile ecosystem balance and preserve healthy soils while also meeting the housing and food needs of growing urban populations. The fast growth of urban centres is also often related to rural-to-urban migration trends, linked to farm workers pushed out of their lands – by unstainable working and living conditions or loss of land altogether – and ending up living in marginal settlements characterised by deep social vulnerability (i.e. economic inequality, social polarisation and diet-related health issues). In short, the complex economic, industrial and agricultural machine that keeps urban centres powered is based on unsustainable planetary ecological footprints and exploitative socio-economic models (for a deeper overview of these issues, see the many contributions in the edited anthology by Tornaghi & Dehaene, 2021).

These issues feature quite high up in the agenda of cities, regions, national governments and international agencies, who see the ramifications of these problems as increasingly interconnected, and a number of strategic documents and objectives have been set up to, allegedly, make some progress against them: the EU Green New Deal, UN-Habitat's New Urban Agenda, the UN Sustainable Development Goals and the Glasgow 'Food and climate' declaration are just a few known examples (see related links in the reference list). As we know, however, progress towards appropriate regulation and national commitments towards shared goals to tackle these problems is either minimal or inexistent, and the efforts currently at play utterly unfit for the challenges ahead.

Nonetheless, and possibly even more so, it is useful to highlight how the cultivation of public space might bring some positive outcomes towards these goals, with the proviso that none of themselves will ever be sufficient or should be intended in substitution of major substantial commitments in many other spheres of intervention. In the next pages, I will begin with offering a few illustrative cases to begin a critical conversation on the role that urban agriculture may play to tackle these issues.

13.2.1 Urban Agriculture for Social Cohesion, Subsistence and Health

The cultivation of food in public space has been claimed to contribute to increase the intake of fresh seasonal foods, to strengthen social cohesion through people's interaction in the neighbourhood and to better human health through diet change, physical exercise and improved human relations.

The 'Back to Front' project in Leeds, a medium city in the West Yorkshire region in England, was promoted in 2010 by the Public Health department of the city council in a socio-economically disadvantaged area of the city – a neighbourhood with among the highest levels of multiple deprivation across the whole country (for other accounts of this project see also Oldroyd & Clavin, 2013). The programme, which was led by a civil servant in the council, partnered with local NGOs, volunteers and academics in a local university, with the aim to help designing food growing spaces in people's front gardens and in fringe or interstitial public spaces. The programme included some mentoring to the people that engaged with the initiative, to support them to acquire food growing skills and to create containers for growing food,[4] using upcycled households' materials, including ordinary milk bottles and other packaging. The programme came at a time when a government reform to the National Health System (NHS) transferred a series of responsibilities related to community health into the hands of local authorities. The change, which came alongside a wave of austerity funding cuts and restructuring, was the drive to invest in prevention programmes and community building, of which the Back to Front project is an example. The central idea of this project was that moving food growing from the back to the front of a house, into the public sphere, or sometimes directly into public space, would be an incentive to create talking points, reduce social isolation and strengthen community cohesion. In the context of austerity politics, the community would become the first point of support for isolated individuals and end up substituting the publicly funded community centres, social centres, children centres and family hubs (and later on a swimming pool and libraries) that were no longer funded and were due to be phased out from public spending budgets.

Similar initiatives have been reported elsewhere, with local authorities recognising and appreciating not only the social cohesion element of community gardening and urban agriculture but also its importance to do physical exercise, increase sun exposure to raise vitamin D levels in the body and enhance intake of fresh food within social groups whose diets (and particularly fruit and veg intake) have been impacted the most by financial difficulties.

While promoting social cohesion and fresh food intake seem worthwhile initiatives, the reality is however more complex. Some civil servants with whom I spoke over the years noted the ongoing lack of resources to maintain adequate support to these initiatives, as well as the wide range of skills that they had to mobilize. So, while the rationale to maintain and promote urban agriculture was to increase community cohesion in the context of growing inequality and social diversity, these initiatives – and particularly community gardens and their surrounding communities – are often highly conflictual, problematic or highly demanding environments that require social workers' skills for mediation between diverse age, gender, cultural and ethnic groups with diverging needs, expectations or desires (see also Veen et al., 2015; Barron, 2018), as well as support with fundraising to acquire needed infrastructure, training and annual consumables. Within the context of austerity politics, however, these initiatives are expected to become self-governing and cost-free for local authorities, while in fact without long-term investment in social

---

[4] Containers for food growing were needed because most people had paved or concreted-over front yards, and the quality of the soil underneath was unknown.

learning and upskilling, they can at best be sustained through shifting of public budgets from one department to another, rather than cutting, or risk becoming yet another contention issue within neighbourhoods that are already challenged and affected by multiple layers of deprivation.

13.2.2 Urban Agriculture for Climate and Economic Resilience

The cultivation of urban public space has also been promoted in relation to climate and economic resilience. While the two – economic and climate resilience – are rather different issues, they also intersect in many ways; hence, I am offering a joint discussion here, particularly with reference to public policies.

One of the most prominent effects of climate change – besides its impact on agricultural productivity and biodiversity preservation – is its impact on price volatility. Sudden prolonged droughts or unpredictable and extreme weather events such as floods and impact on harvest quality and quantity have been seen impacting negatively on the amount of food that countries were willing or able to trade and therefore on demands and prices, with the results that many communities, both in the global north and south, have found themselves struggling to afford food (Kaufman, 2010).

Climate change and economic difficulties are also both connected to rural-to-urban migration, with often the most vulnerable communities of farm workers leaving the farms to land in precarious living conditions in urban contexts, searching for better living and working opportunities, which, however, aren't always there.

In both North and South, local authorities have been promoting urban agriculture to mitigate some of these effects. Offering plots of land in public parks, greenbelts or interstitial urban areas – often unfit for other uses, such as housing – food growing has been a popular choice. However, again, the results can be mixed and contradictory.

I return to the city of Leeds with another significant example. In 2013, the municipality made available a list of public parks and green spaces where food growing would be possible, if a community group would come forward (for other accounts of this event, see also Tornaghi, 2017). These spaces were less regulated than the city community allotments in terms of who, for how long and for what uses grows food there.[5] So, while the city was planning a threefold increase in allotment rents (in the attempt to compensate for government funding cuts that were beginning to

---

[5] Community allotments are the results of historical political negotiations and are regulated nationally with legislation that usually guarantee long leases and affordable prices, but that also prevents these spaces from becoming commercial growing space, by sanctioning that all food produced should be used for member's own consumption. For an overview on the difference between allotments and community gardens see Tornaghi (2019). For an historical overview of allotments, see Crouch and Ward (1988).

painfully impact on other key social services), these green spaces were offered with the hope they would be discharged from the Park Department's direct maintenance and could become places where communities could grow food – potentially also for economic purposes. Besides the fact that an increase in allotment rents on the assumption that allotment holders were a bunch of middle-class people who could afford highly increased costs was wrong and going to impact severely on thousands of families relying on these plots for their fresh food, there were other problems with this manoeuvre. The conditions for undertaking a lease in one of these parks were that no fencing could be erected around the plots; no water collection was to be carried out with structures or tubs; no mulching and no 'messy' looking activity was to be carried out, as these would have 'spoiled' the aesthetic of the park; no animals could be kept on site (neither for direct consumption, not for 'pest' management); and no 'weeds' were to be seen. In short, this would have made very difficult to practice agroecological or permaculture approaches to growing food, which notoriously avoid external inputs and aim to recycle and reuse existing resources in situ and would have made very difficult to ensure a reliable harvest. Obviously, the initiative hasn't been very successful, as the rules weren't based on any solid understanding of what it takes to grow a plant (i.e. water), and because without soil fertility maintenance (composting stations, mulching) and natural ecosystem and pest management (i.e. ducks, frogs, ponds, companion planting), the gardeners would have likely had to rely on noxious, expensive, and soil-damaging industrial agrochemicals to be able to achieve a crop.

It is interesting to compare this case with what another city has done with their public land at a time of financial difficulties and growing social exclusion. The city of Rosario, Argentina, has offered a rather different set of opportunities for urban agriculture. Over the past 20 years, the municipality has invested in resourcing local vulnerable communities and migrants with a farming background with opportunity to access land not only for their own personal consumption but also for their ability to make a living. Over the years, the farmers could count on a municipality-supported seed bank (see Fig. 13.1), on free access to land, on free access to urban organic wastes for soil improvement (Fig. 13.2), on engagement in public events for the promotion of local agroecological food and on market access to commercialise their produce in several markets across the city.

Recognising the multiple benefits to human flourishing, climate mitigation (particularly heatwaves and floods reduction), healthy soil maintenance, protection of bio-cultural diversity and containment of speculative development, the city administration has been acquiring land and regulating farm business in and around cities, phasing out the use of agrochemicals and providing education and coaching to ease the transition to agroecological farming. The urban farming programme has been endorsed by different departments within the public administration and linked to different goals, for example, both economic development, parks/public space maintenance and social programmes, and in so doing maximising their respective resources and supporting each other's goals. The existence of thousands of cultivated parcels across the city, and about 600 baking ovens in public parks, has proved to be a great resource of food during different waves of economic and food crisis

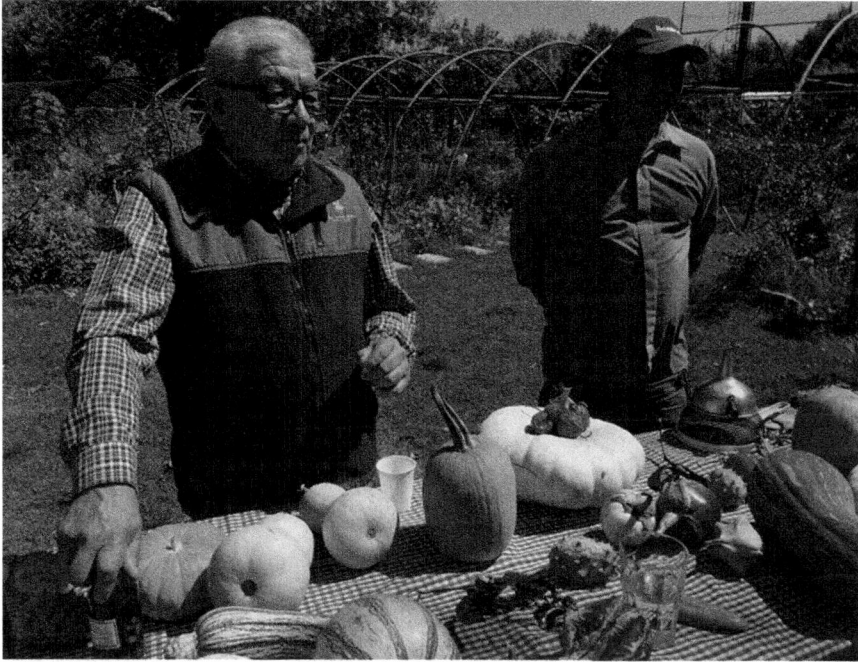

Fig. 13.1 An exhibition of biodiverse crops and seeds at the municipal seed bank of Rosario, Argentina, during a visit from an international delegation of the Urbanising in Place project (February 2019) (Source: Chiara Tornaghi)

since 2002, including the Covid-19 pandemic (for other accounts on Rosario's urban agriculture programme see also Piacentini et al., 2016; Lattuca, 2017; Tornaghi & Dehaene, 2020; Maassen & Galvin, 2021; Hammelman et al., 2022). The case, centred around the provision of public land and public parks to build agroecology-rooted new livelihoods, is in stark contrast with the far too common exploitation of urban agriculture as a rhetorical remedy to the growing urban food poverty, with the expectation that people in need, already burdened by underpaid jobs, long commutes and child and elders care, can take on another task to ensure their own survival.

13.2.3 Common Shortcoming of Urban Planning for Urban Agriculture

As we can see from the examples illustrated in the two sections above, while urban agriculture is engaged and promoted by public authorities with the best intentions, positive results are dependent on municipal intersectoral collaboration, social workers' skills and a deep engagement with long-term social and institutional learning, rather than short-term, money-saving goals.

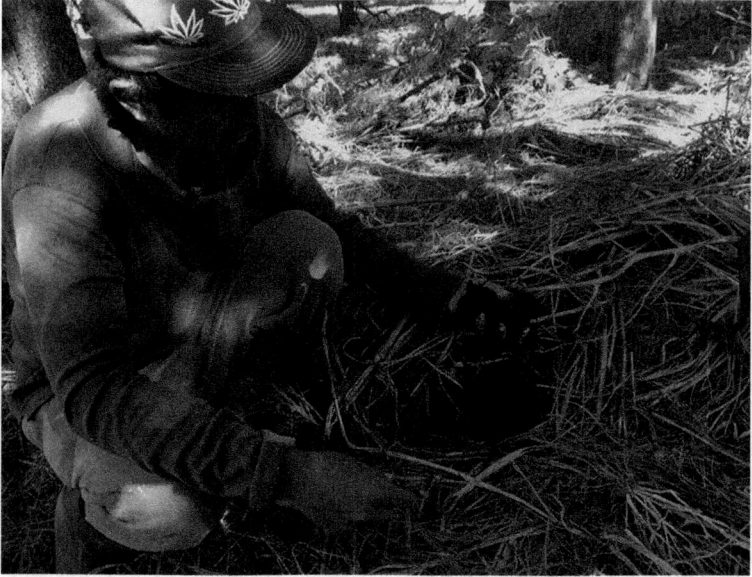

Fig. 13.2 A farmer from the municipal urban and peri-urban agriculture programme of Rosario, showing the high-quality compost made with organic urban waste (urban leaves, urban grass and cow's rumen). Source: Chiara Tornaghi

Over the past years, the multiplication of grassroots initiatives in urban agriculture, alongside institutional concerns for rising diet-related problems, a progressively weakening European farming sector, and research-led debates on the need of a food system approach, has sparked the rise of a number of city networks that have provided support to both municipal actors and public-private partnerships, for the appropriate support and development of food system interventions (i.e. the Milan Urban Food Policy Pact-MUFPP, the Sustainable Food Places coalition in the UK, the Spanish Network of Agroecological Cities, the Organic Cities network in Austria, etc.).

These networks, together with pioneering research associations (i.e. AESOP), have succeeded in further shaping the EU research agenda and making available more funding for research and innovation in this sector. As we speak, a handful of funded research networks are exploring economic and policy opportunities related to urban agriculture.

Despite considerable progress has been made in the past years, including the development of urban agricultural strategies and policy briefs for the inclusion of urban agriculture in the built environment,[6] as of today, these guides remain

---

[6] Some examples are Brighton City Council's guide 'Food Growing and Development. Planning advice note', Sustain's guide 'Food growing in parks. A guide for councils', and Ghent municipality urban agriculture strategy 'Ghent en Garde'. All links are included in the references.

voluntary, non-committing guidelines, which are often de facto, contradicted by non-coherent and self-defeating policies in other municipal sectors, which run opposite aims. Recent research has shown, for example, that the municipality of Ghent, in Belgium, while having developed one of the most acclaimed packages of policies and guides to support sustainable food systems, has also systematically engaged in the sale of public farmland for urban development or biodiversity preservation (Vandermaelen et al., 2022). This is one exemplary case of not-so-unusual incoherent public policies and evidence that current urban planning and land policies remain inappropriate to fully support the promotion of urban agriculture in an ecological and socio-economic justice vein. Here, below, I offer some additional illustrations of areas where this is most apparent.

13.2.4 Contradictory Considerations of Urban Agriculture as a Food-Producing Practice

The food-producing aspects of urban agriculture are acknowledged with significant difference across the public sector, particularly when these bring into question institutional regulation, public investment and service provision.

A strong emphasis is posed on urban agriculture as a new economic activity when this is carried out by new enterprises/businesses through 'innovative' practices often linked to circular economy discourses, such as indoor mushroom cultivation using organic waste as a substrate (i.e. coffee grounds recovered from urban cafes and restaurants), or vertical agriculture and aquaponics in disused (private) former industrial buildings. Under the traction of 'green economic growth', or even the obscure appeal of gentrifying effects and their reverberations on multiple economic activities, these types of urban agriculture are welcomed and sometimes incentivised with support to obtain external funding.[7] When soil-based urban farming activities, however, seek for municipal support to accessing public land, though, they rarely find the same level of enthusiasm, and they find themselves in competition with other (more remunerative) land uses. The ecological value of local production and short food miles remains secondary to land revenues, and land values (and politics) remain strongly connected to speculative powers and development opportunities. The availability of farmland only at full market prices (either, from the onset, or within a short timeframe) means that new local farmers struggle to set up new businesses, given the competition with mainstream food available at a fraction of their costs (Maughan et al., 2021; Tornaghi, 2017). More support tends to be available when urban agriculture is practiced with explicit social benefits, for

---

[7] An exemplar case is the redevelopment of the old abattoir of Anderlecht, in Brussels (see link in reference list), through a mix of urban agriculture and other up-market food initiatives and their explicit gentrifying effects, which were able to obtain European structural development funds despite their negative impact on migrant and vulnerable communities who depended on the popular market pre-existing in the area, for access to culturally appropriate and affordable food.

example, the employment of young offenders, or for community building. Smaller, and non-strategic, pieces of land might be more easily accessed by citizens and community groups when the emphasis is put on crime reduction, social cohesion and physical exercise rather than on its productive and diet-changing power. The assumption that non-remunerated urban agriculture is hobbyist and not leading to significant food intake might be at the basis of municipal lack of engagement with regulation and information (i.e. information campaigns about soil pollutants, soil testing facility or requirements) necessary to practice urban agriculture safely in potentially highly polluted soils. The lack of understanding of, or consideration for, the productive aspects of urban agriculture in these contexts is clearly also at the root of the lack of consideration for the reproduction of soil fertility and soil caring practices, water provision and other factors necessary for the productivity of this practice, as we will discuss further in the point below.

13.2.5   *Invisibility of Soil and Lack of Understanding of the Role of Living Soils and Soil Carers*

Despite 'soil' having surged to one of the key drivers of this year European Research agenda, there is extraordinarily little understanding within municipal planning groups of the role of healthy living soils in agriculture. This means that not only healthy soils are commonly regularly damaged or destroyed by conventional public space practices (e.g. through the regular use of herbicides and pesticides in parks), but the necessary practices needed to maintain and regenerate such soils are often banned, even when urban agriculture is supported in principle. Community gardens in public space, for example, are often limited to growing in mobile structures (i.e. containers), or in temporary spaces, which limits the possibility of a healthy mycorrhizal life and the nourishing exchanges between crops and long-rooted plants, or the planting of permanent crops such as fruit trees and fruit bushes. The conceptualisation of urban agriculture as a mobile practice that can be moved elsewhere when other, more profitable, uses come up (such as building parking lots or new developments), is also a sign of the deep ignorance over the (long!) time it takes to build healthy soils and the role that place attachment plays on people's motivation to cultivate.

13.3   Deepening the Ecological Roots of Urban Agriculture: Considerations for Nurturing an Urban Agroecology

As I have shown in the discussion above, while there is an emerging interest for urban agriculture as a multifunctional practice, municipal and planning approaches that could support it are often contradictory and suboptimal. In this section, I aim to go a bit deeper in the illustration of agroecology and how it can inform municipal planning approaches to the cultivation of public space and public land, in ways that break with the status quo and are more conducive to human and more-than-human equity, justice and health.

13.3.1 Biocultural Diversity: Soil Practices that Address an Expanded Definition of Health

The agroecological cultivation of urban soils (and soils more in general) is based on a deep understanding of the interconnection between healthy soils, healthy plants and healthy people. Agroecological practices are based on the reproduction of soil fertility: this means that the production of food is not only based on healthy and naturally sourced soil inputs (i.e. nitrogen, minerals organic fractions) but that these inputs are sourced locally, and the cultivation practices adopted enable the regeneration/reproduction of these resources or their recovery, through circular, 'closed loops', typically through turning organic 'wastes' into fertility inputs. While in rural setting a whole range of regenerative soil practices can easily be done through the use of animal manures and/or the use of organic fractions coming from woodland management and vegetable production, on-farm closed cycles are very difficult in urban setting, where small plots are often monofunctional (i.e. horticulture, so do not have access to animal manures), or where gardeners and farmers do not have time, space and sometimes knowledge for composting or easy access to these natural soil fertility inputs due to the lack of neighbouring farms. Specific social arrangements are therefore needed to access these from other sources across the city, and farmers would immensely benefit from municipal political will to enable sourcing and distribution, on the model experimented in the municipality of Rosario, Argentina. Planning for urban agroecology could consider the location of different suitable urban organic wastes across the city and enable transportation to the farms or access to appropriate composting sites. Urban municipal waste, for example, green leaves, tree trimmings, grass mowing or food waste from municipal canteens and cafeterias could be diverted towards these composting sites and become a key enabling infrastructure for a thriving urban agroecology, while at the same time reducing urban waste destined to landfill. Municipal (farm)lands could also be strategically used to support circular soil regeneration practices in a landscape in which farming is increasingly fragmented, challenged and endangered by processes of urbanisation.

Plants grown in healthy, fertile, undisturbed, soils (e.g. through no-dig and permaculture approaches in polycultures) can benefit from the network of soil organisms such as mycorrhiza (fungi) living in symbiotic relations with their roots and enabling the exchange of nutrients between plants (Stamets, 2005) (Figs. 13.3 and 13.4).

Such plants are stronger, less prone to diseases and healthier. Research on the effect of cultivations and environmental factors on plants' secondary metabolites has identified that wild plants contain more and/or stronger medicinal compounds

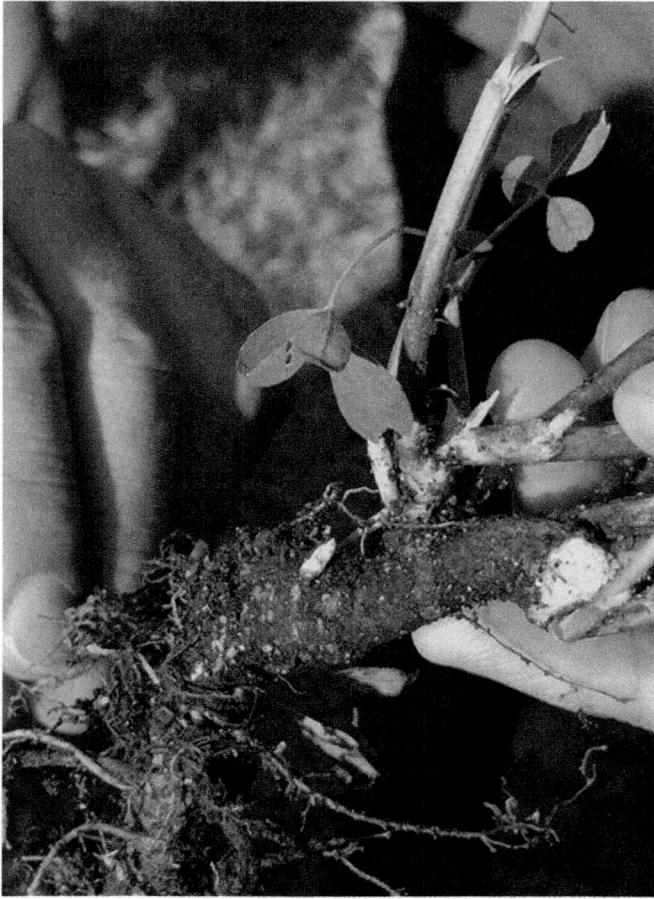

Fig. 13.3 Exploring nitrogen fixing plants' roots and their interaction with mycorrhiza, during a workshop at the Organic Lea urban farm, in London (September 2019) (Source: Chiara Tornaghi)

than conventionally grown plants or greenhouse-grown plants (Clemensen et al., 2020; Ku et al., 2020; Strzemski et al., 2020; Pant et al., 2021): the evidence is aligned with agroecology's philosophy (as well as many indigenous and traditional cosmovisions, from Pacha Mama to Taoism) that soil health, plant health and human health are connected (Tornaghi et al., 2023).

Alongside the centrality of soil health, a second element of urban agroecology for the promotion of human health is its cherishing of cultural and territorial embeddedness and the respect for the knowledge practices, spiritual values and socioeconomic well-being of its practitioners – while recognising them as one among the many soil-dependent 'critters'.

Being practiced in socially just conditions based on principles of equity is essential for agroecology. This means that agroecological projects – whether hobbyist or commercial – will strive for inclusiveness, multicultural diversity and human

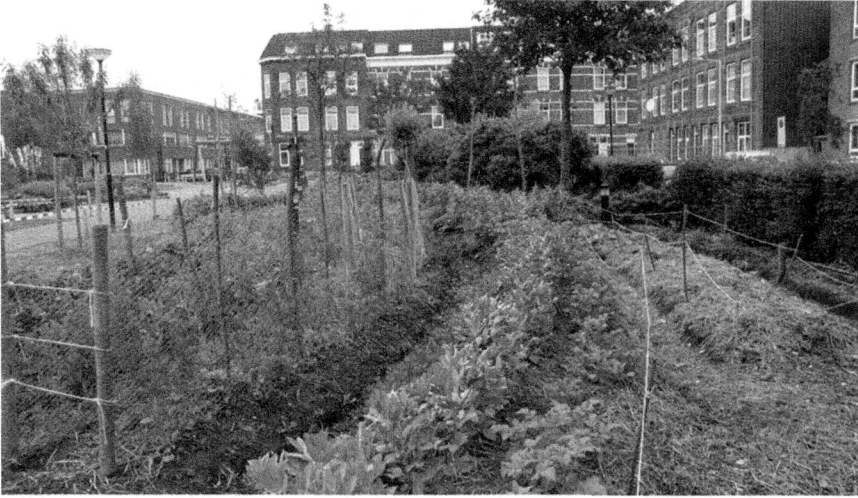

Fig. 13.4 A permaculture-designed open community garden in a public square in Rotterdam (Source: Chiara Tornaghi)

flourishing, rejecting exploitative working conditions and purely profit-oriented endeavours: in short, who grows and who eats count. Acknowledging the lasting impact of colonialism, racism and patriarchy, agroecological practices also strive for restorative and healing work, interweaving the spiritual, embodied and sociocultural reparation together with soil care.

Planning authorities willing to take urban agriculture a step beyond purely productivist or hobbyist community building initiatives, and harness its healing potential, should learn to discern and support initiatives that promote biocultural diversity and more-than-human health through their value orientation and the diversity of knowledge practices deployed around soil and land care.

13.3.2   Knowledge Practices That Heal the Epistemic Rift Between Nature and Society

In the context of a mass deskilling in the realm of food and health (and their interconnection), the urban cultivation of public space through agroecological practices bears the potential to heal the deep knowledge and epistemic rift between society and nature. In their enlightening paper, Schneider and McMichael (2010) have beautifully illustrated how, over the past centuries, humans have grown progressively apart from nature – of which they are part – creating living conditions that have impeded the reproduction of fundamental ecological knowledge needed to respect and maintain the conditions of our own same existence. In short, we have largely forgotten that we have forgotten and normalised unhealthy living conditions, diets and environmental destruction on a global scale. Some of this knowledge, however, still exist within societies where the respect for 'Mother Earth' (through concept such as Pacha Mama, or Buen Vivir) has remained central. It is in these contexts that agroecology as a movement was born, with the intention to fight back against western, colonial, capitalist and patriarchal practices of erasure, which mobilised modernist ideas to label as 'outdated' most ecologically sound cultivating and medicinal practices developed over generations by indigenous people. Healing the epistemic rift and re-building this lost knowledge are often a central element of new urban agroecology initiatives.

As knowledge is always embodied and situated (Geertz, 1983 and Haraway, 1991 in Schneider & McMichael, 2010), the social reproduction of agroecological, food and health knowledge requires spaces where to be put into practice and where different knowledge holders can share it in meaningful and self-directed ways, always in dialogic relations with their environment.

Appreciating that the recovery of knowledge and the healing of rifts within disabling urbanisation (Tornaghi, 2017) is a key challenge for contemporary societies, requiring appropriate time and spaces, municipal authorities could deploy a powerful tool in their hands: public space has an enormous potential to offer an experimental ground, free from market pressures. The availability of public spaces across neighbourhoods, easily accessible to a wider range of communities, means that public authorities hold a fundamental resource for this task. However, sufficient freedom in terms of design and activities needs to be available to local users and residents in these setting, to be able to unfold all the necessary ecological (i.e. composting, mulching, companion planting, etc.) and social activities (i.e. people's gatherings in horizontal participatory processes, training, convivial activities, political and civic engagement, etc.) at the core of urban agroecology. Ensuring that different communities are supported with appropriate infrastructure (i.e. access to water, seeds, availability of urban organic waste, existence of shelter or proximity to a community centre, regular soil testing, or at least at the onset of the project, tools storage, etc) and social support (i.e. social workers to support potentially conflicting communities, support with fundraising, etc), in line with their specific needs, and that these provision do not come in substitution but in addition of existing welfare services will be a social investment, which could harbour the potential to bring multidimensional health benefits.

13.3.3   Reproductive Commons: Land and Food Sharing Practices that Challenge the Commodification of Everything

Alongside the promotion of biocultural diversity and the restorative work to heal the epistemic rift between humans and nature, the cultivation of urban public space can be promoted to foster the reconstruction of reproductive commons: to build and share convivial spaces of social reproduction that challenge the commodification of everything. Urban environments are largely spaces that disable the possibility of peoples to collectively shape their natural environments and build mutual solidarities based on de-commodified access to key resources. Both houses and allotments tend to be individualised spaces, not designed for groups of users sharing these resources. Urban public space and green space tends to be managed in ways that discourage deep forms of engagement and reinterpretations of uses and functions and tend to privilege transient uses. Turning public spaces into urban commons that enable people's agency, sense of belonging and the performance of non-consumerist practices requires to find the right balance between people's appropriation and the maintenance of a certain degree of openness so that a diverse range of communities can benefit from them. While this might seem challenging, the identification of even small patches of land dedicated to communities' self-organisation can be important training grounds where experimental sharing practices can unfold (Fig. 13.5).

The multitude of grassroots initiatives sprouting in marginal, interstitial spaces of the city, from guerrilla grafting to street verges cultivation, from pocket gardens to community gardens, exemplify a need to engage with urban space, but they are far from ideal in terms of soil health and the safety from exposure to urban pollutants.

The availability of existing green leisure spaces as well as disused horticultural infrastructure (i.e. municipal greenhouses) should be considered as a key resource for community-led projects aiming to meaningfully engage with ecological and sociocultural challenge of rebuilding the foundations for socially reproductive commons in the sphere of food and medicine (Figs. 13.5 and 13.6). The right to grow food (Tornaghi, 2017), to meaningfully engage with, and take ownership of, our bodily interaction with nature, should be a reference framework when aiming to support the reconstruction of reproductive commons.

13.4 Conclusions

In this chapter, I have offered some pointers for policy and planning to deepen the ecological and social justice roots of urban agriculture, by fostering an urban agroecology.

I began, in section 13.1, with an overview of the range of claims attached to urban agriculture and the need to understand the fundamental parameters that enable clear and unequivocal positioning in respect to issues of social, economic, ecological and cultural justice.

In Section 13.2, I have highlighted how urban agriculture in public space intersects with contemporary urbanisation challenges and offered a few illustrative cases of how public policy around the cultivation of public space can work in favour or against the abilities of vulnerable urban communities to thrive in the context of disabling urbanisation.

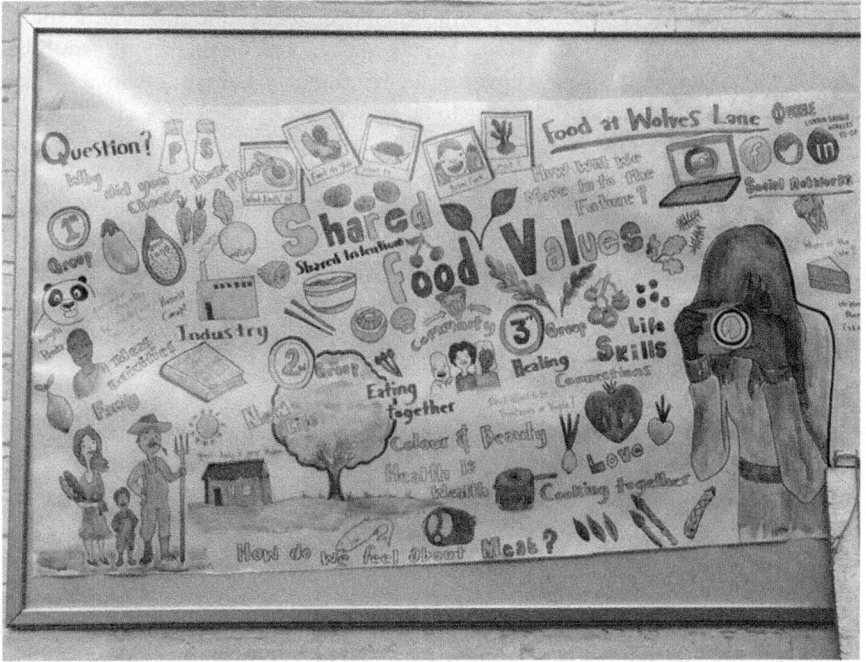

Fig. 13.5 A poster illustrating an exploration of shared food values, at 'Wolves Lane' – a community-managed series of greenhouses and outdoor growing spaces, in London. The poster was decorating the sitting area of the café – open to both local citizens and the grower members of the cooperative project – during a visit of the Urbanising in Place project (September 2019). (Source: Chiara Tornaghi)

In Section 13.3, I discussed three areas where urban planning policy could enable an urban agroecology to thrive: these relate to the promotion of biocultural diversity, the re-germination of reproductive commons and the healing of the epistemic rift between humans and nature.

The successful unfolding of these policies will need: (i) a deeper understanding of the role of healthy soils and thriving soil carers in the web of life, (ii) a shift from productivist to solidarity models in the use of collective resources and an understanding of the long-terms damages of economic growth discourses and (iii) hands-on engagement with decolonial and feminist practices of reproduction of knowledge built on the experience of indigenous and culturally diverse communities.

These three areas are some of the key components of a conceptual model for an alternative model of urbanisation, built on the centrality of soil carer and soil stewardship: a resourceful, reproductive and agroecological urbanism, which I have developed with other colleagues through participatory research with communities of practice across both the Global North and South. (Deh-Tor, 2017, 2021; Tornaghi & Dehaene, 2020, 2021; for further information on this concept see also www.agro-ecologicalurbanism.org). This model aims to be paradigmatically different from capitalist urbanisation, notoriously centred on human and ecological resource

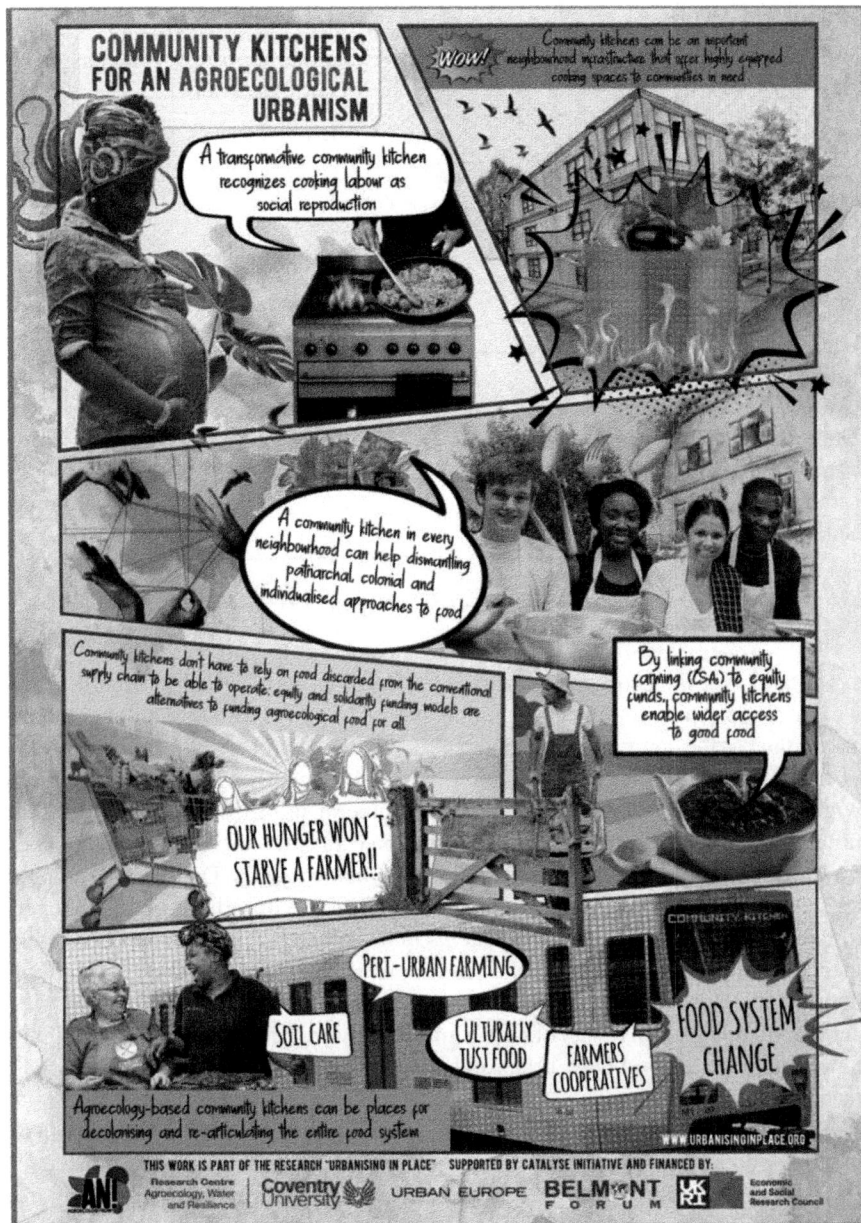

Fig. 13.6 A vision for rebuilding socially reproductive commons: a manifesto for community kitchens as links between producers and consumers. Within the Urbanising in Place project, Community Kitchens were identified as one of the eight building blocks of an agroecological urbanism (Source: Illustration by Kiko Romero, in collaboration with Chiara Tornaghi)

	Building Blocks for an Agroecological Urbanism			
Interrupt logics of substitution (stop land loss)	Agroecological Park	Farming the Fragmented Land		
Embodying an ecology of care and more-than-human solidarities	Territorial Food Hub	Healthy Soil Scape	Community Kitchen	Political Pedagogies for Urban Agroecology
Building resourceful communities through empowering infrastructure	Land and Market Access Incubator		Productive Housing Estate	

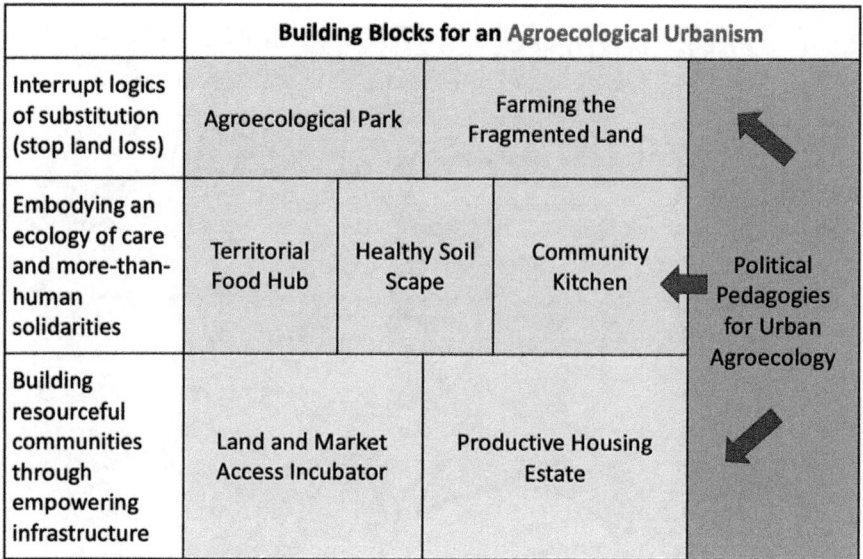

Fig. 13.7 Eight areas of articulation for an agroecological urbanism (Source: Chiara Tornaghi)

exploitation for the economic benefits of a few. The agroecological urbanism that we envision is built around eight building blocks (see Fig. 13.7 for an illustration of one of them – the community kitchen building block-, and Fig. 13.6 for an overview of all of them), or areas of articulation of social relations, which require to break with land speculative logics, to build a resourceful infrastructure for people and farmers and to embrace a value shift centred on care and multi-species solidarity.

An agroecological urbanism offers a programmatic agenda (Dehaene & Tornaghi, 2021) that can guide planning communities to engage in transdisciplinary dialogues to re-articulate urban social arrangements in the sphere of public space and public land (farming the fragmented land, healthy soil scape), the connection between housing and farming (productive housing estate), urban fringes (agroecological park) and a fine grain diversity of public infrastructure at neighbourhood (Community Kitchen, territorial food hub), urban and metropolitan levels (land and market access incubator).

While many of these aspects are in various forms present in a number of policies in cities who engage with sustainable food planning, they are often either treated in silos, accompanied by contradictory policies, or done in ways that are not centred on farmers' needs, and are non-specific to agroecology. We consider this area of re-articulation of socio-spatial relations necessary political pathways to build sustainable urbanisation. All eight areas refer to specific ways to manage and protect natural resources (including urban organic waste), to organise access to fundamental farming infrastructure and to reorganise urban life at different scales, in ways that favour community self-management of land resources, food systems and soil care.

The graphic above (Fig. 13.7) also illustrates and organises these areas of work/political rearticulation alongside three driving value orientations: (i) the need to leave behind the primacy of 'exchange value' over 'use value', which enables the commodification of everything; (ii) the adoption of an ethics of care for humans and non-humans; and (iii) the commitment to resource communities of practice by investing in a social infrastructure as a collective good, in the same way as our current social arrangements provide for many other industries (i.e. transport, parking and logistic infrastructure for mainstream food chains, etc.).

The last building block illustrated in Fig. 13.7 (political pedagogies for urban agroecology) is intentionally illustrated as cross-cutting across these three value orientations, to indicate the necessity to engage in pedagogical and transformational initiatives needed to trigger value shifts.

The departure point for this journey can only be a humble acknowledgement that current urbanisation models are deeply extractive and socio-ecologically catastrophic and that nonetheless we are still gifted with healing power of the many critters of the soil.

Acknowledgements The empirical materials upon which this chapter was built were collected through both personal engagement as scholar activist in urban agriculture and urban agroecology practices in the United Kingdom, as well as in a series of research funded projects. These include the ESRC funded project 'Urban agriculture, social cohesion and environmental justice' (2011–2013; grant no. 224418), the COST-Action project 'Urban Agriculture Europe' (2013–2016), the JPI-Urban Europe, Belmont Forum funded project 'Urbanising in Place' (2018–2022; Project number: 11326801 – and funded in the UK by UKRI/ESRC, grant nr. ES/S002251/1), and the Future-Earth funded project 'Soil Nexus' (2020–2022). Illustration for the Community Kitchen building block of an agroecological urbanism was funded through the Catalyze 1 project (2020–21), funded by Coventry University. Time for writing this chapter was funded through the 'Cultivating Public Space' project, funded by the Research Council of Norway and led by Beata Sirowy. I am thankful to all the farmers/gardeners and civil servants that I have met over the years for their valuable insights and the opportunity to learn from them and the project colleagues with whom many of these ideas have been discussed and/or developed.

References

Abattoir d'Anderlecht, Brussels. https://www.abattoir.be

Agroecological Urbanism. https://www.agroecologicalurbanism.org

Alkon, A., & Agyeman, J. (2011). *Cultivating food justice: Race, class, and sustainability*. MIT Press.

Ambrose, G., Das, K., Fan, Y., & Ramaswami, A. (2020). Is gardening associated with greater happiness of urban residents? A multi-activity, dynamic assessment in the twin-cities region, USA. *Landscape and Urban Planning, 198*, 103776. https://doi.org/10.1016/j.landurbplan.2020.103776

Back to Front project. https://www.backtofront.org.uk/?page_id=131

Barron, J. (2018). *The giving trees: Community orchards as new urban commons*, Doctoral thesis, Carleton University Ottawa, Accessible here [link last accessed 9/9/2022]

Bowen-Siegner, A., Acey, C., & Sowerwine, J. (2020). Producing urban agroecology in the East Bay: From soil health to community empowerment. *Agroecology and Sustainable Food Systems, 44*(5), 566–593.

Brighton City Council. (2011). *PAN 06, Food growing and development. Planning advice note*. (A new version updated in 2020 is available for download here: https://www.brighton-hove.gov.uk/sites/default/files/2020-09/FINAL%20Food%20PAN%202020.pdf

Cadieux, K. V., & Slocum, R. (2015). What does it mean to do food justice? *Journal of Political Ecology, 22*(1), 1–26.

Clemensen, A. K., Provenza, F. D., Hendrickson, J. R., & Grusak, M. A. (2020). Ecological implications of plant secondary metabolites – Phytochemical diversity can enhance agricultural sustainability. *Frontier in sustainable food systems, 4*, 547826.

Crouch, D., & Ward, C. (1988). *The allotment: Its landscape and culture*. Five Leaves.

Deh-Tor, C. M. (2017). From agriculture in the city to an agroecological urbanism: The transformative pathway of urban (political) agroecology. *Urban Agriculture Magazine (RUAF foundation) Issue, 33*, 8–10.

Deh-Tor, C. M. (2021). Food as an urban question, and the foundations of a reproductive, agroecological urbanism. In C. Tornaghi & M. Dehaene (Eds.), *Resourcing an agroecological urbanism: Political, transformational and territorial dimensions*. Chapter 1 (pp. 12–33). Routledge.

Dehaene, M., & Tornaghi C. (2021). Conclusions. The programmatic dimension of an agroecological urbanism. In C. Tornaghi & M. Dehaene (Eds.), *Resourcing an agroecological urbanism: Political, transformational and territorial dimensions*. Routledge.

Dubbeling M. (2013). Urban and peri-urban agriculture and forestry as a strategy for climate change adaptation and disaster risk reduction. In *Disaster risk reduction and resilience building in cities: Focussing on the urban poor. Regional development dialogue* (Vol. 34, No. 1, Spring 2013). United Nations Centre for Regional Development.

Dubbeling, M., van Veenhuizen, R., & Halliday, J. (2019). Urban agriculture as a climate change and disaster risk reduction strategy. *Field Actions Science Reports, The Journal of Field Actions, Issue, 20*, 32–39. https://journals.openedition.org/factsreports/5650

Ebissa, G., & Desta, H. (2022). Review of urban agriculture as a strategy for building a water resilient city. *City and Environment Interactions, 14*, 100081. https://doi.org/10.1016/j.cacint.2022.100081

Engel-Di Mauro, S. (2012). Urban farming: The right to what sort of city? *Capitalism Nature Socialism, 23*, 1–9.

Engel-Di Mauro, S. (2018). Urban Community gardens, commons, and social reproduction: Revisiting Silvia Federici's revolution at point zero. *Gender, Place and Culture, 25*(9), 1379–1390.

Engel-Di Mauro, S. (2021a). Atmospheric sources of trace element contamination in cultivated urban areas: A review. *Journal of Environmental Quality, 50*(1), 38–48.

Engel-Di Mauro, S. (2021b). Soils, industrialised cities, and contaminants: Challenges for an Agroecological urbanism. In C. Tornaghi & M. Dehaene (Eds.), *Resourcing an agroecological urbanism. Political, transformational and territorial dimensions, chapter 6* (pp. 123–142). Routledge.

EU Green New Deal. https://ec.europa.eu/info/strategy/priorities-2019-2024/european-green-deal_en

Galt, R. E., Gray, L. C., & Hurley, P. (2014). Subversive and interstitial food spaces: Transforming selves, societies, and society–environment relations through urban agriculture and foraging. *Local Environment, 19*, 133–146.

Geertz, G. (1983). *Local knowledge: Further essays in interpretive anthropology*. Basic Books.

Ghent food strategy. (2013). *Ghent en garde*. https://ruaf.org/document/gent-en-garde-food-policy/

Glasgow Food and Climate Action Declaration. https://www.glasgowdeclaration.org

Gottlieb, R., & Joshi, A. (2010). *Food justice*. MIT Press.

Graham, A., Das, K., Fan, Y., & Ramaswami, A. (2018). Is gardening associated with greater happiness of urban residents? A multi-activity, dynamic assessment in the twin-cities region, USA. *Landscape and Urban Planning, 198*. https://doi.org/10.1016/j.landurbplan.2020.103776

Hammelman, C. (2018). Urban migrant women's everyday food insecurity coping strategies foster alternative urban imaginaries of a more democratic food system. *Urban Geography, 39*(5), 706–725.

Hammelman, C., Shoffner, E., Cruzat, M., & Lee, S. (2022). Assembling agroecological socionatures: A political ecology analysis of urban and peri-urban agriculture in Rosario, Argentina. *Agriculture and Human Values, 39*, 371–338.

Haraway, D. J. (1991). *Simians, cyborgs, and women: The reinvention of nature*. Routledge.

Heynen, N., Kurtz, H. E., & Trauger, A. (2012). Food justice, hunger, and the city. *Geography Compass, 6*(5), 304–311.

Horst, M., McClintock, N., & Hoey, L. (2017). The intersection of planning, urban agriculture, and food justice: A review of the literature. *Journal of the American Planning Association, 83*(3), 277–295.

Hou, J., Johnson. J. L., & Lawson, L. (2009). *Greening cities, growing communities*. University of Washington Press.

Kaufman J. (2010). The food bubble: How wall street starved millions and got away with it. In *Harper's Magazine*, July. Available at: https://frederickkaufman.typepad.com/files/the-food-bubble-pdf.pdf. Accessed Sept 2022.

Ku, Y.-S., Contador, C. A., Ng, M.-S., Yu, J., Chung, G., & Lam, H.-M. (2020). The effects of domestication on secondary metabolite composition in legumes. *Frontiers in Genetics, 11*, 581357.

Lal, P. (2016). *Appropriating a People's movement: The relationship between gentrification and community gardens in New York city*. Stony Brook University. Available at: https://bit.ly/3astvWn

Lattuca A. (2017). Using agroecological and social inclusion principles in the urban agriculture programme in Rosario, Argentina. *Urban Agriculture Magazine* 33, pp. 51–52. https://www.ruaf.org/using-agroecological-and-social-inclusion-principles-urban-agriculture-programme-rosario-argentina

Lawson, L. (2005). *City bountiful: A century of community gardening in America*. University of California Press.

Lindemann-Matthies, P., & Brieger, H. (2016). Does urban gardening increase aesthetic quality of urban areas? A case study from Germany. *Urban Forestry & Urban Greening, 17*, 33–41.

Lovell, S. (2010). Multifunctional urban agriculture for sustainable land use planning in the United States. *Sustainability, 2*(8), 2499–2522.

Lyson T. A. (2004). *Civic agriculture. Reconnecting Farm, Food and Community*. Tufts University Press.

Maassen, A., & Galvin, M. (2021). *How urban agriculture can hardwire resilience into our cities*. UNFCCC. https://climatechampions.unfccc.int/how-urban-agriculture-can-hardwire-resilience-into-our-cities/

Maughan, N., Pipart, N., Van Dyck, B., & Visser, M. (2021). The potential of bio-intensive market gardening models for a transformative urban agriculture: Adapting SPIN farming to Brussels. In C. Tornaghi & M. Dehaene (Eds.), *Resourcing an agroecological urbanism* (Political, transformational and territorial dimensions, chapter 7) (pp. 143–164). Routledge.

McClintock, N. (2014). Radical, reformist, and garden-variety neoliberal: Coming to terms with urban agriculture's contradictions. *Local Environment, 19*(2), 147–171.

McClintock, N. (2018). Cultivating (a) sustainability capital: Urban agriculture, Ecogentrification, and the uneven valorization of social reproduction. *Annals of the American Association of Geographers, 108*(2), 579–590.

McKay, G. (2011). *Radical Gardening*. Frances Lincoln.

Meenar, M., & Hoover, B. (2012). Community food security via urban agriculture: Understanding people, place, economy, and accessibility from a food justice perspective. *Journal of Agriculture, Food Systems, and Community Development, 3*(1), 143–160.

Mendez, E., Bacon, C. M., Cohen, R., & Glissman, S. (Eds.). (2016). *Agroecology. A transdisciplinary, participatory, and action oriented approach*. CRC Press.

Milan Urban Food Policy Pact-MUFPP. https://www.milanurbanfoodpolicypact.org

Milgroom J. (2021). *Linking food and feminisms: learning from decolonial movements, in AgroecologyNow!* accessible here: https://www.agroecologynow.com/linking-food-and-feminisms/. Accessed 26 Sept 2022.

Nabulo, G., Black, C. R., Craigon, J., & Young, S. D. (2012). Does consumption of leafy veg-etables grown in peri-urban agriculture pose a risk to human health? *Environmental Pollution, 162*, 389–398.

Nicklay, J. A., Cadieux, K. V., Rogers, M. A., Jelinski, N. A., LaBine, K., & Small, G. E. (2020). Facilitating spaces of urban agroecology: A learning framework for community-university part-nerships. *Frontiers in Sustainable Food Systems, 30*. https://doi.org/10.3389/fsufs.2020.00143

Nordahl, D. (2009). *Public produce: The new urban agriculture*. Island Press.

Oldroyd, E., & Clavin, A. A. (2013). Nested scales of design activism: An integrated approach to food growing in inner city Leeds. In A. Viljoen & J. Wiskerke (Eds.), *Sustainable food plan-ning: Evolving theory and practice*. Wageningen Academic Publishers.

Organic Cities network. https://www.organic-cities.eu

Pant, P., Pandey, S., & Dall'Acqua, S. (2021). The influence of environmental conditions on second-ary metabolites in medicinal plants: A literature review. *Chemistry & Biodiversity, 2021*(18), e2100345. https://doi.org/10.1002/cbdv.202100345

Petit-Boix, A., & Apul, D. (2018). From Cascade to bottom-up ecosystem services model: How does social cohesion emerge from urban agriculture? *Sustainability, 10*(4), 998.

Piacentini, R., Feldman, S., Coronel, A., Feldman, N., Vega, M., Moskat, V., Bracalenti, L., Zimmermann, E., Lattuca, A., Biasatti, N., & Dubbeling, M. (2016). Urban and peri-urban agriculture and forestry as a possibility of mitigation and adaptation to climate change. Case study in the city of Rosario and region, Argentina. In S. Nail (Ed.), *Climate change. Lessons from and for cities in LatinAmerica*. Universidad Externado de Colombia.

Pothukuchi, K., & Kaufman, J. L. (2000). The food system: A stranger to the planning field. *Journal of the American Planning Association, 66*(2), 113–124.

Pudup, M. B. (2008). It takes a garden: Cultivating citizen-subjects in organized garden projects. *Geoforum, 39*(3), 1228–1240.

Reynolds, K. (2015). Disparity despite diversity: Social injustice in New York City's urban agri-culture system. *Antipode, 47*(1), 240–259.

Ribeiro, S. M., Bògus, C. M., & Watanabe, H. A. W. (2015). Agroecological urban agriculture from the perspective of health promotion. *Saude e Sociedade, 24*(2), 730–743.

Richardson, T., & Kingsbury, N. (Eds.). (2005). *Vista: The culture and politics of gardens*. Frances Lincoln.

Rosol, M. (2010). Public participation in post-Fordist urban green space governance: The case of community gardens in Berlin. *International Journal of Urban and Regional Research, 34*, 548–563.

Rosset, P., Val, V., Barbosa, L. P., & McCune, N. (2019). Agroecology and La via Campesina II. Peasant agroecology schools and the formation of a sociohistorical and political subject. *Agroecology and Sustainable Food Systems, 43*(7–8), 895–914.

Sbicca, J. (2019). Urban agriculture, revalorization and green gentrification in Denver, Colorado. In T. Barltely (Ed.), *The politics of land* (pp. 149–170). Emerald Publishing Limited.

Scheromm, P., & Javelle, A. (2022). Gardening in an urban farm: A way to reconnect citizens with the soil. *Urban Forestry and Urban Greening, 2022*(72), 1–7.

Schneider, M., & McMichael, P. (2010). Deepening and repairing, the metabolic rift. *The Journal of Peasant Studies, 37*, 461–484.

Spanish Network of Agroecological Cities. https://www.municipiosagroeco.red

Stamets, P. (2005). *Mycelium running. How mushrooms can help save the world*. Ten Speed Press.

Strzemski, M., Dresler, S., Sowa, I., Czubacka, A., Agacka-Mołdoch, M., Płachno, B. J., Granica, S., Feldo, M., & Wójciak-Kosior, M. (2020). The impact of different cultivation systems on the content of selected secondary metabolites and antioxidant activity of *Carlina acaulis* plant material. *Molecules, 25*(1), 146. https://doi.org/10.3390/molecules25010146

Sustain. (2018). *Food growing in parks: A guide for councils*. Available for download at https://www.sustainweb.org/publications/food_growing_in_parks/

Sustainable Food Places coalition (UK). https://www.sustainablefoodplaces.org

Tornaghi, C. (2014). Critical geography of urban agriculture. *Progress in Human Geography, 38*(4), 551–567.

Tornaghi, C. (2017). Urban agriculture in the food-disabling city: (re) defining urban food justice, reimagining a politics of empowerment. *Antipode, 49*(3), 781–801.

Tornaghi, C. (2019). Community gardening. In A. M. Orun (Ed.), *The Wiley Blackwell encyclopedia in urban and regional studies*. Wiley Blackwell. https://doi.org/10.1002/9781118568446.eurs0057

Tornaghi, C., & Dehaene, M. (2020). The prefigurative power of urban political agroecology: Rethinking the urbanisms of agroecological transitions for food system transformation. *Agroecology and Sustainable Food Systems, 44*(5), 594–610.

Tornaghi, C., & Dehaene, M. (Eds.). (2021). *Resourcing an agroecological urbanism. Political, transformational and territorial dimensions*. Routledge.

Tornaghi, C., McAllister, G., Moeller, N., & Pedersen, M. (2023). Building medicinal agroecology: Conceptual grounding for healing of rifts, chapter 1. In Immo Fiebrig (Ed.), *Medicinal agroecology*. Routledge/CRC press.

UN Sustainable Development Goals. https://sdgs.un.org/goals

UN-Habitat, New Urban Agenda. https://unhabitat.org/the-new-urban-agenda-illustrated

Vandermaelen, H., Dehaene, M., Tornaghi, C., Vanempten, E., & Verhoeve, A. (2022). Public land for urban food policy? A critical data-analysis of public land transactions in the Ghent city region (Belgium). *European Planning Studies* – Paper published online open access on 28th July 2022: https://www.tandfonline.com/doi/full/10.1080/09654313.2022.2097860

Veen, E. J., Bock, B. B., Van den Berg, W., Visser, A. J., & Wiskerke, J. S. C. (2015). Community gardening and social cohesion: Different designs, different motivations. *Local Environment, 21*(10), 1271–1287.

Vitiello, D., & Wolf-Powers, L. (2014). Growing food to grow cities? The potential of agriculture for economic and community development in the urban United States. *Community Development Journal, 49*(4), 508–523.

Wakefield, S., Yeudall, F., Taron, C., Reynolds, J., & Skinner, A. (2007). Growing urban health: Community gardening in South-East Toronto. *Health Promotion International, 22*, 92–101.

Walker, S. (2016). Urban agriculture and the sustainability fix in Vancouver and Detroit. *Urban Geography, 37*(2), 163–182.

Weissman, E. (2014). Brooklyn's agrarian questions. *Renewable Agriculture and Food Systems, 30*(1), 92–102.

Wezel, A., Bellon, S., Doré, T., Francis, C., Vallod, D., & David, C. (2009). Agroecology as a science, a movement and a practice. A review. *Agronomy for Sustainable Development, 29*(4), 503–516.

Chapter 14
Reflections: Lessons Learned, Limitations, and the Way Forward for Urban Agriculture in Public Space

Beata Sirowy and Deni Ruggeri

The authors of this volume have contributed a diversity of viewpoints on urban agriculture, its definition, goals, practices, and policy implementation. While there is a range of the types of projects and approaches presented, there seem to be some commonalities in this diversity. First and foremost, our case studies, either in the practical or discoursive realm, seem to suggest that food production alone is seldom a major motive for the integration of urban agriculture in today's cities. This calls for the integration of urban agriculture in a system of multifunctional productive spaces, each making distinct contributions to the well-being of urban dwellers and nonhuman nature – some more focused on individual needs, community-building, education, and health, others focused on reducing the impact of the food systems and increasing the affordability of good quality, locally grown food, some enhancing diversity of urban ecosystems.

In our project, we focused on the role urban agriculture can play in enhancing individual and communal well-being of urban dwellers. On the individual level, it can provide multiple affordances for sustaining capabilities—ways of being and doing people have reasons to value—and offer settings for development of virtues—excellences of character and understanding. On the collective level, urban agriculture can play a crucial role in the realm of community-building, by sustaining civic friendship and activating the kind of mutualism, cooperation, and partnership necessary for the advancement of the right to a humane, livable city.

B. Sirowy (✉)
Department of Urban and Regional Planning, Norwegian University of Life Sciences, Ås, Norway
e-mail: beata.sirowy@gmail.com

D. Ruggeri
Department of Plant Science and Landscape Architecture, University of Maryland, College Park, MD, USA
e-mail: druggeri@umd.edu

© The Author(s) 2024
B. Sirowy, D. Ruggeri (eds.), *Urban Agriculture in Public Space*, GeoJournal Library 132, https://doi.org/10.1007/978-3-031-41550-0_14

311

We started the project with perspectives of philosophy and ethics, envisioning urban agriculture as an arena for human flourishing, and further developed our discussion around the potential for urban agriculture to become an instigator and activator of a transition to a more sustainable and resilient urban society, through the cultivation of livability, health, identity, and community cohesion in every neighborhood. The experiences synthesized in this book seem to suggest that to fully be transformative of a society's capabilities, and those of its individuals, urban agriculture must not only remain accessible to its primary users on the level of a neighbourhood, but able to connect with an audience of secondary and tertiary users of diverse cultural backgrounds, ages, and degrees of abilities through a variety of expressions and ambitions. To illustrate this, the authors in this book assembled a rich kaleidoscope of urban agriculture practices motivated by a variety of goals, beyond yield and consumption of healthy food.

Public space has a unique role to play in actualizing the plethora of benefits of urban agriculture to individual and communal well-being of urban dwellers. Given the role we are asking urban agriculture to play, funding and institutional support needs to be available to integrate it in urban development in a systematic way, on a broad scale. As in some of the cases we have discussed here, the key to the long-term success of urban agriculture is the adequate and stable supply of land, knowledge, and materials. When seen from the point of view of policies and strategic planning, urban agriculture has the advantage to be relatively inexpensive to seed and initiate from the bottom up but harder to sustain without the flow of resources from the top down. This is even more true in public spaces, where professional expertise may be needed to manage the spaces, ensure their productivity, sustain people's participation, and foster continued stewardship. As experiences from some of urban agriculture projects presented in our book suggest, participation of local communities makes the difference in terms of long-term success of urban gardens, increasing their resilience and motivating stewardship. Yet we should not consider permanence of urban agriculture projects as their main criterion of success. Failure may also yield benefits, granting the opportunity to evolve, adapt to changing conditions, or pivot to different cultivation practices for both food and community cultivation.

The Covid-19 pandemic was the ultimate test of urban agriculture and its community and food growing ambitions. Evidence from the CPS research partners seems to suggest that urban agriculture has, in the time of this unprecedented health crisis, strengthened and solidified its presence in the city—at some locations offering opportunities for socially distanced restorative activities, at other locations providing boxes of local produce to the elderly or those most at risk, integrating moments of socially distanced community building and engagement.

We started the project with the goal to find a way to systematically integrate urban agriculture in the dense, Norwegian city. What emerged from the research of the Cultivating Public Space project team were unique stories representing a variety of perspectives and voices on the potentials of urban agriculture to enhance well-being in today's cities, including researchers, policy-makers, educators, activists, growers, managers, and diverse users of urban gardens. Rather than a toolkit of transferable solutions, we have showed the versatility of urban agriculture, its adaptability, and its contribution to urban resilience in the face of uncertainties and challenges like climate change, environmental degradation, growing inequalities, threats to food security, increasing social isolation, and mental health problems in cities, to list but a few.

The findings from our project have demonstrated urban agriculture's impact on people's lives, telling a story of a collective practice that bridges across user groups, giving voice to the marginalized, and helping them exercise, through their hands-on engagement in urban cultivation, their right to landscape. This exemplifies the potential of urban agriculture to reclaim public space and redefine what might be acceptable and even desirable future for it, and for our society.

Urban agriculture is evolving quickly, and there is no way for researchers to keep up with the pace of the change it is facing in our cities and a continuous evolution of its forms. This book represents a milestone in this evolution and a much-needed moment of reflection, storytelling, and documentation. We hope more researchers will pick up where our authors left off and help advance urban agriculture toward becoming even more diverse, integrated, synergistic, and impactful.

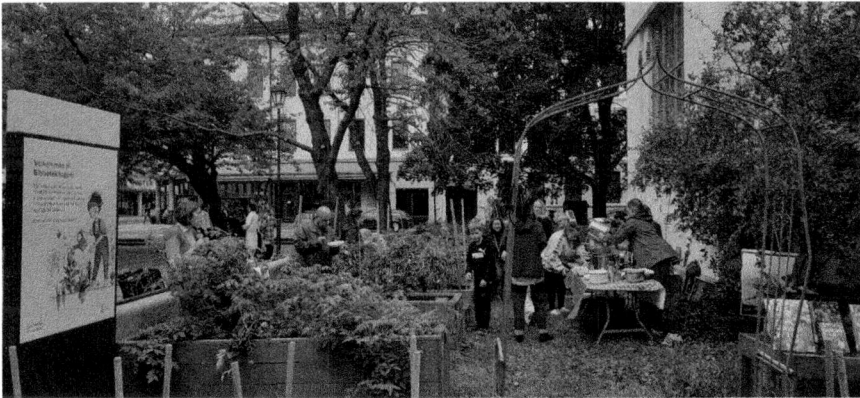

Urban agriculture at Schouss Plaza, Oslo. Photo: B. Sirowy

Index

© The Editor(s) (if applicable) and The Author(s) 2024
B. Sirowy, D. Ruggeri (eds.), *Urban Agriculture in Public Space*, GeoJournal
Library 132, https://doi.org/10.1007/978-3-031-41550-0